Management of Degenerative Cervical Myelopathy and Spinal Cord Injury

Management of Degenerative Cervical Myelopathy and Spinal Cord Injury

Editors

Allan R. Martin
Aria Nouri

MDPI • Basel • Beijing • Wuhan • Barcelona • Belgrade • Manchester • Tokyo • Cluj • Tianjin

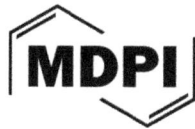

Editors
Allan R. Martin
University of California
USA

Aria Nouri
Geneva University Hospitals
Switzerland

Editorial Office
MDPI
St. Alban-Anlage 66
4052 Basel, Switzerland

This is a reprint of articles from the Special Issue published online in the open access journal *Journal of Clinical Medicine* (ISSN 2077-0383) (available at: https://www.mdpi.com/journal/jcm/special_issues/Cervical_Myelopathy_Spinal_Cord_Injury).

For citation purposes, cite each article independently as indicated on the article page online and as indicated below:

LastName, A.A.; LastName, B.B.; LastName, C.C. Article Title. *Journal Name* **Year**, *Volume Number*, Page Range.

ISBN 978-3-0365-5625-3 (Hbk)
ISBN 978-3-0365-5626-0 (PDF)

© 2022 by the authors. Articles in this book are Open Access and distributed under the Creative Commons Attribution (CC BY) license, which allows users to download, copy and build upon published articles, as long as the author and publisher are properly credited, which ensures maximum dissemination and a wider impact of our publications.

The book as a whole is distributed by MDPI under the terms and conditions of the Creative Commons license CC BY-NC-ND.

Contents

Khadija Soufi, Aria Nouri and Allan R. Martin
Degenerative Cervical Myelopathy and Spinal Cord Injury: Introduction to the Special Issue
Reprinted from: *J. Clin. Med.* **2022**, *11*, 4253, doi:10.3390/jcm11154253 1

Thorsten Jentzsch, David W. Cadotte, Jefferson R. Wilson, Fan Jiang, Jetan H. Badhiwala, Muhammad A. Akbar, Brett Rocos, Robert G. Grossman, Bizhan Aarabi, James S. Harrop and Michael G. Fehlings
Spinal Cord Signal Change on Magnetic Resonance Imaging May Predict Worse Clinical In- and Outpatient Outcomes in Patients with Spinal Cord Injury: A Prospective Multicenter Study in 459 Patients
Reprinted from: *J. Clin. Med.* **2021**, *10*, 4778, doi:10.3390/jcm10204778 9

Talia C. Oughourlian, Chencai Wang, Noriko Salamon, Langston T. Holly and Benjamin M. Ellingson
Sex-Dependent Cortical Volume Changes in Patients with Degenerative Cervical Myelopathy
Reprinted from: *J. Clin. Med.* **2021**, *10*, 3965, doi:10.3390/jcm10173965 23

Katharina Wolf, Marco Reisert, Saúl Felipe Beltrán, Jan-Helge Klingler, Ulrich Hubbe, Axel J. Krafft, Nico Kremers, Karl Egger and Marc Hohenhaus
Spinal Cord Motion in Degenerative Cervical Myelopathy: The Level of the Stenotic Segment and Gender Cause Altered Pathodynamics
Reprinted from: *J. Clin. Med.* **2021**, *10*, 3788, doi:10.3390/jcm10173788 37

Samuel Sommaruga, Joaquin Camara-Quintana, Kishan Patel, Aria Nouri, Enrico Tessitore, Granit Molliqaj, Shreyas Panchagnula, Michael Robinson, Justin Virojanapa, Xin Sun, Fjodor Melnikov, Luis Kolb, Karl Schaller, Khalid Abbed and Joseph Cheng
Clinical Outcomes between Stand-Alone Zero-Profile Spacers and Cervical Plate with Cage Fixation for Anterior Cervical Discectomy and Fusion: A Retrospective Analysis of 166 Patients
Reprinted from: *J. Clin. Med.* **2021**, *10*, 3076, doi:10.3390/jcm10143076 53

Agnieszka Wincek, Juliusz Huber, Katarzyna Leszczyńska, Wojciech Fortuna, Stefan Okurowski, Krzysztof Chmielak and Paweł Tabakow
The Long-Term Effect of Treatment Using the Transcranial Magnetic Stimulation rTMS in Patients after Incomplete Cervical or Thoracic Spinal Cord Injury
Reprinted from: *J. Clin. Med.* **2021**, *10*, 2975, doi:10.3390/jcm10132975 63

Zdenek Kadanka Jr., Zdenek Kadanka Sr., Rene Jura and Josef Bednarik
Vertigo in Patients with Degenerative Cervical Myelopathy
Reprinted from: *J. Clin. Med.* **2021**, *10*, 2496, doi:10.3390/jcm10112496 79

Zdenek Kadanka Jr., Zdenek Kadanka Sr., Tomas Skutil, Eva Vlckova and Josef Bednarik
Walk and Run Test in Patients with Degenerative Compression of the Cervical Spinal Cord
Reprinted from: *J. Clin. Med.* **2021**, *10*, 927, doi:10.3390/jcm10050927 91

Kalum Ost, W. Bradley Jacobs, Nathan Evaniew, Julien Cohen-Adad, David Anderson and David W. Cadotte
Spinal Cord Morphology in Degenerative Cervical Myelopathy Patients; Assessing Key Morphological Characteristics Using Machine Vision Tools
Reprinted from: *J. Clin. Med.* **2021**, *10*, 892, doi:10.3390/jcm10040892 103

Jamie R. F. Wilson, Jetan H. Badhiwala, Ali Moghaddamjou, Albert Yee, Jefferson R. Wilson and Michael G. Fehlings
Frailty Is a Better Predictor than Age of Mortality and Perioperative Complications after Surgery for Degenerative Cervical Myelopathy: An Analysis of 41,369 Patients from the NSQIP Database 2010–2018
Reprinted from: *J. Clin. Med.* **2020**, *9*, 3491, doi:10.3390/jcm9113491 . . . . **121**

Arash Ghaffari-Rafi, Catherine Peterson, Jose E. Leon-Rojas, Nobuaki Tadokoro, Stefan F. Lange, Mayank Kaushal, Lindsay Tetreault, Michael G. Fehlings and Allan R. Martin
The Role of Magnetic Resonance Imaging to Inform Clinical Decision-Making in Acute Spinal Cord Injury: A Systematic Review and Meta-Analysis
Reprinted from: *J. Clin. Med.* **2021**, *10*, 4948, doi:10.3390/jcm10214948 . . . . **137**

Xiaoyu Yang, Aref-Ali Gharooni, Rana S. Dhillon, Edward Goacher, Edward W. Dyson, Oliver Mowforth, Alexandru Budu, Guy Wynne-Jones, Jibin Francis, Rikin Trivedi, Marcel Ivanov, Sashin Ahuja, Kia Rezajooi, Andreas K. Demetriades, David Choi, Antony H. Bateman, Quraishi Nasir, Vishal Kumar, Manjul Tripathi, Sandeep Mohindra, Erlick A. Pereira, Giles Critchley, Michael G. Fehlings, Peter J. A. Hutchinson, Benjamin M. Davies and Mark R. N. Kotter
The Relative Merits of Posterior Surgical Treatments for Multi-Level Degenerative Cervical Myelopathy Remain Uncertain: Findings from a Systematic Review
Reprinted from: *J. Clin. Med.* **2021**, *10*, 3653, doi:10.3390/jcm10163653 . . . . **171**

Melissa Lannon and Edward Kachur
Degenerative Cervical Myelopathy: Clinical Presentation, Assessment, and Natural History
Reprinted from: *J. Clin. Med.* **2021**, *10*, 3626, doi:10.3390/jcm10163626 . . . . **185**

Ji Tu, Jose Vargas Castillo, Abhirup Das and Ashish D. Diwan
Degenerative Cervical Myelopathy: Insights into Its Pathobiology and Molecular Mechanisms
Reprinted from: *J. Clin. Med.* **2021**, *10*, 1214, doi:10.3390/jcm10061214 . . . . **197**

Khadija H. Soufi, Tess M. Perez, Alexis O. Umoye, Jamie Yang, Maria Burgos and Allan R. Martin
How Is Spinal Cord Function Measured in Degenerative Cervical Myelopathy? A Systematic Review
Reprinted from: *J. Clin. Med.* **2022**, *11*, 1441, doi:10.3390/ jcm11051441 . . . . **223**

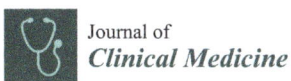

Editorial

Degenerative Cervical Myelopathy and Spinal Cord Injury: Introduction to the Special Issue

Khadija Soufi [1], Aria Nouri [2] and Allan R. Martin [1,*]

[1] Department of Neurosurgery, University of California, Davis, CA 95817, USA; khsoufi@ucdavis.edu
[2] Division of Neurosurgery, Geneva University Hospitals, 1205 Geneva, Switzerland; arianouri9@gmail.com
* Correspondence: armartin@ucdavis.edu

Damage to the spinal cord (SC) can arise from either traumatic or non-traumatic spinal cord injury (SCI). Non-traumatic forms of SCI include degenerative cervical myelopathy (DCM) in which spinal degeneration secondary to age-related degeneration of the discs, ligaments, and vertebrae of the cervical spine causes cord compression, resulting in varying degrees of neurological dysfunction. On the other hand, traumatic spinal cord injury (tSCI) is principally due to immediate mechanical insult resulting in sudden onset motor, sensory and autonomic dysfunction, and secondary injury mechanisms resulting from the resulting inflammation. Both DCM and tSCI share similar pathological and molecular characteristics including neuro-inflammation, axonal degeneration, and alpha-motor neuron degeneration and result in similar patterns of anterograde and retrograde remodeling of synaptic pathways [1,2]. MRI-based imaging studies have found similarities in the degeneration of the dorsal and lateral columns and in degrees of remote SC pathology [1,2]. In addition, patients with either DCM or non-myelopathic SC compression are predisposed to tSCI from even a minor trauma, as the compressed SC is more vulnerable to dynamic forces and kinking, particularly in hyperextension injuries; this type of tSCI is commonly termed 'central cord syndrome' and presents with quadriparesis that affects upper extremities more than lower extremities [3]. The relationship between DCM and tSCI is still being elucidated in the literature and could offer a means to study SCI by assessing the large population of individuals with DCM that frequently have stable or slowly progressive disease.

Both traumatic and non-traumatic SCI are anatomically and physiologically complex pathologies that present with variable symptoms and severity including numbness, impaired hand dexterity, weakness, unsteady gait, and sphincter dysfunction [1,2]. Traditionally, physician administered outcome measures such as mJOA and Nurick, and patient reported NDI, have been used to classify DCM severity, while tSCI studies typically report ASIA Impairment Scale (AIS) and the ISNCSCI, which includes high reliability and objective interpretation of findings. However, the ISNCSCI is not sensitive to subtle SC dysfunction such as hand incoordination or gait imbalance, which are subjectively captured by DCM outcome measures (e.g., mJOA) [4]. Both pathologies impair patients' mobility, strength, and coordination, significantly affecting patients' quality of life, resulting in a significant healthcare burden as the leading cause of SC dysfunction. Over the past few years, there has been increased research on clinical course, diagnosis, treatment threshold, and patient outcomes which have guided the establishment of treatment and diagnosis guidelines. However, there remains significant knowledge gaps, and, as a consequence, practice guidelines have been formed with limited strength of evidence, indicating a continued need for further investigation.

The present Special Issue is dedicated to presenting current research topics in DCM and SCI in an attempt to bridge gaps in knowledge for both of the two main forms of SCI. The issue consists of fourteen studies, of which the majority were on DCM, the more common pathology, while three studies focused on tSCI. This issue includes two narrative reviews, three systematic reviews and nine original research papers. Areas of research

Citation: Soufi, K.; Nouri, A.; Martin, A.R. Degenerative Cervical Myelopathy and Spinal Cord Injury: Introduction to the Special Issue. *J. Clin. Med.* **2022**, *11*, 4253. https://doi.org/10.3390/jcm11154253

Received: 5 July 2022
Accepted: 19 July 2022
Published: 22 July 2022

Publisher's Note: MDPI stays neutral with regard to jurisdictional claims in published maps and institutional affiliations.

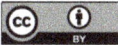

Copyright: © 2022 by the authors. Licensee MDPI, Basel, Switzerland. This article is an open access article distributed under the terms and conditions of the Creative Commons Attribution (CC BY) license (https://creativecommons.org/licenses/by/4.0/).

covered include image studies, predictive modeling, prognostic factors, and multiple systemic or narrative reviews on various aspects of these conditions. These articles include the contributions of a diverse group of researchers with various approaches to studying SCI coming from multiple countries, including Canada, Czech Republic, Germany, Poland, Switzerland, United Kingdom, and the United States.

The pathological impacts of DCM and tSCI are not limited to the SC; downstream and upstream neural pathways have been shown to significantly affect cortical volume with an increased connectivity within sensorimotor and pain related cortical regions which may affect patient perceived pain and symptom burden over time [5]. Oughourlian et al. [5] were one of the first to assess sex related differences in cerebral cortex changes, utilizing a vertex level linear model (n = 85). They found significant differences between male and female DCM patients, including significantly less grey matter volume (GMV) changes in females over a broader range of cortical areas compared to their male counterparts despite no differences between GMV volumetric differences amongst controls. These changes were also correlated with mJOA and in the future could be used to further understand role of sex-hormones and prognostic factors in pathogenesis of DCM. Wolf et al. [6] also found gender related differences in SC motion patterns amongst men with stenosis at the C5/C6 or C6/C7 levels and no relationship between cervical joint motion to severity of the stenosis indicating the need for further assessment of gender differences in pathological features of DCM. On assessment of outcome measures for DCM, Kadanka et al. [7], showed that the standardized 10 m walk/run test can assess motor and balance abnormalities in both classic DCM patients and non-myelopathic degenerative cervical cord compression (NMDCC) patients, which has a 40% prevalence in 60+ age groups in European/American subpopulation. This was the first study assessing such changes in NMDCC patients and the 10 m walk/run test closely correlated with mJOA, which could allow for early detection of DCM before permanent neurodegeneration occurs.

In terms of surgical prognostic factors, Wilson et al. [8] challenged the previously used parameter of age and found that frailty as scored by the MFI-5 has the largest effect size and is more likely to predict peri-operative adverse events including mortality, readmission or re-operation, length of hospital stay, and recovery location. This study utilized information from over 41,000 DCM patients who underwent a variety of surgical treatments with the majority (70.8%) of single or two-level pathology providing strong evidence to incorporate frailty tests such as MFI-5 in clinical practice instead of less reliable measures such as age.

Image-oriented research by Jentzsch et al. [9] assessed potential surgical prognostic factors found on MRI for prospectively collected data for 459 patients who had prior SCI and found that SC signal change is a significant predictor (109%) of adverse events including neurologic impairment and decreased ambulation initially and at follow-up one year later. These findings are in agreement with the 14 small (n < 100) prospective studies summarized by Jentzsch et al. in the paper which found further negative prognostic association between pre-operative SC signal change and post-operative clinical outcomes. The implications of this study are significant and highlight the need for further research on other imaging based prognostic factors through large prospective, long-term, and confounder-controlled studies.

Building on this concept, Ost et al. [10] explored the predictive modeling of MR imaging of 328 DCM patients and found that metrics such as cross-sectional area, eccentricity, and solidity were not correlated with mJOA disease severity, and with the variations appearing to be due to patient-specific parameters. This highlights the complexity of DCM and the need for further integrated approaches to modeling efforts. Imaging data is one of many core tenets to management and surgical decision making for DCM, however, assessing severity and progression continues to rely on physical and neurological measures. The authors additionally conclude that future efforts that utilize more complex models, normalize metrics per-patient, and assess healthy control variations could overcome the limitations of the current model used by Ost et al.

Beyond conservative management and close monitoring, surgical decompression is the main-stay treatment for DCM and a variety of surgical approaches and interventions have been utilized. Appropriate selection of surgical intervention is based on patient characteristics, disease pathology, and risk factors. Sommaruga et al. [11] compared the surgical outcomes including Bazaz dysphagia score, Nurick grade, and hospital stay between stand-alone zero-profile implants and more traditionally used cervical plating in anterior cervical discectomy and fusion. The study, consisting of 116 patients, found a shorter hospital course and operation time for stand-alone implants; however, neurologic and dysphagia outcomes were similar across both groups. This study adds to the growing literature on differences between various anterior surgical treatments.

On a similar note, Wincek et al. [12] studied repetitive transcranial magnetic stimulation (rTMS) and kinesiotherapy across an average of 5 months in 26 patients with incomplete SCI and found significant improvements including reduced upper extremity spasticity, motor unit recruitment and efferent neural transmission. These findings are a promising therapeutic method for enhancing outcomes in patients with incomplete SCI and addressing neurodegenerative changes in DCM. However, this area remains in its infancy.

Many patients with DCM present with uncommon symptoms and, due to the older age and complex anatomy of DCM involving both SC and brain, present with a variety of unexplained symptoms. Previous literature included cervical vertigo as a symptom which was discussed by Kadanka et al. [13] through a patient case series ($n = 38$) on vertigo in DCM patients which found alternate etiology, indicating the importance of appropriately assessing the symptoms that may occur in DCM and considering alternate diagnoses.

This Special Issue also includes three systematic reviews. The first of these, by Ghaffari-Rafi et al. [14], assessed the role and impact of obtaining an MRI in acute SCI on clinical outcomes and decision making. Of the 32 studies included, MR imaging frequently identified pathologies such as spinal cord compression, ligamentous injury, and epidural hematoma that altered the acute management of SCI, including the need for surgery, timing of surgery, and the surgical approach (anterior vs. posterior). MRI also showed good to excellent diagnostic accuracy for various types of ligamentous injury and epidural hematoma, but poor accuracy for fracture detection. This systematic review and meta-analysis strengthens the argument that obtaining MRI is important in cases of acute SCI, while highlighting knowledge gaps on cost-effectiveness and impact on outcomes.

Yang et al. [15] provided a comprehensive systematic review of posterior approaches to multi-level DCM, highlighting that the variation of study designs, outcomes, and limited direct comparison of techniques has led to lack of high-level evidence to guide surgical approach to management of DCM. Amongst the limited studies that directly compared surgical techniques, there were many contradictory findings, emphasizing the need for future RCT or prospective multi-center studies, which are currently underway in the UK with POLYFIX-DCM trial (Posterior LaminectomY and FIXation for DCM).

Lannon et al. [16] summarized the clinical presentation, treatment, and natural history of DCM in their manuscript. Of note, there are no pathognomonic signs for DCM, but rather a constellation of symptoms, physical exam findings, and imaging features that all typically have a slowly progressive course. Imaging findings classically include the absence of a cerebrospinal fluid signal on T2-weighted images, T2 signal hyperintensity, and rarely "snake eyes appearance", with symmetric circular foci in the gray matter. Additionally, DCM tends to involve progressive neurological deterioration amongst 20% to 62% of patients within 3–6 years. On the other hand, Tu et al. [17] comprehensively discussed the physical exam sensitivity and specificity, commonly used radiographic measures, and T1 vs. T2 MRI findings. Tu et al. also comprehensively summarized the associated genetic polymorphisms, impact of microbiome and molecular features involved in the pathogenesis of disc degeneration, SC dysfunction, axonal injury, and the role and impact of various cell lines on disease course. This study highlighted multiple molecular and micro-structural knowledge gaps, as well as the limited methods to assess degenerative cervical myelopathy appropriately and extensively.

Recognizing the limitations and variability of current outcome measures utilized to study DCM, Soufi et al. [4], assessed the number, quality, and variety of outcome measures currently used in the literature through a systematic review on 148 studies. A total of 39% percent of studies utilized single outcome measures with an average of 2.36 outcome measures used in the studies, with no studies specifically assessing key functions including dorsal column sensory pathway or respiratory, bowel, and sexual function. Objective physical testing of neurological function was rarely utilized, with questionnaires representing 92% (320/349) of all outcome measures utilized, emphasizing the need for a concerted effort in more accurately quantifying neurological dysfunction in DCM, for the purpose of improving diagnosis, measuring severity, and monitoring patients for deterioration.

It was the intention of this Special Issue to address a wide range of topics regarding DCM and SCI. This project was pursued by the Journal of Clinical Medicine Editorial Board with the hope of contributing new research to help tackle these two prevalent and disabling clinical disorders. We would like to thank the various authors and peer-reviewers for helping to amass this unique body of work (Table 1).

Table 1. Summary of published papers in this Special Issue.

Authors	Purpose	Study Design	Main Results	Conclusions
Jentzsch et al. [9]	Investigate whether baseline MRI features predicted the clinical course of the disease utilizing the prospective North American Clinical Trials Network (NACTN) registry	Prospective observational	There were more adverse events in patients with SC signal change (230 (65.0%) vs. 47 (44.8%), $p < 0.001$; odds ratio (OR) = 2.09 (95% confidence interval (CI) 1.31–3.35), $p = 0.002$). The length of stay was longer in patients with SC signal change (13.0 (IQR 17.0) vs. 11.0 (IQR 14.0), $p = 0.049$) and there was no difference between the groups in mortality.	MRI SC signal change may predict adverse events and length of hospital stay.
Oughourlian et al. [5]	Investigate the role of sex differences on the structure of the cerebral cortex in DCM and determine how structural differences may relate to clinical measures of neurological function.	Cross-sectional cohort study	Males demonstrated a significant positive correlation between grey matter volume (GMV) and mJOA score, in which patients with worsening neurological symptoms exhibited decreasing GMV primarily across somatosensory and motor related cortical regions. Females exhibited a similar association, across a broader range of cortical areas including those involved in pain processing. In sensorimotor regions, female patients consistently showed smaller GMV compared with male patients, independent of mJOA score.	Results from the current study suggest strong sex-related differences in cortical volume in patients with DCM, which may reflect hormonal influence or differing compensation mechanisms.
Wolf et al. [6]	Hypothesized that we could reproduce similar patterns of spinal cord motion at the different levels of cervical stenosis among DCM patients presenting with monosegmental stenosis.	Monocentric, prospective, matched-pair-controlled study	Age and severity of stenosis did not relate to spinal cord motion. Spinal cord motion was focally increased at a level of stenosis among patients with stenosis at C4/C5 ($n = 14$), C5/C6 ($n = 33$), and C6/C7 ($n = 10$) ($p < 0.033$). Gender was a significant predictor of higher spinal cord dynamics among men with stenosis at C5/C6 ($p = 0.048$) and C6/C7 ($p = 0.033$).	Gender-related effects lead to dynamic alterations among men with stenosis at C5/C6 and C6/C7. The missing relation of motion to severity of stenosis underlines a possible additive diagnostic value of spinal cord motion analysis in DCM
Sommaruga et al. [11]	Investigate differences in surgical outcomes between SA (stand-alone zero-profile implants) and CP (cervical plating) in ACDF	Retrospective Case series	No significant difference in neurological outcome or rates of dysphagia between SA and CP, and that both lead to overall improvement of symptoms (NDI).	Two approaches have comparable outcomes. Further clinical studies needed to assess.
Wincek et al. [12]	Investigated the long-term effect of the rTMS protocol at frequencies ranging from 20 to 25 Hz and a stimulus strength that was 70–80% of the resting motor threshold in patients with C2–Th12 iSCI	Prospective Cohort Study	The application of rTMS at 20–25 Hz reduced spasticity in the upper extremity muscles, improved the recruitment of motor units in the upper and lower extremity muscles, and slightly improved the transmission of efferent neural impulses within the spinal pathways in patients with C2–Th12 iSCI	Results support the hypothesis about the importance of rTMS therapy and possible involvement of the residual efferent pathways including propriospinal neurons in the recovery of the motor control of iSCI patients
Kadanka et al. [13]	To assess the prevalence and cause of vertigo in patients with degenerative cervical myelopathy (DCM)	Retrospective cross-sectional observational study	Symptoms of vertigo were described by 18 patients (47%) of patients. Causes of vertigo included: orthostatic dizziness in eight (22%), hypertension in five (14%), benign paroxysmal positional vertigo in four (11%) and psychogenic dizziness in one patient (3%).	Despite the high prevalence of vertigo in DCM, the etiology in all cases could be attributed to causes outside cervical spine and related nerve structures.
Kadanka et al. [7]	Assess 10 m walk and run test capability of detecting early gait impairment in a non-myelopathic degenerative cervical cord compression (NMDCC)	Cross-sectional observational cohort study	Walking/running time/velocity, number of steps and cadence of walking/running were recorded; analysis also disclosed abnormalities in 66.7% of NMDCC subjects. More significant differences in DCM patients	Standardized 10 m walk/run test has the capacity to disclose locomotion abnormalities in NMDCC subjects.
Ost et al. [10]	To evaluate the current state of a computational models such as Spinal Cord Toolbox (SCT) automated process	Image Analysis Study	Metrics extracted from these automated methods are insufficient to reliably predict disease severity	Although modeling techniques are still in their infancy, future models of DCM severity could greatly improve automated clinical diagnosis and outcomes.

Table 1. *Cont.*

Authors	Purpose	Study Design	Main Results	Conclusions
Wilson et al. [8]	Define effects of age and frailty on outcomes following surgical intervention for DCM.	Ambispective	Age and frailty have a significant effect on all outcomes, but the MFI-5 has the largest effect size. Increasing frailty correlated significantly with the risk of perioperative adverse events, longer hospital stay, and risk of a non-home discharge destination.	Measures of frailty have a greater effect size and a higher discriminative value to predict adverse events than age alone.
Gaffari-Rafi et al. [14]	Critically evaluate evidence regarding the role of MRI to influence decision-making and outcomes in acute SCI.	Systemic Review	A total of 32 studies were identified and consistently concluded that MRI was useful prior to surgical treatment (13 studies) and after surgery to assess decompression (two studies), but utility before/after closed reduction of cervical dislocations was unclear (three studies).	MRI is safe and frequently identifies findings alter clinical management in acute SCI, although direct evidence of its impact on outcomes is lacking
Yang et al. [15]	Assess the reporting of study design and characteristics in multi-level degenerative cervical myelopathy (DCM) treated by posterior surgical approaches	Systemic Review	Laminoplasty was described in 56 studies (75%), followed by laminectomy with (36%) and without fusion (16%). Most studies were conducted in Asia (84%), in the period of 2016–2019 (51%), of which laminoplasty was studied predominantly. Twelve (16%) prospective studies and 63 (84%) retrospective studies were identified.	Heterogeneity in the reporting of study and sample characteristics exists, as well as in clinical and radiographic outcomes, with a paucity of studies with a higher level of evidence. Future studies are needed to elucidate the clinical effectiveness of posterior surgical treatments.
Soufi et al. [4]	Assess the neurological, functional, and quality of life (QoL) outcome measures currently in use to quantify impairment in DCM	Systemic Review	The most commonly used instruments were subjective functional scales including the Japanese Orthopedic Association (JOA) (71 studies), modified JOA (mJOA) (66 studies), Neck Disability Index (NDI) (54 studies), and Nurick (39 studies). A total of 92% (320/349) of all outcome measures were questionnaires, whereas objective physical testing of neurological function (strength, gait, balance, dexterity or sensation) made up 8% (29/349). Studies utilized an average of 2.36 outcomes measures, while 58 studies (39%) utilized only a single outcome measure.	Clinical decision-making and future clinical studies in DCM should employ a combination of subjective and objective assessments to capture the multitude of spinal cord functions to improve clinical management and inform practice guidelines.
Lannon et al. [16]	Summarize current clinical understanding of presentation, pathophysiology, diagnosis, natural history, and surgical management for DCM	Narrative Review	DCM is a common clinical entity with increasing prevalence. Patients with clinically progressive myelopathic symptoms and correlating radiographic evidence of cord compression should be referred for surgical evaluation if it is within the patient's care goals to prevent further neurologic deterioration	Early diagnosis and surgical management may improve neurologic and overall, outcomes for these patients and, importantly, prevent progressive deterioration
Tu et al. [17]	Discuss epidemiological, diagnostic, pathophysiological, risk factors, molecular features, treatment, and future directions in the management of DCM	Narrative Review	The pathophysiology of the disease is not completely understood, and several mechanisms have been postulated to explain it. The key for successfully treating DCM could be partly J. Clin. Med. 2021, 10, 1214 18 of 25 hidden in the huge array of interactions that take place and have been mentioned in our review.	Given the fact that the aged population in the world is continuously increasing, DCM is posing a formidable challenge that needs urgent attention.

Author Contributions: Conceptualization, A.R.M. and A.N.; data curation, K.S.; Writing—original draft preparation, K.S.; writing—review and editing, A.R.M., A.N. and K.S.; supervision, A.R.M. and A.N. All authors have read and agreed to the published version of the manuscript.

Funding: This research received no external funding.

Conflicts of Interest: The authors declare no conflict of interest.

References

1. David, G.; Vallotton, K.; Hupp, M.; Curt, A.; Freund, P.; Seif, M. Extent of cord pathology in the lumbosacral enlargement in non-traumatic versus traumatic spinal cord injury. *J. Neurotrauma* **2022**, *39*, 639–650. [CrossRef] [PubMed]
2. David, G.; Mohammadi, S.; Martin, A.R.; Cohen-Adad, J.; Weiskopf, N.; Thompson, A.; Freund, P. Traumatic and nontraumatic spinal cord injury: Pathological insights from neuroimaging. *Nat. Rev. Neurol.* **2019**, *15*, 718–731. [CrossRef] [PubMed]
3. Seif, M.; David, G.; Huber, E.; Vallotton, K.; Curt, A.; Freund, P. Cervical cord neurodegeneration in traumatic and non-traumatic spinal cord injury. *J. Neurotrauma* **2020**, *37*, 860–867. [CrossRef] [PubMed]
4. Soufi, K.H.; Perez, T.M.; Umoye, A.O.; Yang, J.; Burgos, M.; Martin, A.R. How Is Spinal Cord Function Measured in Degenerative Cervical Myelopathy? A Systematic Review. *J. Clin. Med.* **2022**, *11*, 1441. [CrossRef] [PubMed]
5. Oughourlian, T.C.; Wang, C.; Salamon, N.; Holly, L.T.; Ellingson, B.M. Sex-Dependent Cortical Volume Changes in Patients with Degenerative Cervical Myelopathy. *J. Clin. Med.* **2021**, *10*, 3965. [CrossRef] [PubMed]
6. Wolf, K.; Reisert, M.; Beltrán, S.F.; Klingler, J.-H.; Hubbe, U.; Krafft, A.J.; Kremers, N.; Egger, K.; Hohenhaus, M. Spinal Cord Motion in Degenerative Cervical Myelopathy: The Level of the Stenotic Segment and Gender Cause Altered Pathodynamics. *J. Clin. Med.* **2021**, *10*, 3788. [CrossRef] [PubMed]
7. Kadanka Jr, Z.; Kadanka Sr, Z.; Skutil, T.; Vlckova, E.; Bednarik, J. Walk and Run Test in Patients with Degenerative Compression of the Cervical Spinal Cord. *J. Clin. Med.* **2021**, *10*, 927. [CrossRef] [PubMed]
8. Wilson, J.; Badhiwala, J.; Moghaddamjou, A.; Yee, A.; Wilson, J.; Fehlings, M. Frailty is a better predictor than age of mortality and perioperative complications after surgery for degenerative cervical myelopathy: An analysis of 41,369 patients from the nsqip database 2010–2018. *J. Clin. Med.* **2020**, *9*, 3491. [CrossRef] [PubMed]
9. Jentzsch, T.; Cadotte, D.W.; Wilson, J.R.; Jiang, F.; Badhiwala, J.H.; Akbar, M.A.; Rocos, B.; Grossman, R.G.; Aarabi, B.; Harrop, J.S.; et al. Spinal Cord Signal Change on Magnetic Resonance Imaging May Predict Worse Clinical In- and Outpatient Outcomes in Patients with Spinal Cord Injury: A Prospective Multicenter Study in 459 Patients. *J. Clin. Med.* **2021**, *10*, 4778. [CrossRef] [PubMed]
10. Ost, K.; Jacobs, W.; Evaniew, N.; Cohen-Adad, J.; Anderson, D.; Cadotte, D. Spinal cord morphology in degenerative cervical myelopathy patients; assessing key morphological characteristics using machine vision tools. *J. Clin. Med.* **2021**, *10*, 892. [CrossRef] [PubMed]
11. Sommaruga, S.; Camara-Quintana, J.; Patel, K.; Nouri, A.; Tessitore, E.; Molliqaj, G.; Panchagnula, S.; Robinson, M.; Virojanapa, J.; Sun, X.; et al. Clinical Outcomes between Stand-Alone Zero-Profile Spacers and Cervical Plate with Cage Fixation for Anterior Cervical Discectomy and Fusion: A Retrospective Analysis of 166 Patients. *J. Clin. Med.* **2021**, *10*, 3076. [CrossRef] [PubMed]
12. Wincek, A.; Huber, J.; Leszczyńska, K.; Fortuna, W.; Okurowski, S.; Chmielak, K.; Tabakow, P. The long-term effect of treatment using the transcranial magnetic stimulation rTMS in patients after incomplete cervical or thoracic spinal cord injury. *J. Clin. Med.* **2021**, *10*, 2975. [CrossRef] [PubMed]
13. Kadanka, Z.; Kadanka, Z.; Jura, R.; Bednarik, J. Vertigo in patients with degenerative cervical myelopathy. *J. Clin. Med.* **2021**, *10*, 2496. [CrossRef] [PubMed]
14. Ghaffari-Rafi, A.; Peterson, C.; Leon-Rojas, J.E.; Tadokoro, N.; Lange, S.F.; Kaushal, M.; Tetreault, L.; Fehlings, M.G.; Martin, A.R. The Role of Magnetic Resonance Imaging to Inform Clinical Decision-Making in Acute Spinal Cord Injury: A Systematic Review and Meta-Analysis. *J. Clin. Med.* **2021**, *10*, 4948. [CrossRef]
15. Yang, X.; Gharooni, A.A.; Dhillon, R.S.; Goacher, E.; Dyson, E.W.; Mowforth, O.; Budu, A.; Wynne-Jones, G.; Francis, J.; Trivedi, R.; et al. The relative merits of posterior surgical treatments for multi-level degenerative cervical myelopathy remain uncertain: Findings from a systematic review. *J. Clin. Med.* **2021**, *10*, 3653. [CrossRef]
16. Lannon, M.; Kachur, E. Degenerative Cervical myelopathy: Clinical presentation, assessment, and natural history. *J. Clin. Med.* **2021**, *10*, 3626. [CrossRef]
17. Tu, J.; Castillo, J.V.; Das, A.; Diwan, A. Degenerative cervical myelopathy: Insights into its pathobiology and molecular mechanisms. *J. Clin. Med.* **2021**, *10*, 1214. [CrossRef]

Article

Spinal Cord Signal Change on Magnetic Resonance Imaging May Predict Worse Clinical In- and Outpatient Outcomes in Patients with Spinal Cord Injury: A Prospective Multicenter Study in 459 Patients

Thorsten Jentzsch [1,2,3], David W. Cadotte [4], Jefferson R. Wilson [1,5], Fan Jiang [1,2], Jetan H. Badhiwala [1,2], Muhammad A. Akbar [1,2], Brett Rocos [1,2], Robert G. Grossman [6], Bizhan Aarabi [7], James S. Harrop [8] and Michael G. Fehlings [1,2,*]

1. Division of Neurosurgery, Department of Surgery, University of Toronto, Toronto, ON M5T 2S8, Canada; thorsten.jentzsch@gmail.com (T.J.); jefferson.wilson@unityhealth.to (J.R.W.); fan.jiang@uhn.ca (F.J.); jetan.badhiwala@mail.utoronto.ca (J.H.B.); muhammad.akbar@mail.utoronto.ca (M.A.A.); brett.rocos@sickkids.ca (B.R.)
2. Division of Neurosurgery, Toronto Western Hospital, University Health Network, Toronto, ON M5G 2C4, Canada
3. Department of Orthopedics, Balgrist University Hospital, University of Zurich, 8008 Zurich, Switzerland
4. Division of Neurosurgery, Department of Clinical Neurosciences, University of Calgary Combined Spine Program, Hotchkiss Brain Institute, University of Calgary, Calgary, AB T2N 1N4, Canada; david.cadotte@ucalgary.ca
5. Division of Neurosurgery, St. Michael's Hospital, University Health Network, Toronto, ON M5T 2S8, Canada
6. Department of Neurosurgery, Houston Methodist Hospital, Houston, TX 77030, USA; RGrossman@houstonmethodist.org
7. Department of Neurosurgery, University of Maryland Medical Center and R Adams Cowley Shock Trauma Center, Baltimore, MD 21201, USA; BAarabi@som.umaryland.edu
8. Departments of Neurological Surgery and Orthopedic Surgery, Thomas Jefferson University, Philadelphia, PA 19107, USA; james.harrop@jefferson.edu
* Correspondence: michael.fehlings@uhn.ca; Tel.: +1-(416)-603-5801

Abstract: Prognostic factors for clinical outcome after spinal cord (SC) injury (SCI) are limited but important in patient management and education. There is a lack of evidence regarding magnetic resonance imaging (MRI) and clinical outcomes in SCI patients. Therefore, we aimed to investigate whether baseline MRI features predicted the clinical course of the disease. This study is an ancillary to the prospective North American Clinical Trials Network (NACTN) registry. Patients were enrolled from 2005–2017. MRI within 72 h of injury and a minimum follow-up of one year were available for 459 patients. Patients with American Spinal Injury Association impairment scale (AIS) E were excluded. Patients were grouped into those with ($n = 354$) versus without ($n = 105$) SC signal change on MRI T2-weighted images. Logistic regression analysis adjusted for commonly known a priori confounders (age and baseline AIS). Main outcomes and measures: The primary outcome was any adverse event. Secondary outcomes were AIS at the baseline and final follow-up, length of hospital stay (LOS), and mortality. A regression model adjusted for age and baseline AIS. Patients with intrinsic SC signal change were younger (46.0 (interquartile range (IQR) 29.0 vs. 50.0 (IQR 20.5) years, $p = 0.039$). There were no significant differences in the other baseline variables, gender, body mass index, comorbidities, and injury location. There were more adverse events in patients with SC signal change (230 (65.0%) vs. 47 (44.8%), $p < 0.001$; odds ratio (OR) = 2.09 (95% confidence interval (CI) 1.31–3.35), $p = 0.002$). The most common adverse event was cardiopulmonary (186 (40.5%)). Patients were less likely to be in the AIS D category with SC signal change at baseline (OR = 0.45 (95% CI 0.28–0.72), $p = 0.001$) and in the AIS D or E category at the final follow-up (OR = 0.36 (95% CI 0.16–0.82), $p = 0.015$). The length of stay was longer in patients with SC signal change (13.0 (IQR 17.0) vs. 11.0 (IQR 14.0), $p = 0.049$). There was no difference between the groups in mortality (11 (3.2%) vs. 4 (3.9%)). MRI SC signal change may predict adverse events and overall LOS in the SCI population. If present, patients are more likely to have a worse baseline clinical presentation (i.e., AIS) and in- or outpatient clinical outcome after one year. Patients with SC signal change may benefit from earlier, more aggressive treatment strategies and need to be educated about an unfavorable prognosis.

Keywords: spinal cord injuries; magnetic resonance imaging; MRI; neurology; paralysis; walking; outcome

Key Points

1. This is a report on a prospective registry with an exceptionally large sample size of 459 traumatic spinal cord injury patients and a long follow-up for trauma populations;

2. Spinal cord (SC) signal change on initial magnetic resonance imaging may be an independent predictor of adverse events after controlling for age and baseline neurological impairment (odds ratio of 2.09 for adverse events; odds ratios of 0.45 and 0.36 for ambulation at baseline and final follow-up, respectively);

3. Patients with SC signal change may benefit from earlier, more aggressive treatment strategies and need to be educated about an unfavorable prognosis.

1. Introduction

Spinal cord (SC) injury (SCI) is a devastating event and risk factors for the clinical outcome play an important role in patient management and education. The prevalence of traumatic SCI ranges from 236–1009 per million [1], but is likely underestimated due to a high mortality rate at the time of injury and limited diagnosis. One of the highest incidences of SCI is found in the United States, with 54 cases per million per year [2], while low rates have been reported for Spain with 8 cases per million population [3]. The levels of injury vary and incomplete tetraplegia (34%) is more common than complete paraplegia (25%), complete tetraplegia (22%), and incomplete paraplegia (17%) [4].

Physicians struggle with providing optimal care, defining the resources they need, and explaining the prognosis due to limited available data. Although magnetic resonance imaging (MRI) is a powerful imaging modality, there has been a lack of evidence regarding prospective MRI assessment and potential clinical outcomes [5–18]. A limited number of studies have reported on the association between SC intraparenchymal signal change and the clinical outcome [5–8,11,13–19], but these studies have been limited by small sample sizes with heterogeneous populations. Further, these reports also lacked long-term follow-up [5,10], inclusion of injuries to the entire spine [6], patients with an ossified posterior longitudinal ligament (OPLL) [7,8,14], SCI without radiographic abnormality (SCIWORA) [11], upper extremity impairment [16], and postoperative imaging assessment [19].

Therefore, this study aimed to investigate whether baseline MRI features predicted the clinical course of the disease. To definitively understand this relationship, a large, prospective patient cohort with SCI was examined. Based on preliminary understandings of SCI and radiological findings, it was hypothesized that MRI-assessed SC signal change at baseline would be a predictor for increased in- and outpatient adverse events and worse functional outcomes.

2. Materials and Methods

This is a study based on data from the prospective North American Clinical Trials Network (NACTN) registry [20,21], with prospective collection of imaging data and pre-determined clinical endpoints after ethical approval (CAPCR-ID: 05-0626) and with informed consent. NACTN, established in 2004, is a consortium of international neurosurgical institutions. The database is registered on ClinicalTrials.gov (accessed on 13 October 2021) [22]. NACTN's goals are to organize a multicenter network and provide a large database with which to study and improve the course of disease and adverse events of SCI.

Patients were enrolled into the NACTN database from June 2005 to March 2017. Neurologically intact patients and those with American Spinal Injury Association impairment scale (AIS) E were excluded. Patients were included if MRI was performed within 72 h of the SCI and a minimum clinical follow-up evaluation at one year was available, of which 459 patients met these criteria. Patients were grouped into those with (n = 354) versus (vs.) without (n = 105) SC signal change detected on their MRI immediately after injury. MRI SC signal change was defined as sagittal and/or axial T2-weighted signal change, read by trained radiologists and entered into the database by each participating site [23]. The MRI scanner type and field strength varied depending on the institution. SC signal change was chosen as it is thought to represent injury to the SC, which likely has implications for clinical function.

The primary outcome was the presence of one or more adverse events. The definition of an adverse event was that offered by Jiang et al. [24], including all adverse events recorded by the participating centers consisting of cardiopulmonary, pulmonary embolus, deep vein thrombosis, gastrointestinal and genitourinary, hematologic, skin, systemic infection, urinary tract infection, wound infection, neurological deterioration, hardware failure, and other (unspecified) adverse events.

The secondary outcome measures were: baseline and final AIS at the last follow-up [4], length of hospital stay, and mortality.

An extensive literature search was also undertaken for previous literature on prospective studies about acute SCI, MRI, and complications (Table 1. PubMed.gov was searched with the terms "prospective, acute spinal cord injury, magnetic resonance imaging, complications".

Table 1. Excluded studies of previous literature on prospective studies about acute spinal cord injury, magnetic resonance imaging, and complications (n = 41) [25–51].

Exclusion Criterion	Studies (n)
No acute SCI	9 [25–33]
No MRI of the spine	6 [34–39]
Experimental study	4 [40–43]
Case report	2 [44,45]
Focus on brain injury	2 [46,47]
Heterogenous study population (not exclusively SCI patients)	1 [48]
Metastatic SC compression	1 [49]
Neurological condition (amyotrophic lateral sclerosis)	1 [50]
No association between imaging and clinical outcome	1 [51]

Note: PubMed.gov (accessed on 31 August 2020) search with the terms "prospective, acute spinal cord injury, magnetic resonance imaging, complications".

Data are given in absolute numbers with percentages (%) and medians with interquartile ranges (IQRs). For univariate analysis, the Wilcoxon rank sum and chi-squared tests were used. For multivariate analysis, logistic regression models were chosen due to the categorical nature of the data. AIS was categorized into AIS D (ambulatory) vs. AIS A-C (non-ambulatory). The analysis adjusted for commonly known a priori confounders (instead of a preliminary analysis for predictor identification), age, and baseline AIS, and included 435 patients due to missing data in the age category (n = 24). Surgery was not included in the analysis since this would have reduced the patient number even further. Of note, even when including this variable, the results did not change substantially. The performance of the model was acceptable according to the goodness-of-fit test by Hosmer-Lemeshow. We also calculated the sensitivity, specificity, positive predictive value (PPV), negative predictive value (NPV), likelihood ratios (LRs) and area under the curve. p-values < 5% were considered significant. In a post hoc power calculation, the power was 96.0% (considering the adverse events in each SC signal change group (65.0% (n = 354) vs. 44.8% (n = 105)) and an alpha of 5.0%). Analyses were carried out using Stata (version IC 13.1; StataCorp LP, College Station, TX, USA).

3. Results

SCI traumatic patients with MRI SC signal change were younger (46.0 (interquartile range (IQR)) 29.0 vs. 50.0 (IQR 20.5) years, $p = 0.039$). There were no differences in the other baseline variables, i.e., gender (females: 65 (19.1%) vs. 21 (20.0%), $p = 0.831$), body mass index (25.9 (IQR 5.9) vs. 25.8 (7.0), $p = 0.708$), smoking (95 (27.8%) vs. 20 (19.6%), $p = 0.098$), comorbidities (138 (40.1%) vs. 42 (40.0%), $p = 0.983$), mechanism of injury (fall: 132 (39.1%) vs. 49 (49.5%), $p = 0.116$), and injury location (cervical: 273 (78.5%) vs. 88 (84.6%), $p = 0.388$) (Table 2).

Table 2. Baseline data for spinal cord injury patients stratified by radiographic spinal cord signal change ($n = 459$).

		Spinal Cord T2 Signal Change				
		Yes ($n = 355$)		No ($n = 105$)		
Variable		Median	(IQR)	Median	(IQR)	p-Value *
Age ($n = 435$)		46.0	(29.0)	50.0	(20.5)	0.039
Gender (n = 446), n (%)						0.831
	Female	65	(19.1)	21	(20.0)	
	Male	277	(81.0)	84	(80.0)	
BMI ($n = 422$)		25.9	(5.9)	25.8	(7.0)	0.708
Smoker ($n = 444$), n (%)		95	(27.8)	20	(19.6)	0.098
Comorbidities ($n = 449$), n (%)		138	(40.1)	42	(40.0)	0.983
Mechanism of injury ($n = 437$), n (%)						0.116
	Fall	132	(39.1)	49	(49.5)	
	Motor vehicle accident	154	(45.4)	34	(34.3)	
	Sports	32	(9.5)	7	(7.1)	
	Other (assault, blast)	20	(5.9)	9	(9.1)	
Injury location ($n = 452$), n (%)						0.169
	Cervical	273	(78.5)	88	(84.6)	
	Thoracic and lumbosacral conus	75	(21.5)	16	(15.4)	

* Wilcoxon rank sum or chi-squared test. Abbreviations: n (absolute number); IQR (interquartile range); % (percent); BMI (body mass index).

Adverse events were observed in 277 (60.4%) patients. The most common adverse event was cardiopulmonary (186 (40.5%)). There were more adverse events in patients with SC signal change (230 (65.0%) vs. 47 (44.8%), $p < 0.001$) (Table 3). These differences remained significant in a logistic regression model (odds ratio (OR) = 2.09 (95% confidence interval (CI) 1.32–3.35), $p = 0.002$), indicating that patients with SC signal change were 109% more likely to develop an adverse event than patients without SC signal change, when controlling for other factors (Table 4). The sensitivity of the SC signal change for adverse events was 83.0% and the specificity was 31.9%. The PPV was 64.9% and the NPV was 55.2%. The positive LR was 1.22 (95% CI 1.09–1.36) and the negative LR was 0.53 (0.38–0.75). The area under the curve was 0.57 (95% CI 0.53–0.62).

Patients with SC signal change at baseline had significantly worse neurologic injuries (OR = 0.45 (95% CI 0.28–0.72), $p = 0.001$) and final follow-ups (OR = 0.36 (95% CI 0.16–0.82), $p = 0.015$) when adjusting for age (OR = 1.00 (95% CI 0.99–1.02), $p = 0.379$ and OR = 1.03 (95% CI 1.01–1.05), $p < 0.001$, respectively). This indicated that patients with SC signal change were 55% and 64% less likely to be in the AIS D category at baseline and AIS D or E category at final follow-up after one year, respectively, than patients without SC signal change.

Table 3. Clinical outcome data for spinal cord injury patients stratified by radiographic spinal cord signal change (n = 459).

	Spinal Cord T2 Signal Change				
	Yes (n = 354)		No (n = 105)		
Variable	Median	(IQR)	Median	(IQR)	p-Value *
Adverse events, n (%) [†]	230	(65.0)	47	(44.8)	<0.001
Cardiopulmonary	157	(68.3)	29	(61.7)	0.383
Pulmonary embolus	12	(5.2)	2	(4.3)	0.784
DVT	16	(7.0)	2	(4.3)	0.494
Systemic	11	(4.8)	5	(10.6)	0.117
UTI	45	(19.6)	7	(14.9)	0.455
GI and GU	28	(12.2)	5	(10.6)	0.767
Wound infection	5	(2.2)	3	(6.4)	0.116
Hematology	78	(33.9)	16	(34.0)	0.986
Skin	35	(15.2)	6	(12.7)	0.666
Neurological	60	(26.1)	12	(25.5)	0.937
Hardware failure	3	(1.3)	3	(1.3)	0.431
Other (unspecified)	143	(62.2)	22	(46.8)	0.050
AIS D					
Baseline	175	(49.7)	72	(68.6)	0.001
AIS D or E					
Follow-up	288	(81.1)	97	(92.4)	0.006
Length of stay (n = 442)	13.0	(17.0)	11.0	(14.0)	0.049
Death (n = 443), n (%)	11	(3.2)	4	(3.9)	0.767

* Wilcoxon rank sum or chi-squared test; [†] It was possible that patients experienced more than one adverse event, and other (unspecified) refers to adverse events that were not further specified. Abbreviations: n (absolute number); IQR (interquartile range); % (percent); DVT (deep vein thrombosis); UTI (urinary tract infection); GI (gastrointestinal); GU (genitourinary), AIS (American Spinal Injury Association impairment scale).

Table 4. Logistic regression model for adverse events in spinal cord injury patients (n = 435).

Variable	OR	95% CI	p-Value *
Spinal cord T2 signal change	2.09	(1.31–3.35)	0.002
Age	1.00	(0.99–1.01)	0.598
AIS D at baseline	0.36	(0.24–0.55)	<0.001

* Wald test. Note: This logistic regression model included all shown variables (adverse events, spinal cord T2 signal change, age, and AIS D at baseline) (pseudo R2 = 0.066). The analysis adjusted for commonly known a priori confounders (instead of a preliminary analysis for predictor identification), age, and AIS D at baseline. Age and AIS D were chosen as they are known to influence the outcome (e.g., younger patients and AIS D (i.e., ambulatory) patients are less likely to have an unfavorable outcome after spinal cord injury compared to elderly patients and AIS A-C (non-ambulatory) patients) [52,53]. Importantly, the other potential predictors (Table 2) did not show any statistical associations in the univariate analysis, confirming our choice of a priori confounders. Abbreviations: OR (odds ratio); % (percent); CI (confidence interval); AIS (American Spinal Injury Association impairment scale).

The length of stay was significantly longer in patients with SC signal change (13 (IQR 17.0) vs. 11 (IQR 14.0), p = 0.049). There was no difference in mortality (11 (3.2%) vs. 4 (3.9%), p = 0.767) (Table 2).

The results of the literature search on prospective studies about acute SCI, MRI, and complications are shown in Table 5 and Table S1 in Supplementary Material.

Table 5. Previous literature on prospective studies about acute spinal cord injury, magnetic resonance imaging, and adverse events (n = 41) [5–18].

Study Number	Author(s)	Patients (n)	Aim	Main Finding	Age Mean	Age (SD)	Limitation
1	Rutges et al. [5]	19	Change during first three postoperative weeks	1. SC edema length increased within first 48 h, but decreased thereafter 2. Hematoma in all AIS-A and B patients	57.2	(15.1)	Short-term follow-up (three weeks)
2	Martinez-Pérez et al. [6]	86	Radiologic findings for neurologic prognosis	Edema > 36 mm and facet dislocation predicted worse neurological outcome	47.6	na	Limited patient number and cervical spine only
3	Gu et al. [7]	36	Outcome predictors in patients with OPLL	High-intensity zones (vs low-intensity zones) were associated with worse outcomes (mJOA improvement of 2.5 (SD 2.8) vs. 6.3 (1.5) points)	53.5	(13.3)	Limited to OPLL
4	Kwon et al. [8]	38	Outcome predictors in patients with OPLL	Higher intramedullary signal intensity grade and space available for cord were associated with worse outcomes	62.7	na	Limited to OPLL
5	Freund et al. [9]	13 (18 controls)	Neuronal degeneration above the lesion level	1. Rapid decline in cross-sectional spinal cord area 2. Decreased cross-sectional SC loss was associated with improved SCIM scores	46.9	(20.2)	Limited patient number
6	Maeda et al. [10]	88	Extraneural soft-tissue damage and clinical relevance in patients without bone injury	Association between anterior longitudinal disruption, disc damage, and prevertebral hyperintensity with AIS motor score	64	na	Short-follow-up (mean six months (range of one to seven months))
7	Machino et al. [11]	100	Occurrence rate of ISI and PVH in patients with cervical SCIWORA	1. ISI and PVH in 92% and 90%, respectively 2. ISI and PVH in 100% each in AIS A and B patients. 3. Negative correlation between ISI and preoperative JOA score and recovery rate of JOA score	55	na	Limited to SCIWORA

Table 5. Cont.

Study Number	Author(s)	Patients (n)	Aim	Main Finding	Age Mean	Age (SD)	Limitation
8	Miyanji et al. [12]	100	MRI association with neurologic status	1. MSCC and lesion length was associated with complete motor and sensory SCI 2. Edema, hemorrhage, cord swelling, stenosis, and soft-tissue injury associated with complete SCI 3. MSCC and MCC correlated with baseline AIS motor scores 4. MSCC, cord swelling, and hemorrhage predictive of neurological outcome 5. Cord swelling and hemorrhage correlated with AIS score after controlling for baseline neurologic assessment	45	na	Limited number of patients
9	Boldin et al. [13]	29	Investigated spinal cord hemorrhage and length of hematoma as predictors of recovery	1. Hemorrhage > 4 mm was associated with complete injury 2. Edema and hematoma length were longer in AIS A patients	43.5	18.1	Limited patient number
10	Koyanagi et al. [14]	28	Radiographic and clinical findings in patients with OPLL	1. Intramedullary hyperintensity and paravertebral soft tissue injuries in all four patients with Frankel grades A and B, in 80% with Frankel C, and 56% in Frankel D 2. Paravertebral soft tissue injuries were also associated with Frankel grades A–C	63.0	na	Limited to OPLL
11	Takahashi et al. [15]	43	Investigated association between image findings and clinical outcome	1. Baseline low-intensity T2 signal was associated with poor prognosis 2. High-intensity signal after 2–3 weeks was associated with permanent paralysis	63.4	na	Limited patient number

Table 5. *Cont.*

Study Number	Author(s)	Patients (n)	Aim	Main Finding	Age Mean	Age (SD)	Limitation
12	Ishida and Tominaga [16]	22	Evaluated MRI predictors for good neurologic recovery in patients with only upper extremity impairment	1. Absence of abnormal signal intensity was best predictor of neurologic recovery	45.9	na	Limited patient number
13	Koyanagi et al. [17]	42	MRI predictors of worse outcome in patients without fracture or dislocation	Intramedullary hyperintensity on T2-weighted images was associated with more severe neurological deficits	58.9	na	No results on association between MRI and clinical outcome
14	Shimada and Tokioka [18]	75	MRI findings and clinical outcomes	1. T2-weighted images were associated with severity of spinal cord damage and clinical outcome 2. Best time for imaging is at time of injury and two to three weeks later	54.7	na	Limited patient number

Note 1: PubMed.gov (accessed on 31 August 2020) search with the terms "prospective, acute spinal cord injury, magnetic resonance imaging, adverse events"; Note 2: The variables used for MRI and clinical outcome evaluation are heterogenous. Previous studies most commonly described SC edema [5,6,13] ("signal intensity" [7,8,11,14–18]) in their MRI evaluation, but also hematoma [5,13], space available for cord [8], cross-sectional SC area [9], anterior longitudinal disruption [10], disc damage [10], prevertebral hyperintensity [10,11], maximum spinal cord compression [12], lesion length [12], cord swelling [12], stenosis [12], soft-tissue injury [12], and maximum canal compromise [12]. They often focused on the AIS grade [5,6,13,18] in their clinical evaluation, but also mentioned the mJOA [7] and JOA [11], AIS motor score [8,10,12,16], spinal cord independence measure [9], Frankel grade [14], incomplete and complete paralysis [15,17]. Abbreviations: n (absolute number); SD (standard deviation); SC (spinal cord); h (hours); AIS (American Spinal Injury Association impairment scale); mm (millimeters); na (not applicable); vs. (versus); OPLL (ossification of posterior longitudinal ligament); mJOA (modified Japanese Orthopedic Association); SCIM (spinal cord independence measure); ISI (increased signal intensity); PVH (prevertebral hyperintensity); SCIWORA (spinal cord injury without radiographic abnormality); MRI (magnetic resonance imaging); MSCC (maximum spinal cord compression); MCC (maximum canal compromise).

4. Discussion
4.1. Main Findings

This ancillary study on the prospective NACTN registry [20] reviewed 459 patients with a relatively long follow-up in a trauma population of at least one year. The data showed that SC signal change on the initial MRI after traumatic SCI is an independent predictor of adverse events, as defined by Jiang et al. [24]. This factor remained significant even after controlling for age and baseline AIS impairment, and patients with SC signal change were 109% more likely to suffer an adverse event. SC signal change is consistent with significant neurologic impairment in that 55% were ambulatory at baseline and were 64% less likely to be ambulatory at the final follow-up. The length of stay in the hospital was also longer in patients with SC signal change, but there was no difference in mortality. The SC signal intensity appears to be a rapid and accurate method with which to assess the predicted outcome, tailor the treatment options (e.g., early surgery), and educate the patient, so as to potentially alter the actual outcome.

The initial mechanical force acting on the SC is the primary injury. These injuries are mostly due to impact with persistent compression (e.g., bone fracture fragments) but can also be due to impact with transient compression (e.g., hyperextension injury). These forces damage the SC pathways and blood vessels, which leads to secondary injuries by several mechanisms, such as vascular malfunctioning (acute phase), Wallerian degeneration (subacute phase), and glial scarring (chronic phase), as summarized by Alizadeh et al. [54]. In the authors' opinion, it is very important to obtain and carefully assess initial MRIs after traumatic SCI to make general predictions of the patient's immediate and long-term outcome.

4.2. Current Knowledge and Addition of Our Findings

The previous literature on the predictive nature of SC signal change for the clinical baseline and outcome in patients with SCI is sparse. A detailed literature search of SCI and MRI signal change was performed with a systematic review [5–18,25–51] (Tables 1 and 5). Fourteen studies met the inclusion criteria, as defined as being prospective and examining acute SCI, MRI, and adverse events [5–18]. Aside from the limited number of studies and their lack of controlling for confounders such as age [5–18], the available reports are limited by short-term follow-up (5, 10), a smaller sample size [9,12,13,15,17,18], cervical spine only [6], OPLL [7,8,14], SCIWORA [11], and upper extremity impairment [16].

Herein, the previous literature on associations between imaging findings and clinical outcomes is described. Rutges et al. [5] investigated the MRI signal change during the first three postoperative weeks (n = 19). They reported that the SC T2 signal increased within the first 48 h but decreased thereafter. Martínez-Pérez et al. [6] described the radiologic findings for the neurological prognosis (n = 86). They noted that a T2 signal > 36 millimeters (mm) and facet dislocation predicted a worse neurological outcome. Gu et al. [7] and Kwon et al. [8] studied radiological outcome predictors in SCI patients with ossified posterior longitudinal ligament (OPLL) (n = 36 and n = 38, respectively). The authors reported that high-intensity zones and a higher intramedullary signal intensity grade, as well as space available for the cord, were associated with worse outcomes. Freund et al. [9] investigated neuronal degeneration above the SCI lesion level (n = 13 and 18 controls). The authors found a rapid decline in cross-sectional spinal cord area and an association between decreased cross-sectional SC loss and improved SC independence. Maeda et al. [10] reported extraneural soft-tissue damage and clinical relevance in patients without bone injury (n = 88). They showed an association between anterior longitudinal disruption, disc damage, and prevertebral hyperintensity with AIS motor scores. Machino et al. [11] reported the occurrence rate of increased signal intensity (ISI) and prevertebral hyperintensity (PVH) in patients with cervical SCI without radiographic abnormality (SCIWORA) (n = 100). They found that ISI and PVH were common (92% and 90%, respectively), particularly in AIS A-B patients (100% each), and noted a negative correlation between the ISI and preoperative Japanese Orthopedic Association (JOA) score as well as its recovery rate. Miyanji et al. [12]

studied MRI associations with the neurologic status ($n = 100$). These authors reported that the maximum SC compression and lesion length were associated with complete motor and sensory SCI. Further, they noted that edema, hemorrhage, cord swelling, stenosis, and soft-tissue injury were associated with complete SCI. Boldin et al. [13] investigated SCI hemorrhage and the length of hematoma as predictors of recovery ($n = 29$). They reported a hemorrhage >4 mm to be associated with complete injury. The edema and hematoma length were also longer in AIS A patients. Koyanagi et al. [14] investigated radiographic and clinical findings in patients with OPLL. Their results showed intramedullary hyperintensity and paravertebral soft tissue injuries in all four patients with Frankel grades A and B, in 80% with Frankel C, and 56% in Frankel D. Takahashi et al. [15] studied the association between image findings and clinical outcomes ($n = 43$). They reported that a baseline low-intensity T2 signal was associated with a poor prognosis. A high-intensity signal after two to three weeks was also associated with permanent paralysis. Ishida and Tominaga [16] evaluated MRI predictors for neurological recovery in patients with only upper-extremity impairment ($n = 22$). Their results showed that an absence of abnormal signal intensity was the best predictor of neurological recovery. Koyanagi et al. [17] reported on MRI predictors of the worse outcomes in patients without a fracture or dislocation ($n = 42$). Intramedullary hyperintensity on T2-weighted images was associated with more severe neurological deficits. Shimada and Tokioka [18] investigated MRI findings and clinical outcomes. Their results showed that T2-weighted images were associated with the severity of spinal cord damage and clinical outcome.

This study is limited by the inherent issues with registries and the heterogeneity of the SCI population. Since multiple institutions are involved, the exact timing of the MRI, the type and setting of the MRI scanner, and the availability and validity of data regarding the clinical assessments may vary. Future studies may add other potential predictor variables, such as corticosteroid use and comorbidities in their regression models. Although we controlled for age in the final regression model and there were no statistical differences in the mechanism of injury, the cohort with SC signal change was younger and included more motor vehicle accidents. Future studies should focus on this issue. Subsequent studies may also investigate different MRI findings, such as tissue bridges [55], the benefit of early surgical intervention in patients with SC signal change, and the use and prediction of subsequent MRIs and longer follow-ups. Another limitation is that many adverse events were not specified in detail, thus limiting further sub-analysis or assessment of the actual severity of adverse events. Future studies should focus on specifying adverse events in as much detail as possible. Furthermore, cervical SCI accounts for almost 80% of cases in this study, while the number of thoracic SCI cases was low. This constitutes a substantial limitation of this study, which analyzed the entire SCI spectrum, based on this composition. Future studies could opt to include more thoracic SCI cases.

5. Conclusions

MRI SC signal change may predict the clinical course of disease in patients after acute traumatic SCI. If signal change is present, patients are more likely to have a lower baseline clinical presentation as well as a decreased in- or outpatient clinical outcome after one year. Therefore, patients with SC signal change may benefit from earlier and more aggressive treatment strategies and need to be educated about an unfavorable prognosis.

Supplementary Materials: The following are available online at https://www.mdpi.com/article/10.3390/jcm10204778/s1, Table S1: Excluded studies of previous literature on prospective studies about acute spinal cord injury, magnetic resonance imaging, and complications ($n = 41$), References S1: Supplementary references.

Author Contributions: T.J. and M.G.F., idea, conception and design, acquisition of data, analysis and interpretation of data, and drafting the manuscript; M.A.A. and B.R., acquisition, analysis, and interpretation of data, F.J., J.H.B., D.W.C., J.R.W., R.G.G., B.A. and J.S.H., acquisition of data. All authors have read and agreed to the published version of the manuscript.

Funding: No specific funding supported this work.

Institutional Review Board Statement: The study was conducted according to the guidelines of the Declaration of Helsinki, and approved by the University Health Network Research Ethics Board (CAPCR-ID: 05-0626 approved on 9 November 2005).

Informed Consent Statement: Informed consent was obtained from all individuals who participated in the study.

Data Availability Statement: All data is reported in this study.

Acknowledgments: The NACTN SCI Registry is supported by the US Army Medical Research Acquisition Activity (USAMRAA) under Contract No. W81XWH-16-C-0031 and earlier Department of Defense Awards. M.G.F. is supported by the Gerry and Tootsie Halbert Chair in Neural Repair and Regeneration and the DeZwirek Family Foundation.

Conflicts of Interest: The authors declare that they have no competing interest.

References

1. Cripps, R.A.; Lee, B.; Wing, P.; Weerts, E.; Mackay, J.; Brown, D. A global map for traumatic spinal cord injury epidemiology: Towards a living data repository for injury prevention. *Spinal Cord* **2010**, *49*, 493–501. [CrossRef] [PubMed]
2. Dixon, G.S.; Danesh, J.N.; Caradoc-Davies, T.H. Epidemiology of Spinal Cord Injury in New Zealand. *Neuroepidemiology* **1993**, *12*, 88–95. [CrossRef] [PubMed]
3. Biering-Sørensen, F.; Pedersen, V.; Clausen, S. Epidemiology of spinal cord lesions in Denmark. *Spinal Cord* **1990**, *28*, 105–118. [CrossRef] [PubMed]
4. Kirshblum, S.C.; Burns, S.P.; Biering-Sørensen, F.; Donovan, W.; Graves, D.; Jha, A.; Johansen, M.; Jones, L.; Krassioukov, A.; Mulcahey, M.; et al. International standards for neurological classification of spinal cord injury (Revised 2011). *J. Spinal Cord Med.* **2011**, *34*, 535–546. [CrossRef]
5. Rutges, J.P.H.J.; Kwon, B.K.; Heran, M.; Ailon, T.; Street, J.T.; Dvorak, M.F. A prospective serial MRI study following acute traumatic cervical spinal cord injury. *Eur. Spine J.* **2017**, *26*, 2324–2332. [CrossRef]
6. Martínez-Pérez, R.; Cepeda, S.; Paredes, I.; Alen, J.F.; Lagares, A. MRI Prognostication Factors in the Setting of Cervical Spinal Cord Injury Secondary to Trauma. *World Neurosurg.* **2017**, *101*, 623–632. [CrossRef]
7. Gu, J.; Guan, F.; Zhu, L.; Guan, G.; Chi, Z.; Li, W.; Yu, Z. Predictors of Surgical Outcome in Acute Spinal Cord Injury Patients with Cervical Ossification of the Posterior Longitudinal Ligament. *World Neurosurg.* **2016**, *90*, 364–371. [CrossRef]
8. Kwon, S.Y.; Shin, J.J.; Lee, J.H.; Cho, W.H. Prognostic factors for surgical outcome in spinal cord injury associated with ossification of the posterior longitudinal ligament (OPLL). *J. Orthop. Surg. Res.* **2015**, *10*, 1–9. [CrossRef]
9. Freund, P.; Weiskopf, N.; Ashburner, J.; Wolf, K.; Sutter, R.; Altmann, D.R.; Friston, K.; Thompson, A.; Curt, A. MRI investigation of the sensorimotor cortex and the corticospinal tract after acute spinal cord injury: A prospective longitudinal study. *Lancet Neurol.* **2013**, *12*, 873–881. [CrossRef]
10. Maeda, T.; Ueta, T.; Mori, E.; Yugue, I.; Kawano, O.; Takao, T.; Sakai, H.; Okada, S.; Shiba, K. Soft-Tissue Damage and Segmental Instability in Adult Patients With Cervical Spinal Cord Injury Without Major Bone Injury. *Spine* **2012**, *37*, E1560–E1566. [CrossRef]
11. Machino, M.; Yukawa, Y.; Ito, K.; Nakashima, H.; Kanbara, S.; Morita, D.; Kato, F. Can magnetic resonance imaging reflect the prognosis in patients of cervical spinal cord injury without radiographic abnormality? *Spine* **2011**, *36*, E1568–E1572. [CrossRef]
12. Miyanji, F.; Furlan, J.C.; Aarabi, B.; Arnold, P.M.; Fehlings, M.G. Acute Cervical Traumatic Spinal Cord Injury: MR Imaging Findings Correlated with Neurologic Outcome—Prospective Study with 100 Consecutive Patients1. *Radiology* **2007**, *243*, 820–827. [CrossRef]
13. Boldin, C.; Raith, J.; Fankhauser, F.; Haunschmid, C.; Schwantzer, G.; Schweighofer, F. Predicting Neurologic Recovery in Cervical Spinal Cord Injury With Postoperative MR Imaging. *Spine* **2006**, *31*, 554–559. [CrossRef]
14. Koyanagi, I.; Iwasaki, Y.; Hida, K.; Imamura, H.; Fujimoto, S.; Akino, M. Acute Cervical Cord Injury Associated with Ossification of the Posterior Longitudinal Ligament. *Neurosurgery* **2003**, *53*, 887–892. [CrossRef]
15. Takahashi, M.; Harada, Y.; Inoue, H.; Shimada, K. Traumatic cervical cord injury at C3–4 without radiographic abnormalities: Correlation of magnetic resonance findings with clinical features and outcome. *J. Orthop. Surg.* **2002**, *10*, 129–135. [CrossRef]
16. Ishida, Y.; Tominaga, T. Predictors of Neurologic Recovery in Acute Central Cervical Cord Injury with Only Upper Extremity Impairment. *Spine* **2002**, *27*, 1652–1657. [CrossRef]
17. Koyanagi, I.; Iwasaki, Y.; Hida, K.; Akino, M.; Imamura, H.; Abe, H. Acute cervical cord injury without fracture or dislocation of the spinal column. *J. Neurosurg. Spine* **2000**, *93*, 15–20. [CrossRef]
18. Shimada, K.; Tokioka, T. Sequential MR studies of cervical cord injury: Correlation with neurological damage and clinical outcome. *Spinal Cord* **1999**, *37*, 410–415. [CrossRef]
19. Aarabi, B.; Sansur, C.A.; Ibrahimi, D.M.; Simard, J.M.; Hersh, D.; Le, E.; Diaz, C.; Massetti, J.; Akhtar-Danesh, N. Intramedullary Lesion Length on Postoperative Magnetic Resonance Imaging is a Strong Predictor of ASIA Impairment Scale Grade Conversion Following Decompressive Surgery in Cervical Spinal Cord Injury. *Neurosurgery* **2016**, *80*, 610–620. [CrossRef]

20. Grossman, R.G.; Toups, E.G.; Frankowski, R.F.; Burau, K.D.; Howley, S. North American Clinical Trials Network for the Treatment of Spinal Cord Injury: Goals and progress. *J. Neurosurg. Spine* **2012**, *17*, 6–10. [CrossRef]
21. Grossman, R.G.; Frankowski, R.F.; Burau, K.D.; Toups, E.G.; Crommett, J.W.; Johnson, M.M.; Fehlings, M.; Tator, C.H.; Shaffrey, C.I.; Harkema, S.J.; et al. Incidence and severity of acute complications after spinal cord injury. *J. Neurosurg. Spine* **2012**, *17*, 119–128. [CrossRef]
22. ClinicalTrials.gov. Spinal Cord Injury Registry—NACTN (NACTN). 2005. Available online: http://clinicaltrials.gov/ct2/show/NCT00178724?term=NACTN&recr=Open&cond=spinal+cord+injury&rank=1 (accessed on 13 October 2021).
23. Rhee, J.; Tetreault, L.A.; Chapman, J.R.; Wilson, J.R.; Smith, J.S.; Martin, A.R.; Dettori, J.R.; Fehlings, M.G. Nonoperative Versus Operative Management for the Treatment Degenerative Cervical Myelopathy: An Updated Systematic Review. *Glob. Spine J.* **2017**, *7* (Suppl. 3), 35S–41S. [CrossRef]
24. Jiang, F.; Jaja, B.N.; Kurpad, S.N.; Badhiwala, J.H.; Aarabi, B.; Grossman, R.G.; Harrop, J.S.; Guest, J.D.; Schär, R.T.; Shaffrey, C.I.; et al. Acute Adverse Events After Spinal Cord Injury and Their Relationship to Long-term Neurologic and Functional Outcomes: Analysis From the North American Clinical Trials Network for Spinal Cord Injury. *Crit. Care Med.* **2019**, *47*, e854–e862. [CrossRef]
25. Giannarini, G.; Kessler, T.M.; Roth, B.; Vermathen, P.; Thoeny, H.C. Functional Multiparametric Magnetic Resonance Imaging of the Kidneys Using Blood Oxygen Level Dependent and Diffusion-Weighted Sequences. *J. Urol.* **2014**, *192*, 434–439. [CrossRef]
26. Katsumi, K.; Yamazaki, A.; Watanabe, K.; Ohashi, M.; Shoji, H. Can Prophylactic Bilateral C4/C5 Foraminotomy Prevent Postoperative C5 Palsy After Open-Door Laminoplasty? *Spine* **2012**, *37*, 748–754. [CrossRef]
27. Ichihara, D.; Okada, E.; Chiba, K.; Toyama, Y.; Fujiwara, H.; Momoshima, S.; Nishiwaki, Y.; Hashimoto, T.; Ogawa, J.; Watanabe, M.; et al. Longitudinal magnetic resonance imaging study on whiplash injury patients: Minimum 10-year follow-up. *J. Orthop. Sci.* **2009**, *14*, 602–610. [CrossRef]
28. Marquardt, G.; Setzer, M.; Szelenyi, A.; Seifert, V.; Gerlach, R. Significance of serial S100b and NSE serum measurements in surgically treated patients with spondylotic cervical myelopathy. *Acta Neurochir.* **2009**, *151*, 1439–1443. [CrossRef]
29. Como, J.J.; Thompson, M.A.; Anderson, J.S.; Shah, R.R.; Claridge, J.A.; Yowler, C.J.; Malangoni, M.A. Is magnetic resonance imaging essential in clearing the cervical spine in obtunded patients with blunt trauma? *J. Trauma* **2007**, *63*, 544–549. [CrossRef]
30. Summers, B.; Malhan, K.; Cassar-Pullicino, V. Low back pain on passive straight leg raising: The anterior theca as a source of pain. *Spine* **2005**, *30*, 342–345. [CrossRef]
31. Ishibe, T.; Takahashi, S. Respiratory Dysfunction in Patients with Chronic-Onset Cervical Myelopathy. *Spine* **2002**, *27*, 2234–2239. [CrossRef]
32. Friedman, D.; Flanders, A.; Thomas, C.; Millar, W. Vertebral artery injury after acute cervical spine trauma: Rate of occurrence as detected by MR angiography and assessment of clinical consequences. *Am. J. Roentgenol.* **1995**, *164*, 443–447. [CrossRef] [PubMed]
33. Tosi, L.; Righetti, C.; Terrini, G.; Zanette, G. Atypical syndromes caudal to the injury site in patients following spinal cord injury. A clinical, neurophysiological and MRI study. *Spinal Cord* **1993**, *31*, 751–756. [CrossRef] [PubMed]
34. Bush, L.; Brookshire, R.; Roche, B.; Johnson, A.; Cole, F.; Karmy-Jones, R.; Long, W.; Martin, M.J. Evaluation of Cervical Spine Clearance by Computed Tomographic Scan Alone in Intoxicated Patients with Blunt Trauma. *JAMA Surg.* **2016**, *151*, 807. [CrossRef] [PubMed]
35. Arija-Blázquez, A.; Ceruelo-Abajo, S.; Díaz-Merino, M.S.; Godino-Duran, J.A.; Martínez-Dhier, L.; Martin, J.L.R.; Florensa-Vila, J. Effects of electromyostimulation on muscle and bone in men with acute traumatic spinal cord injury: A randomized clinical trial. *J. Spinal Cord Med.* **2013**, *37*, 299–309. [CrossRef]
36. Sabre, L.; Tomberg, T.; Kõrv, J.; Kepler, J.; Kepler, K.; Linnamägi, Ü.; Asser, T. Brain activation in the acute phase of traumatic spinal cord injury. *Spinal Cord* **2013**, *51*, 623–629. [CrossRef]
37. Kim, K.; Mishina, M.; Kokubo, R.; Nakajima, T.; Morimoto, D.; Isu, T.; Kobayashi, S.; Teramoto, A. Ketamine for acute neuropathic pain in patients with spinal cord injury. *J. Clin. Neurosci.* **2013**, *20*, 804–807. [CrossRef]
38. Kelly, J.; O'Briain, D.; Kelly, G.; Mc Cabe, J. Imaging the spine for tumour and trauma—A national audit of practice in Irish hospitals. *Surgeon* **2012**, *10*, 80–83. [CrossRef]
39. Hiersemenzel, L.-P.; Curt, A.; Dietz, V. From spinal shock to spasticity: Neuronal adaptations to a spinal cord injury. *Neurology* **2000**, *54*, 1574–1582. [CrossRef]
40. Wang-Leandro, A.; Hobert, M.K.; Alisauskaite, N.; Dziallas, P.; Rohn, K.; Stein, V.M.; Tipold, A. Spontaneous acute and chronic spinal cord injuries in paraplegic dogs: A comparative study of in vivo diffusion tensor imaging. *Spinal Cord* **2017**, *55*, 1108–1116. [CrossRef]
41. Wang-Leandro, A.; Siedenburg, J.; Hobert, M.; Dziallas, P.; Rohn, K.; Stein, V.; Tipold, A. Comparison of Preoperative Quantitative Magnetic Resonance Imaging and Clinical Assessment of Deep Pain Perception as Prognostic Tools for Early Recovery of Motor Function in Paraplegic Dogs with Intervertebral Disk Herniations. *J. Veter Intern. Med.* **2017**, *31*, 842–848. [CrossRef]
42. Dickomeit, M.; Jaggy, A.; Forterre, F.; Gorgas, D.; Lang, J.; Spreng, D. Incidence of spinal compressive lesions in chondrodystrophic dogs with abnormal recovery after hemilaminectomy for treatment of thoracolumbar disc disease: A prospective magnetic resonance imaging study. *Vet. Surg.* **2010**, *39*, 165–172. [CrossRef]
43. Nout, Y.S.; Mihai, G.; Tovar, C.A.; Schmalbrock, P.; Bresnahan, J.C.; Beattie, M.S. Hypertonic saline attenuates cord swelling and edema in experimental spinal cord injury: A study utilizing magnetic resonance imaging. *Crit. Care Med.* **2009**, *37*, 2160–2166. [CrossRef]

44. Liu, H.M.; Dong, C.; Zhang, Y.Z.; Tian, Y.Y.; Chen, H.X.; Zhang, S.; Li, N.; Gu, P. Clinical and imaging features of spinal cord type of neuro Behçet disease: A case report and systematic review. *Medicine* **2017**, *96*, e7958. [CrossRef]
45. Takahata, S.; Shirado, O.; Minami, A.; Oda, H. Quadriparesis due to acute collapse of a seemingly stabilized C5/6 segment in a patient with rheumatoid arthritis—A case report. *Orthopedics* **2008**, *31*, 401.
46. Tolonen, A.; Turkka, J.; Salonen, O.; Ahoniemi, E.; Alaranta, H. Traumatic brain injury is under-diagnosed in patients with spinal cord injury. *Acta Derm. Venereol.* **2007**, *39*, 622–626. [CrossRef]
47. Hadjipavlou, A.; Tosounidis, T.; Gaitanis, I.; Kakavelakis, K.; Katonis, P. Balloon kyphoplasty as a single or as an adjunct procedure for the management of symptomatic vertebral haemangiomas. *J. Bone Jt. Surgery. Br. Vol.* **2007**, *89*, 495–502. [CrossRef]
48. Awad, B.I.; Carmody, M.A.; Lubelski, D.; El Hawi, M.; Claridge, J.A.; Como, J.J.; Mroz, T.E.; Moore, T.A.; Steinmetz, M.P. Adjacent Level Ligamentous Injury Associated with Traumatic Cervical Spine Fractures: Indications for Imaging and Implications for Treatment. *World Neurosurg.* **2015**, *84*, 69–75. [CrossRef]
49. McGivern, U.; Drinkwater, K.; Clarke, J.; Locke, I. A Royal College of Radiologists National Audit of Radiotherapy in the Treatment of Metastatic Spinal Cord Compression and Implications for the Development of Acute Oncology Services. *Clin. Oncol.* **2014**, *26*, 453–460. [CrossRef]
50. Santos, J.M.G.; Blanquer, M.; del Río, S.T.; Iniesta, F.; Espuch, J.G.; Pérez-Espejo, M.Á.; Martínez, S.; Moraleda, J.M. Acute and chronic MRI changes in the spine and spinal cord after surgical stem cell grafting in patients with definite amyotrophic lateral sclerosis: Post-infusion injuries are unrelated with clinical impairment. *Magn. Reson. Imaging* **2013**, *31*, 1298–1308. [CrossRef]
51. Lamothe, G.; Müller, F.; Vital, J.-M.; Goossens, D.; Barat, M. Evolution of spinal cord injuries due to cervical canal stenosis without radiographic evidence of trauma (SCIWORET): A prospective study. *Ann. Phys. Rehabil. Med.* **2011**, *54*, 213–224. [CrossRef]
52. DeVivo, M.J.; Kartus, P.L.; Rutt, R.D.; Stover, S.L.; Fine, P.R. The Influence of Age at Time of Spinal Cord Injury on Rehabilitation Outcome. *Arch. Neurol.* **1990**, *47*, 687–691. [CrossRef]
53. Kaminski, L.; Cordemans, V.; Cernat, E.; M'Bra, K.I.; Mac-Thiong, J.-M. Functional Outcome Prediction after Traumatic Spinal Cord Injury Based on Acute Clinical Factors. *J. Neurotrauma* **2017**, *34*, 2027–2033. [CrossRef]
54. Alizadeh, A.; Dyck, S.M.; Karimi-Abdolrezaee, S. Traumatic Spinal Cord Injury: An Overview of Pathophysiology, Models and Acute Injury Mechanisms. *Front. Neurol.* **2019**, *10*, 282. [CrossRef]
55. Pfyffer, D.; Vallotton, K.; Curt, A.; Freund, P. Tissue bridges predict neuropathic pain emergence after spinal cord injury. *J. Neurol. Neurosurg. Psychiatry* **2020**, *91*, 1111–1117. [CrossRef]

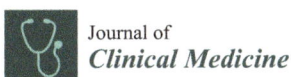

Article

Sex-Dependent Cortical Volume Changes in Patients with Degenerative Cervical Myelopathy

Talia C. Oughourlian [1,2,3], Chencai Wang [1,2], Noriko Salamon [2], Langston T. Holly [4,*] and Benjamin M. Ellingson [1,2,3,5]

1. UCLA Center for Computer Vision and Imaging Biomarkers, David Geffen School of Medicine, University of California Los Angeles, Los Angeles, CA 90024, USA; toughourlian@mednet.ucla.edu (T.C.O.); chencaiwang@mednet.ucla.edu (C.W.); bellingson@mednet.ucla.edu (B.M.E.)
2. Department of Radiological Sciences, David Geffen School of Medicine, University of California Los Angeles, Los Angeles, CA 90095, USA; nsalamon@mednet.ucla.edu
3. Neuroscience Interdepartmental Graduate Program, David Geffen School of Medicine, University of California Los Angeles, Los Angeles, CA 90095, USA
4. Department of Neurosurgery, David Geffen School of Medicine, University of California Los Angeles, Los Angeles, CA 90095, USA
5. Department of Psychiatry and Biobehavioral Sciences, David Geffen School of Medicine, University of California Los Angeles, Los Angeles, CA 90095, USA
* Correspondence: lholly@mednet.ucla.edu; Tel.: +1-(310)-319-3475

Abstract: Degenerative cervical myelopathy (DCM) is a progressive condition characterized by degeneration of osseocartilaginous structures within the cervical spine resulting in compression of the spinal cord and presentation of clinical symptoms. Compared to healthy controls (HCs), studies have shown DCM patients experience structural and functional reorganization in the brain; however, sex-dependent cortical differences in DCM patients remains largely unexplored. In the present study, we investigate the role of sex differences on the structure of the cerebral cortex in DCM and determine how structural differences may relate to clinical measures of neurological function. T1-weighted structural MRI scans were acquired in 85 symptomatic and asymptomatic patients with DCM and 90 age-matched HCs. Modified Japanese Orthopedic Association (mJOA) scores were obtained for patients. A general linear model was used to determine vertex-level significant differences in gray matter volume (GMV) between the following groups (1) male HCs and female HCs, (2) male patients and female patients, (3) male patients and male HCs, and (4) female patients and female HCs. Within patients, males exhibited larger GMV in motor, language, and vision related brain regions compared to female DCM patients. Males demonstrated a significant positive correlation between GMV and mJOA score, in which patients with worsening neurological symptoms exhibited decreasing GMV primarily across somatosensory and motor related cortical regions. Females exhibited a similar association, albeit across a broader range of cortical areas including those involved in pain processing. In sensorimotor regions, female patients consistently showed smaller GMV compared with male patients, independent of mJOA score. Results from the current study suggest strong sex-related differences in cortical volume in patients with DCM, which may reflect hormonal influence or differing compensation mechanisms.

Keywords: degenerative cervical myelopathy; cervical spondylosis; cervical spine degeneration; sex differences; MRI; cortical volume

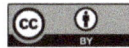

1. Introduction

Degenerative cervical myelopathy (DCM) is a chronic condition involving the progressive deterioration of osseocartilaginous structures within the cervical spine resulting in compression of the spinal cord [1,2]. DCM often occurs as a consequence of age-related degeneration of the spine and is the most common spinal cord impairment in people over the age of 55 [3]. Spinal cord compression can lead to weakness in the upper limbs, loss of fine motor skills, and/or limb dyscoordination [1,4].

Chronic narrowing of the spinal canal from cervical spondylosis not only induces structural and functional alterations within the spinal cord, but also leads to changes within the brain as well [1]. Studies have shown that, when compared to healthy subjects, DCM patients exhibit significant reductions in cortical volume in somatosensory, motor, and cerebellar cortices [5–7]. Furthermore, patients demonstrate increased anatomical and functional connectivity within sensorimotor and pain related brain regions associated with patient symptom severity [8,9], possibly due to compensatory mechanisms resulting from spinal cord neuronal atrophy [5,6,8–11]. Although these previous studies have identified unique anatomic features associated with DCM, the potential of sex as a biological variable in this disease remains largely unexplored.

Numerous studies suggest sex hormones influence neuroprotective and inflammatory responses to neurotrauma. Following brain injury, damaged neurons release glutamate resulting in excess intracellular calcium, thus triggering several pathological events including loss of dendritic spines, axonal myelin damage, mitochondrial dysfunction, and neuronal cell death, further leading to glial cell activation and neuroinflammation [12]. Sex hormone receptors are expressed in neurons, glia, and immune cells; and directly influence cellular responses to central nervous system (CNS) injury [13]. Preclinical studies have demonstrated neuroprotective effects of testosterone, estrogen, and progesterone [12–18]. In traumatic brain injury (TBI), investigators reported significant sex-specific differences in overall brain damage, sex hormone receptor gene expression, and proinflammatory responses to hormone treatment [19–21]. A clinical study found serum sex hormone levels were altered after TBI; furthermore higher levels of testosterone were correlated with a higher probability of recovery [22]. Differences in sex hormones may influence a patient's response to neurotrauma within the spinal cord [23], consequently affecting compensatory changes within the brain.

The investigation of sex as a biological variable has become a priority of the National Institutes of Health and other federal funding sources due to its potential impact on disease pathogenesis and treatment. In the present study, we sought to investigate the role of sex differences on brain structure in degenerative cervical myelopathy and to determine how those structural differences are related to measures of neurological function as measured using the modified Japanese Orthopedic Association (mJOA) score. We tested the hypotheses that (1) sex-dependent differences in GMV exist between patients and healthy controls in sensorimotor and pain related brain regions, and (2) there is a sex-dependent association between GMV and mJOA within sensorimotor cortices in patients with DCM.

2. Materials and Methods

2.1. Patient Population

A total of 85 patients were prospectively enrolled from 2016 to 2021 in a cross-sectional study including brain and spinal cord imaging as well as a neurological examination. Patients were recruited from an outpatient neurosurgery clinic and exhibited spinal cord compression with evidence of spinal cord deformation, mass effect, and no visible cerebrospinal fluid signal around the spinal cord at the site of maximal compression on MRI. Patients and healthy controls were excluded if they had neurological or neurocognitive impairment or significant psychiatric comorbidities. All patients signed Institutional Review Board-approved consent forms, and all analyses were performed in compliance with the Health Insurance Portability and Accountability Act (HIPAA). The patient cohort consisted of 52 males and 33 females ranging in age from 31 to 81 years with a mean age of 58.5 years for males and 58 years for females. All patients underwent brain and spinal cord imaging at UCLA. The modified Japanese Orthopedic Association (mJOA) score was used as a measure of neurological function [24]. The mJOA scoring scale ranges from 0 to 18, where lower scores represent a worse neurological impairment and an mJOA score of 18 represents no impairment of neurological function. Patient demographic data is summarized in Table 1.

Table 1. Cohort demographics. Age is provided in mean years ± the standard deviation, minimum and maximum years, and *p*-value of Wilcoxon-Mann-Whitney test between age of males and females. The modified Japanese Orthopedic Association (mJOA) score is provided in mean score ± the standard deviation, minimum and maximum scores, and *p*-value of Wilcoxon-Mann-Whitney test between scores of males and females. * = HCs were categorized with an mJOA score of 18 due to their healthy neurological status.

Subject Population	Number of Subject (Male/Female)	Age (Male/Female) (min, max) *p-Value*	mJOA (Male/Female) (min, max) *p-Value*
DCM Patients	85 (52/33)	(58.5 ± 11.6/58.0 ± 10.7) (31, 81) $p = 0.8068$	(15.0 ± 2.7/15.6 ± 2.4) (9, 18) $p = 0.3885$
Healthy Controls	90 (53/37)	(58.7 ± 6.4/59.8 ± 6.3) (45, 70) $p = 0.4076$	18 *

2.2. Healthy Control Population

A total of 90 age-matched healthy control (HC) volunteers were included from the Parkinson's Progression Markers Initiative (PPMI) data repository (www.ppmiinfo.org/data, access date 5 February 2021 [25]. (For up-to-date information on this database, visit www.ppmiinfo.org. PPMI—a public-private partnership—is funded by the Michael J. Fox Foundation for Parkinson's Research and funding partners, including (list the full names of all of the PPMI funding partners found at www.ppmiinfo.org/fundingpartners) (access date 5 February 2021). Study investigators completed the PPMI Data Use and Biospecimen Use Agreements. The HC cohort used consisted of 53 males and 37 females ranging in age from 45 to 70 years with a mean age of 59.1 years. Male or female HCs between the ages of 45 and 70 with T1-weighted brain images were included. Exclusion criteria implemented by the PPMI investigators consisted of (1) significant neurological or psychiatric disorder at the time of study participation, (2) first degree relative with idiopathic Parkinson's Disease, (3) a Montreal Cognitive Assessment (MoCA) score of 26 or less, (4) women who are pregnant, planning to become pregnant, or lactating at time of study, (5) use of medication that may interfere with dopamine transporter SPECT imaging, and (6) use of investigational drug or device within 60 days prior to study participation [25]. Due to the above exclusion criteria, the healthy control subjects included in this study were categorized as neurologically asymptotic and assigned an mJOA score of 18. HC demographic data was also summarized in Table 1.

2.3. MR Imaging Acquisition

For the patient cohort, high-resolution 1 mm 3-dimensional (3D) T1-weighted structural MRIs were acquired on a 3T MR scanner (Siemens Prisma or Trio; Siemens Healthcare, Erlangen, Germany) using a 3D magnetization-prepared rapid gradient-echo (MPRAGE) sequence in either the coronal, sagittal, or axial orientation, with a repetition time (TR) of 2300 to 2500 ms, a minimum echo time (TE), an inversion time (TI) of 900 to 945 ms, a flip angle of 9° to 15°, FOV = 240 × 320 mm and matrix size of 240 × 320, slice thickness = 1 mm. For the HC cohort, high-resolution 3-dimensional (3D) T1-weighted structural MRIs were acquired on a 3T MR scanner using a 3D T1-weighted sequence (e.g., MPRAGE or SPGR) with a slice thickness = 1.5 mm or less with no interslice gap. All other parameters including repetition (TR) and echo (TE) time were specific to site scanner manufacturer recommendations for a T1-weighted, 3D sequence.

2.4. Image Processing and Analysis

Cortical segmentation and computation of GMV were performed using FreeSurfer (https://surfer.nmr.mgh.harvard.edu/fswiki, access date 1 May 2021 on the T1-weighted images described above [26]. Processed brain surfaces were smoothed with a full-width half-maximum of 10 mm, then registered to a standard space defined by the Desikan-Killiany-Tourville (DKT) atlas [27]. Whole-brain cortical volume analysis was completed using FreeSurfer. A general linear model (GLM) was used to determine vertex-level significant differences in GMV between the following groups: (1) male HCs and female HCs, (2) male patients and female patients, (3) male patients and male HCs, and (4) female patients and female HCs. To control for the influence of age on GMV, age was included as a covariate in morphometric analyses [28,29]. When comparing GMV between male patients and female patients, both age and mJOA score were included as covariates. To evaluate the association between sex, cortical volume, and neurological deficit, a GLM was used to determine vertex-level significant correlations between GMV and mJOA score in (A) male patients and HCs, and (B) female patients and HCs. Following the overlapping of significant clusters observed in the male group and significant clusters observed in the female group, we identified common cortical regions showing significant correlations between GMV and mJOA in both male and female groups. Additionally, average GMVs for each individual subject were extracted from the mutually significant clusters and corrected for subject age. In the male patient group and the female patient group, linear regression analyses were performed between age corrected average GMV and mJOA score within sensorimotor and pain related brain regions. In addition, linear regression analyses were used to identify differences in GMV and mJOA slope and intercept between male and female patients. Healthy controls were excluded in regression analyses. Regression analyses were performed using MATLAB (Release 2018a, MathWorks, Natick, MA, USA) and GraphPad Prism software (Version 7.0c GraphPad Software, San Diego, CA, USA). The vertex-wise level of significance was set at $p < 0.05$, with multiple comparisons correction performed by using Monte Carlo permutations with a significance level of $p < 0.05$.

3. Results

3.1. Subject Characteristics

As summarized in Table 1, the patient cohort consisted of 52 males with a mean age of 58.5 ± 11.6 years and 33 females with a mean age of 58.0 ± 10.7 years. There was no significant difference in age between male patients and female patients (Wilcoxon-Mann-Whitney test, $p = 0.8068$). The mJOA scores within the cohort ranged from 9 to 18 with a mean score of 15.0 ± 2.7 for male patients and 15.6 ± 2.4 for female patients. Of the 85 total study patients, 19 had asymptomatic spinal cord compression (mJOA = 18), 38 presented with mild myelopathy ($15 \leq$ mJOA ≤ 17), 19 exhibited moderate myelopathy ($12 \leq$ mJOA ≤ 14), and 9 patients were categorized with severe myelopathy (mJOA ≤ 11). No significant difference in mJOA score was observed between male and female patients (Wilcoxon-Mann-Whitney test, $p = 0.3885$).

The HC cohort consisted of 53 males with a mean age of 58.7 ± 6.4 years and 37 females with a mean age of 59.8 ± 6.3 years. There was no significant difference in age between male and female HCs (Wilcoxon-Mann-Whitney test, $p = 0.4076$). Additionally, no significant difference in age was found between the patient cohort and the HC cohort (Mann-Whitney test, $p = 0.9206$). Due to lack of neurological impairment, all HC participants had an mJOA score of 18.

3.2. Sex-Dependent Cortical Volumetric Differences

Results from the whole-brain cortical volume analysis revealed no significant difference in GMV between males and females within the HC cohort, but significant differences in GMV between male and female within patients with DCM. We observed that male DCM patients compared to female patients (Figure 1A, Table 2) exhibited significantly larger GMV in the caudal middle frontal, superior temporal, transverse temporal, and lingual gyrus of the left hemisphere, as well as in the precentral gyrus, insula, and lingual gyrus of the right hemisphere. Additionally, when controlling for mJOA, male DCM patients demonstrated significantly larger GMV than female patients in the bilateral lateral occipital gyri, left superior temporal gyrus, right insula, right middle temporal gyrus, and right lingual gyrus (Figure 1B, Table 2).

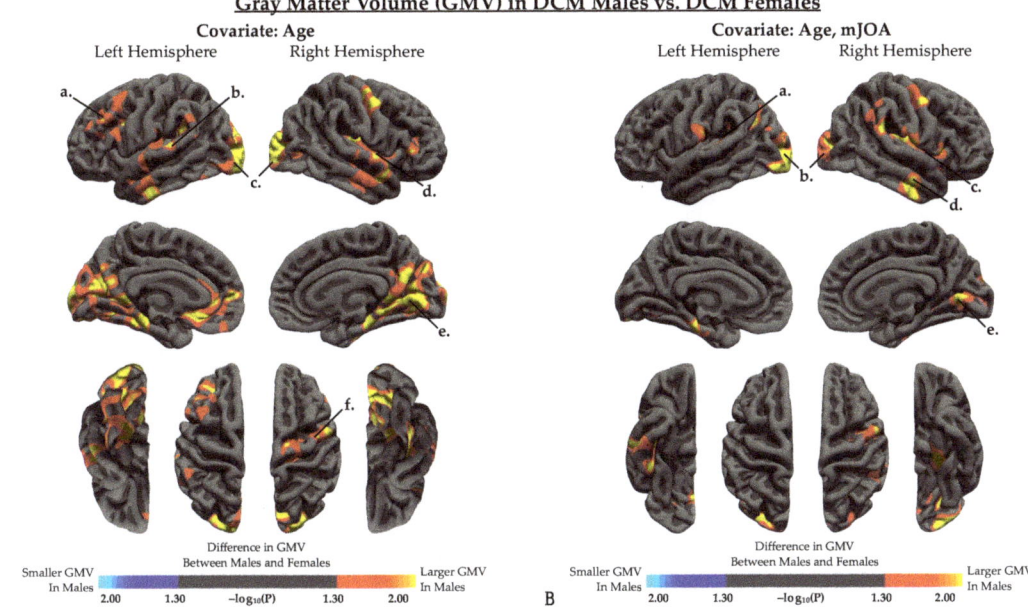

Figure 1. Whole brain analysis comparing gray matter volume (GMV) between DCM males and DCM females after regressing out the effects of (**A**) age and (**B**) both age and mJOA score. (**A**,**B**) Red-yellow color denotes larger GMV in males, while blue-light blue color denotes smaller GMV in males compared to females. (**A**) When controlling for age, regions with significant differences in GMV were identified in the *a*, left rostral middle frontal gyrus; *b*, left superior temporal gyrus; *c*, bilateral lateral occipital cortex; *d*, right insular cortex; *e*, right lingual gyrus; and *f*, right precentral gyrus. (**B**) When controlling for both age and mJOA, regions with significant differences in GMV were identified in the *a*, left superior temporal gyrus; *b*, bilateral lateral occipital cortex; *c*, right insular cortex; *d*, right middle temporal gyrus; and *e*, right lingual gyrus. Significant clusters were determined by thresholding based on statistical significance ($p < 0.05$).

Table 2. Summary of regions showing significant difference in gray matter volume (GMV) between DCM males and DCM females.

Cortical Regions	Covariate	Left Hemisphere		Right Hemisphere	
		p Value	Surface Cluster Size	*p* Value	Surface Cluster Size
Caudal Middle Frontal	Age	0.0035	456.56	-	-
Cuneus	Age	0.0405	1009.85	-	-
Fusiform	Age	0.0006	1178.84	<0.0001	1730.3
Insula	Age	0.0015	443.74	<0.0001	1175.08
Lateral Occipital	Age	0.0006	3119.09	0.0007	2424.42
Lingual	Age	<0.0001	1050.38	0.0032	1698.96
Middle Temporal	Age	<0.0001	339.04	<0.0001	652.45
Parahippocampal	Age	0.0028	529.01	<0.0001	402.56
Precentral	Age	0.0403	56.35	0.0129	1715.10
Postcentral	Age	0.0048	55.24	-	-
Rostral Middle Frontal	Age	0.0001	949.68	0.0360	68.95
Superior Temporal	Age	<0.0001	290.82	0.0024	797.12
Supramarginal	Age	<0.0001	613.04	-	-
Inferior Parietal	Age, mJOA	0.0048	471.79	0.0621	85.62

Table 2. *Cont.*

Cortical Regions	Covariate	Left Hemisphere		Right Hemisphere	
		p Value	Surface Cluster Size	*p* Value	Surface Cluster Size
Inferior Temporal	Age, mJOA	-	-	<0.0001	640.1
Insula	Age, mJOA	0.0168	24.63	<0.0001	1118.52
Lateral Occipital	Age, mJOA	0.0019	2160.62	0.0014	1302.23
Lingual	Age, mJOA	<0.0001	389.34	0.0001	565.68
Middle Temporal	Age, mJOA	-	-	0.0002	250.46
Parahippocampal	Age, mJOA	0.0076	414.86	-	-
Pericalcarine	Age, mJOA	0.1354	90.56	0.0527	538.2
Postcentral	Age, mJOA	0.0013	30.06	0.0038	479.84
Precentral	Age, mJOA	-	-	0.0042	965.98
Superior Temporal	Age, mJOA	<0.0001	370.66	0.0003	179.34
Supramarginal	Age, mJOA	<0.0001	171.87	0.0076	712.19

Male DCM patients displayed significantly larger gray matter volume (GMV) in the left parahippocampal gyrus, left paropercularis, right lateral occipital cortex, and right lingual gyrus compared with male HCs (Figure 2A, Table 3). On the contrary, female DCM patients exhibited significantly smaller GMV compared with female HCs, specifically in the left pericalcarine cortex and right lingual gyrus (Figure 2B, Table 3).

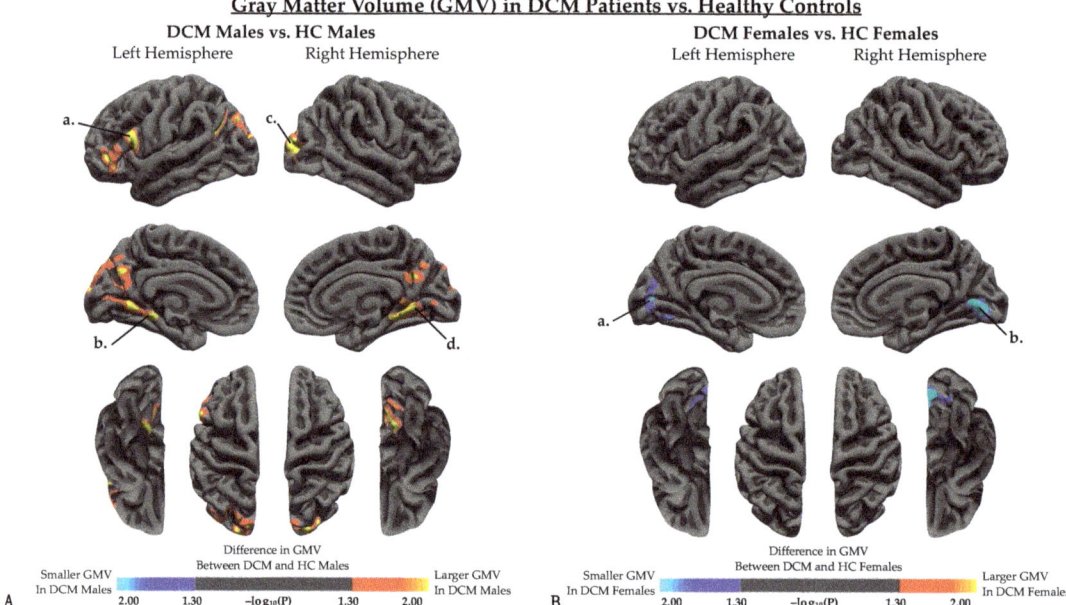

Figure 2. Whole brain analysis comparing gray matter volume (GMV) between DCM patients and healthy controls when regressing out the effect of age in (**A**) males and (**B**) females. (**A**) Red-yellow color denotes larger GMV in DCM males, while blue-light blue color denotes smaller GMV in DCM males compared to HC males. When controlling for age, regions with significant differences in GVM were identified in the *a*, left parsopercularis; *b*, left parahippocampal gyrus; *c*, right lateral occipital cortex; and *d*, left lingual gyrus. (**B**) Red-yellow color denotes larger GMV in DCM females, while blue-light blue color denotes smaller GMV in DCM males compared to HC females. When controlling for both age and mJOA, regions with significant differences in GMV were identified in the *a*, left pericalcarine cortex; and *b*, right lingual gyrus. Significant clusters were determined by thresholding based on statistical significance ($p < 0.05$).

Table 3. Summary of regions showing significant difference in gray matter volume (GMV) between patients and healthy controls.

Cortical Regions	Group	Left Hemisphere		Right Hemisphere	
		p Value	Surface Cluster Size	*p* Value	Surface Cluster Size
Cuneus	Males	0.0004	380.97	0.0292	95.29
Inferior Parietal	Males	0.8914	966.31	0.4102	93.41
Isthmus Cingulate	Males	0.2006	30.38	0.0250	296.28
Lateral Occipital	Males	0.2161	337.21	0.0608	1094.64
Lingual	Males	0.0283	737.72	0.0378	848.74
Parahippocampal	Males	0.1567	138.26	0.1132	109.2
Pars Opercularis	Males	0.2592	506.63	-	-
Pars Triangularis	Males	0.4047	623.99	-	-
Pericalcarine	Males	0.0049	412.39	0.0020	18.51
Precuneus	Males	0.0533	736.32	0.0311	396.69
Superior Parietal	Males	0.3403	950.17	0.0371	116.98
Lingual	Females	0.1318	323.52	0.0016	957.86
Pericalcarine	Females	0.0050	417.95	0.0001	323.6

3.3. Interaction between Cortical Volume and mJOA Scores

When examining the effect of sex on the association between GMV and mJOA score (Figure 3, Table 4), both males (Figure 3A) and females (Figure 3B) demonstrated a significant positive correlation between GMV and mJOA score across multiple cortical regions. Female subjects demonstrated associations between GMV and mJOA in similar regions to male subjects, but regions in female subjects appeared to extend across a broader area of the brain perhaps suggesting more widespread cortical changes in females. Mutually significant regions with a positive correlation between GMV and mJOA common for both males and females are illustrated in Figure 4A. Within DCM patients only (excluding HCs), males and females demonstrated significant correlations between age corrected GMV and mJOA within similar regions, but the degree of change (i.e., slope of the regression line) and overall GMV (i.e., intercept of regression line) were different between males and females within the left superior frontal ($p = 0.0013$), right superior frontal ($p = 0.0301$), left paracentral ($p < 0.0001$), right rostral middle frontal ($p < 0.0001$), left precentral ($p < 0.0001$), and right precentral ($p < 0.0001$) gyri, as well as the anterior, isthmus, and posterior cingulate cortex, the insula, and the precuneus (Figure 4B, Table 5).

Table 4. Summary of regions showing significant positive correlation between gray matter volume (GMV) and mJOA score.

Cortical Regions	Group	Left Hemisphere			Right Hemisphere		
		p Value	T Score	Surface Cluster Size	*p* Value	T Score	Surface Cluster Size
Caudal Middle Frontal	Male	0.0147	2.4808	931.02	0.0001	4.0121	574.47
Cuneus	Male	0.0001	4.0905	901.29	<0.0001	4.2566	1024.76
Inferior Parietal	Male	0.0003	3.7056	177.33	-	-	-
Isthmus Cingulate	Male	0.0056	2.8325	274.58	0.0107	2.5992	194.44
Lingual	Male	0.0323	2.1702	47.57	0.0014	3.2878	682.61
Middle Temporal	Male	-	-	-	0.0018	3.1981	536.62
Paracentral	Male	0.0038	2.9585	325.61	0.0007	3.5082	616.92
Pericalcarine	Male	0.0004	3.6829	498.08	0.0008	3.4660	1016.29
Postcentral	Male	0.0065	2.7768	838.30	0.0005	3.6186	1484.26
Precentral	Male	0.0027	3.0707	519.88	0.0003	3.7609	1448.52
Precuneus	Male	0.0007	3.4827	922.63	0.0002	3.9008	1591.98
Rostral Middle Frontal	Male	0.0063	2.7869	1346.88	<0.0001	4.6934	1227.85
Superior Frontal	Male	0.0002	3.9345	3468.21	0.0001	3.9840	2102.31
Superior Parietal	Male	0.0003	3.7857	957.57	0.0001	4.0080	612.55
Superior Temporal	Male	0.0012	3.3395	912.92	0.0006	3.5349	1166.35
Supramarginal	Male	0.0001	4.1949	345.84	0.0012	3.3300	531.18
Caudal Anterior Cingulate	Female	0.0038	3.0027	418.91	<0.0001	4.1818	479.93
Caudal Middle Frontal	Female	0.0164	2.4607	580.33	<0.0001	3.5973	1444.70

Table 4. Cont.

		Left Hemisphere			Right Hemisphere		
Cortical Regions	Group	p Value	T Score	Surface Cluster Size	p Value	T Score	Surface Cluster Size
Cuneus	Female	0.0017	3.2730	873.88	<0.0001	4.1733	1049.93
Inferior Parietal	Female	0.0082	2.7241	1190.14	-	-	-
Insula	Female	0.0007	3.5679	1047.41	0.0018	3.2477	1134.00
Isthmus Cingulate	Female	0.0004	3.7128	489.74	0.0015	3.3082	327.50
Lingual	Female	0.0190	2.4029	741.95	0.0004	3.7339	1733.44
Middle Temporal	Female	-	-	-	<0.0001	5.3954	1139.43
Paracentral	Female	0.0001	4.2580	1188.91	0.0001	4.1773	1065.10
Pericalcarine	Female	0.0056	2.8602	533.04	0.0001	4.0976	1144.62
Postcentral	Female	0.0005	3.6730	1839.21	<0.0001	4.3079	2904.11
Posterior Cingulate	Female	0.0017	3.2702	354.79	-	-	-
Precentral	Female	0.0004	3.7429	2635.05	<0.0001	4.5894	2441.22
Precuneus	Female	0.0003	3.8012	2157.81	0.0002	4.0130	1517.61
Rostral Anterior Cingulate	Female	-	-	-	0.0001	4.0743	215.08
Rostral Middle Frontal	Female	0.0104	2.6356	219.43	0.0001	4.2596	1726.86
Superior Frontal	Female	<0.0001	4.3678	4436.93	<0.0001	5.0532	4684.97
Superior Parietal	Female	0.0004	3.7294	2221.67	0.0003	3.8566	1024.18
Superior Temporal	Female	<0.0001	4.6447	1161.84	0.0003	3.8598	976.21
Supramarginal	Female	0.0023	3.1696	115.25	0.0011	3.4254	1135.15

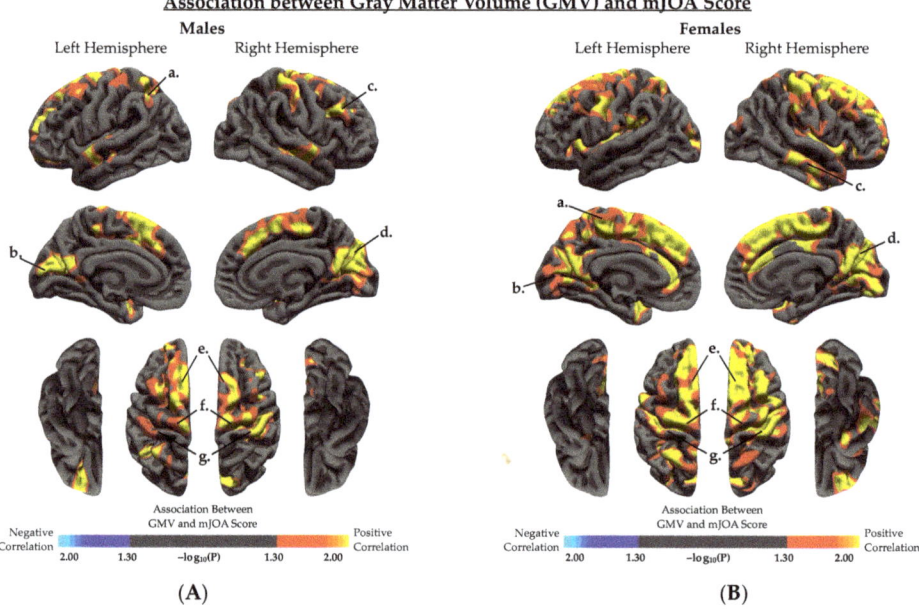

Figure 3. Association between gray matter volume (GMV) and mJOA score in (**A**) DCM and HC males, and (**B**) DCM and HC females, regressing out the effect of age. (**A,B**) Red-yellow color indicated a positive association between GMV and mJOA score, while blue-light blue color indicated negative association between GMV and mJOA score. (**A**) In males, regions with significant association between GMV and mJOA were identified in several regions including the *a*, left inferior parietal cortex; *b*, left pericalcarine cortex; *c*, right rostral middle frontal gyrus; *d*, right cuneus; *e*, bilateral superior frontal gyrus; *f*, bilateral precentral gyrus; and *g*, bilateral postcentral gyrus. (**B**) In females, regions with significant association between GMV and mJOA were identified in several regions including the *a*, left paracentral gyrus; *b*, left pericalcarine and lingual gyrus; *c*, right middle temporal gyrus; *d*, right cuneus and pericalcarine cortex; *e*, bilateral superior frontal gyrus; *f*, bilateral precentral gyrus; and *g*, bilateral postcentral gyrus. Significant clusters were determined by thresholding based on statistical significance ($p < 0.05$).

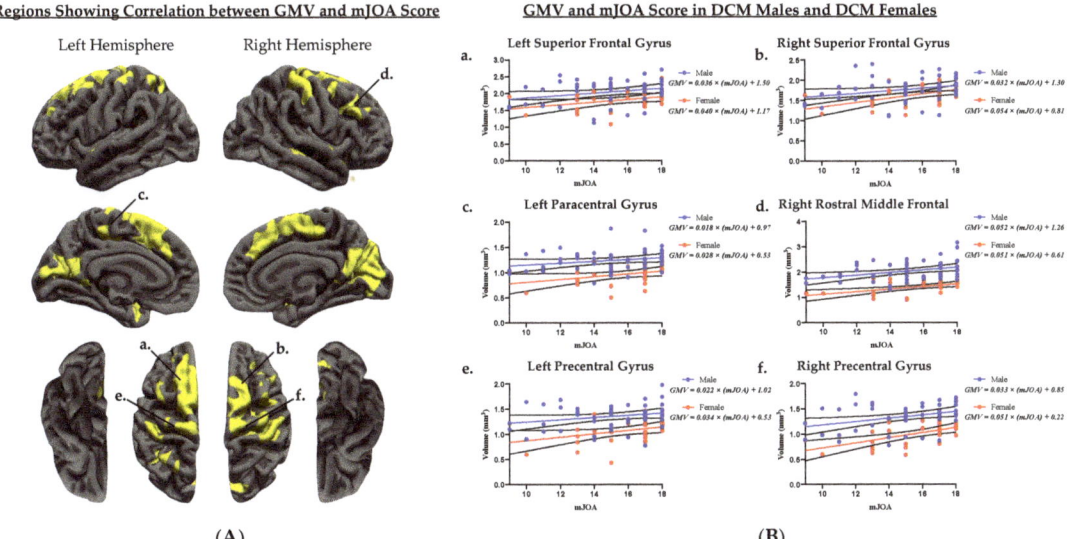

Figure 4. (**A**) Cortical regions with significant positive association between gray matter volume (GMV) and mJOA score in both males and females. (**A**) Age corrected average GMV was extracted from mutually significant cortical regions and (**B**) are plotted against patient mJOA score in DCM males and DCM females. ROI regions include the *a*, left superior frontal gyrus; *b*, right superior frontal gyrus; *c*, left paracentral gyrus; *d*, right rostral middle frontal gyrus; *e*, left precentral gyrus; and *f*, right precentral gyrus. (**B**) Age corrected average GMV and mJOA plots include simple linear regression for male patients (blue line) and female patients (red line). The light blue region denotes the 95% confidence interval for male patients and the pink region denotes the 95% confidence interval for female patients.

Table 5. Regression analyses quantifying the association between average gray matter volume (GMV) and mJOA score for regions found significant in both sexes. LH denotes left hemisphere and RH denotes right hemisphere. The table includes the following: mutually significant anatomical region, surface area of cortical region of interest (ROI), *p*-value evaluating whether male and female linear fits are significantly different in slope and y-intercept, *p*-value evaluating whether a linear relationship occurs between average GMV and mJOA score in males, *p*-value evaluating whether a linear relationship occurs between average GMV and mJOA score in females, goodness of fit for males, and goodness of fit for females.

Region	Size of ROI (mm^2)	Comparison of Male & Female Fits *p*-Value	Male Simple Linear Regression *p*-Value	Female Simple Linear Regression *p*-Value	Male R^2	Female R^2
LH Paracentral	322.69	<0.0001	0.0954	0.0543	0.05462	0.1143
RH Paracentral	518.81	0.8711	0.0379	0.0218	0.08336	0.1583
LH Postcentral	674.12	0.9319	0.1626	0.1628	0.03862	0.06187
RH Postcentral	1414.2	0.1601	0.0571	0.0237	0.0705	0.1544
LH Precentral	439.37	<0.0001	0.0762	0.0473	0.06152	0.121
RH Precentral	1205.41	<0.0001	0.0102	0.001	0.1248	0.2986
LH Superior Frontal	2874.67	0.0013	0.0469	0.0515	0.0767	0.1169
RH Superior Frontal	1894.1	0.0301	0.0452	0.004	0.0778	0.2382
LH Rostral Middle Frontal	150.27	0.9753	0.1075	0.1016	0.05099	0.0841
RH Rostral Middle Frontal	473.04	<0.0001	0.0063	0.0027	0.1398	0.2561
LH Superior Parietal	698.91	0.0556	0.0255	0.0273	0.09588	0.1476
RH Superior Parietal	308.98	<0.0001	0.0623	0.041	0.06777	0.1279

Table 5. Cont.

Region	Size of ROI (mm²)	Comparison of Male & Female Fits p-Value	Male Simple Linear Regression p-Value	Female Simple Linear Regression p-Value	Male R²	Female R²
LH Supramarginal	144.22	<0.0001	**0.0029**	**0.0413**	0.1638	0.1275
RH Supramarginal	341.88	**0.0005**	0.0656	0.0845	0.06618	0.09296
LH caudal ACC	22.44	<0.0001	0.2588	0.107	0.02543	0.08163
RH caudal ACC	2.18	<0.0001	0.492	**0.0159**	0.00949	0.1736
RH rostral ACC	43.86	<0.0001	0.1569	**0.009**	0.03968	0.2003
LH isthmus Cingulate	227.99	<0.0001	0.2472	**0.0242**	0.02669	0.1535
RH isthmus Cingulate	107.14	<0.0001	0.3069	0.0996	0.02087	0.08505
LH posterior Cingulate	61.68	<0.0001	0.5837	**0.0184**	0.006048	0.1666
LH Insula	55.35	<0.0001	0.7624	0.0534	0.001845	0.1151
RH Insula	40.95	<0.0001	0.443	0.2181	0.01182	0.04851
LH Precuneus	855.31	<0.0001	**0.0398**	0.0525	0.0818	0.116
RH Precuneus	1421.53	<0.0001	0.0686	0.0732	0.06477	0.09986

4. Discussion

The present study demonstrates significant sex-related differences in cortical volume in patients with degenerative cervical myelopathy. Prior to this investigation, the role of sex on brain structure in DCM remained largely understudied. Our findings may foster further investigation and understanding of the influence of sex and sex hormones on supraspinal plasticity following spinal cord injury.

4.1. Cortical Volumetric Differences in HCs Are Not Sex Dependent

The current study found no statistically significant differences in GMV between HC males and females. Literature investigating sex-related differences in cortical morphometry of the healthy brain remains controversial, with some studies reporting significant sex-related differences in GMV and others citing no significant difference [30–33]. To address these inconsistencies, Sanchis-Segura et al. examined how the number, size, and direction of sex differences in regional GMV vary depending on how total intercranial volume (TIV) is statistically controlled; and they concluded that when TIV effects are properly accounted for, sex differences in GMV are relatively small in healthy adults [34].

4.2. Sex-Dependent Cortical Volumetric Differences in Patients

When investigating volumetric differences within patients, we found male patients exhibited larger GMV in various regions compared to female patients, including motor, language, and pain related cortices. Previous studies have revealed DCM patients exhibit functional and morphological alterations within primary motor and sensorimotor cortices when compared to age-matched HCs [11,35,36]. We suspect patients experience alterations in such brain regions due to hormonal, neuroinflammatory, and neuronal compensatory differences between sexes [23]. Preclinical studies of spinal cord injury (SCI), stroke, and traumatic brain injury (TBI) have shown sex steroids, particularly 17-estradiol, estrogen, progesterone, and testosterone, can provide neuroprotective, pro-myelination, and anti-inflammatory effects resulting in improved tissue sparing and motor function [12–18].

In humans with acute traumatic SCI, administration of progesterone and vitamin D was associated with better functional recovery and outcome [17]. Interestingly, preclinical studies have shown testosterone treatment also provides neuroprotective benefits following SCI, but in the clinical setting about 43–57% of male patients experience low levels of testosterone following SCI, and low levels of testosterone were associated with severity of injury [14,22,37,38]. Sex-dependent volumetric differences observed within DCM patients and between patients and HCs may be driven by variations in hormone levels. In the male group, DCM patients exhibited larger GMV in regions involved in memory, vision, and language. Female patients exhibited fewer alterations than male patients when compared to healthy counterparts, a possible indication of the neuroprotective effects of normal or elevated progesterone and estrogen levels.

Furthermore, significant positive associations between GMV and mJOA scores were found in both male and female groups primarily across somatosensory and motor related cortical regions. Such findings are consistent with previous reports in which cortical alterations and cerebral reorganization were correlated with neurological function, proposing a compensatory relationship between cortical alterations and symptom progression in patients with cervical spondylosis [5,10,35]. A positive association between GMV and mJOA appears to confirm that patients with worsening neurological symptoms exhibit decreasing GMV across sensorimotor related cortices. Females exhibited an association between GMV and mJOA across a broader range of brain regions compared with male patients, including regions believed to be involved in pain processing [39]. Independent of mJOA, female patients consistently showed lower GMV than males within various regions involved in sensorimotor function. Our results reflect the possible influence of sex hormones on cerebral compensatory mechanisms and disease progression between males and females with DCM. Based on these novel preliminary studies, future investigations that evaluate supraspinal microstructural and functional alterations are warranted and will provide additional insight into the role of sex hormones in DCM neural plasticity.

4.3. Limitations and Future Direction

Although our patient and healthy control cohorts were well matched in terms of age and numbers of male and female subjects, it is important to note the healthy control subjects were acquired retrospectively from an image repository. Therefore, collection of age- and gender-matched HCs with brain and spinal cord imaging and mJOA testing is warranted for validating our findings and future studies. Furthermore, collection and inclusion of additional clinical and demographic information, such as handedness, disease duration, and medical comorbidities, will contribute to analyses of cortical structure in future studies. Additionally, measurement and assessment of serum sex hormones in relation to sex and neurological function would greatly benefit our understanding of the mechanisms underlying sexual dimorphism in DCM.

5. Conclusions

To the best of our knowledge this is the first study to investigate sex differences in cortical volume in patients with DCM. Results suggest males with DCM exhibit significantly larger GMV compared to female DCM patients in various brain regions, and DCM patients exhibit significant sex-related differences in the association between GMV and neurological function, particularly in brain areas involved in sensorimotor function.

Author Contributions: Conceptualization, B.M.E. and L.T.H.; methodology, B.M.E., C.W. and T.C.O.; software, C.W.; validation, N.S. and L.T.H.; formal analysis, T.C.O. and C.W.; investigation, T.C.O.; resources, L.T.H.; writing—original draft preparation, T.C.O.; writing—review and editing, T.C.O., C.W., L.T.H. and B.M.E.; visualization, T.C.O.; supervision, B.M.E. and L.T.H.; funding acquisition, B.M.E. and L.T.H. All authors have read and agreed to the published version of the manuscript.

Funding: This research was funded by the National Institutes of Health (NIH) and the National Institute of Neurological Disorders and Stroke (NINDS), grand number R01NS078494.

Institutional Review Board Statement: The study was conducted according to the guidelines of the Declaration of Helsinki and approved by the Institutional Review Board of the University of California, Los angeales (#11-001876 approved 12 September 2020).

Informed Consent Statement: Informed consent was obtained from all subjects involved in the study.

Data Availability Statement: Data will be made available upon request from investigators.

Acknowledgments: We kindly thank the patients and their families for participating in our study. We also thank the Parkinson's Progression Markers Initiative (PPMI) for providing imaging data for our healthy control cohort.

Conflicts of Interest: The authors declare no conflict of interest.

References

1. Theodore, N. Degenerative Cervical Spondylosis. *N. Engl. J. Med.* **2020**, *383*, 159–168. [CrossRef]
2. Tracy, J.A.; Bartleson, J.D. Cervical Spondylotic Myelopathy. *Neurology* **2010**, *16*, 176–187. [CrossRef] [PubMed]
3. Binder, A.I. Cervical spondylosis and neck pain. *BMJ* **2007**, *334*, 527–531. [CrossRef] [PubMed]
4. Karadimas, S.K.; Erwin, W.M.; Ely, C.G.; Dettori, J.R.; Fehlings, M. Pathophysiology and Natural History of Cervical Spondylotic Myelopathy. *Spine* **2013**, *38*, S21–S36. [CrossRef]
5. Woodworth, D.C.; Holly, L.T.; Mayer, E.A.; Salamon, N.; Ellingson, B.M. Alterations in Cortical Thickness and Subcortical Volume are Associated with Neurological Symptoms and Neck Pain in Patients with Cervical Spondylosis. *Neurosurgery* **2018**, *84*, 588–598. [CrossRef] [PubMed]
6. Jütten, K.; Mainz, V.; Schubert, G.A.; Gohmann, R.F.; Schmidt, T.; Ridwan, H.; Clusmann, H.; Mueller, C.A.; Blume, C. Cortical volume reductions as a sign of secondary cerebral and cerebellar impairment in patients with degenerative cervical myelopathy. *NeuroImage Clin.* **2021**, *30*, 102624. [CrossRef] [PubMed]
7. Yang, Q.; Xu, H.; Zhang, M.; Wang, Y.; Li, D. Volumetric and functional connectivity alterations in patients with chronic cervical spondylotic pain. *Neuroradiology* **2020**, *62*, 995–1001. [CrossRef]
8. Holly, L.T.; Wang, C.; Woodworth, D.C.; Salamon, N.; Ellingson, B.M. Neck disability in patients with cervical spondylosis is associated with altered brain functional connectivity. *J. Clin. Neurosci.* **2019**, *69*, 149–154. [CrossRef]
9. Woodworth, D.C.; Holly, L.T.; Salamon, N.; Ellingson, B.M. Resting-State Functional Magnetic Resonance Imaging Connectivity of the Brain Is Associated with Altered Sensorimotor Function in Patients with Cervical Spondylosis. *World Neurosurg.* **2018**, *119*, e740–e749. [CrossRef]
10. Wang, C.; Laiwalla, A.; Salamon, N.; Ellingson, B.M.; Holly, L.T. Compensatory brainstem functional and structural connectivity in patients with degenerative cervical myelopathy by probabilistic tractography and functional MRI. *Brain Res.* **2020**, *1749*, 147129. [CrossRef]
11. Holly, L.T.; Dong, Y.; Albistegui-DuBois, R.; Marehbian, J.; Dobkin, B. Cortical reorganization in patients with cervical spondylotic myelopathy. *J. Neurosurg. Spine* **2007**, *6*, 544–551. [CrossRef]
12. Kövesdi, E.; Szabó-Meleg, E.; Abrahám, I.M. The Role of Estradiol in Traumatic Brain Injury: Mechanism and Treatment Potential. *Int. J. Mol. Sci.* **2020**, *22*, 11. [CrossRef]
13. Elkabes, S.; Nicot, A. Sex steroids and neuroprotection in spinal cord injury: A review of preclinical investigations. *Exp. Neurol.* **2014**, *259*, 28–37. [CrossRef]
14. Byers, J.S.; Huguenard, A.; Kuruppu, D.; Liu, N.-K.; Xu, X.-M.; Sengelaub, D.R. Neuroprotective effects of testosterone on motoneuron and muscle morphology following spinal cord injury. *J. Comp. Neurol.* **2012**, *520*, 2683–2696. [CrossRef] [PubMed]
15. Sengelaub, D.R.; Han, Q.; Liu, N.-K.; Maczuga, M.A.; Szalavari, V.; Valencia, S.A.; Xu, X.-M. Protective Effects of Estradiol and Dihydrotestosterone following Spinal Cord Injury. *J. Neurotrauma* **2018**, *35*, 825–841. [CrossRef] [PubMed]
16. Zendedel, A.; Mönnink, F.; Hassanzadeh, G.; Zaminy, A.; Ansar, M.M.; Habib, P.; Slowik, A.D.; Kipp, M.; Beyer, C. Estrogen Attenuates Local Inflammasome Expression and Activation after Spinal Cord Injury. *Mol. Neurobiol.* **2017**, *55*, 1364–1375. [CrossRef] [PubMed]
17. Aminmansour, B.; Asnaashari, A.; Rezvani, M.; Ghaffarpasand, F.; Noorian, S.M.A.; Saboori, M.; Abdollahzadeh, P. Effects of progesterone and vitamin D on outcome of patients with acute traumatic spinal cord injury; a randomized, double-blind, placebo controlled study. *J. Spinal Cord Med.* **2015**, *39*, 272–280. [CrossRef] [PubMed]
18. Garcia-Ovejero, D.; González, S.; Paniagua-Torija, B.; Lima, A.; Molina-Holgado, E.; De Nicola, A.F.; Labombarda, F. Progesterone Reduces Secondary Damage, Preserves White Matter, and Improves Locomotor Outcome after Spinal Cord Contusion. *J. Neurotrauma* **2014**, *31*, 857–871. [CrossRef] [PubMed]
19. Wagner, A.K.; McCullough, E.H.; Niyonkuru, C.; Ozawa, H.; Loucks, T.; Dobos, J.A.; Brett, C.A.; Santarsieri, M.; Dixon, C.E.; Berga, S.L.; et al. Acute Serum Hormone Levels: Characterization and Prognosis after Severe Traumatic Brain Injury. *J. Neurotrauma* **2011**, *28*, 871–888. [CrossRef]
20. Gölz, C.; Kirchhoff, F.P.; Westerhorstmann, J.; Schmidt, M.; Hirnet, T.; Rune, G.M.; Bender, R.A.; Schäfer, M.K. Sex hormones modulate pathogenic processes in experimental traumatic brain injury. *J. Neurochem.* **2019**, *150*, 173–187. [CrossRef]
21. Sarkaki, A.; Haddad, M.K.; Soltani, Z.; Shahrokhi, N.; Mahmoodi, M. Time- and Dose-Dependent Neuroprotective Effects of Sex Steroid Hormones on Inflammatory Cytokines after a Traumatic Brain Injury. *J. Neurotrauma* **2013**, *30*, 47–54. [CrossRef]
22. Zhong, Y.H.; Wu, H.Y.; He, R.H.; Zheng, B.E.; Fan, J.Z. Sex Differences in Sex Hormone Profiles and Prediction of Consciousness Recovery After Severe Traumatic Brain Injury. *Front. Endocrinol.* **2019**, *10*, 261. [CrossRef]
23. Stewart, A.N.; MacLean, S.M.; Stromberg, A.J.; Whelan, J.P.; Bailey, W.M.; Gensel, J.C.; Wilson, M.E. Considerations for Studying Sex as a Biological Variable in Spinal Cord Injury. *Front. Neurol.* **2020**, *11*, 802, ARTN 597689fneur.2020.597689. [CrossRef]

24. Yonenobu, K.; Abumi, K.; Nagata, K.; Taketomi, E.; Ueyama, K. Interobserver and Intraobserver Reliability of the Japanese Orthopaedic Association Scoring System for Evaluation of Cervical Compression Myelopathy. *Spine* **2001**, *26*, 1890–1894. [CrossRef] [PubMed]
25. Imaging Data Parkinson's Progression Markers Initiative (PPMI). Available online: https://onlinelibrary.wiley.com/doi/pdfdirect/10.1002/acn3.644 (accessed on 30 August 2021).
26. Fischl, B.; Sereno, M.I.; Dale, A.M. Cortical Surface-Based Analysis: II: Inflation, Flattening, and a Surface-Based Coordinate System. *NeuroImage* **1999**, *9*, 195–207. [CrossRef] [PubMed]
27. Desikan, R.S.; Ségonne, F.; Fischl, B.; Quinn, B.T.; Dickerson, B.C.; Blacker, D.; Buckner, R.L.; Dale, A.M.; Maguire, R.; Hyman, B.T.; et al. An automated labeling system for subdividing the human cerebral cortex on MRI scans into gyral based regions of interest. *NeuroImage* **2006**, *31*, 968–980. [CrossRef]
28. Lemaitre, H.; Goldman, A.L.; Sambataro, F.; Verchinski, B.A.; Meyer-Lindenberg, A.; Weinberger, D.R.; Mattay, V.S. Normal age-related brain morphometric changes: Nonuniformity across cortical thickness, surface area and gray matter volume? *Neurobiol. Aging* **2012**, *33*, 617.e1–617.e9. [CrossRef] [PubMed]
29. Salat, D.H.; Buckner, R.L.; Snyder, A.Z.; Greve, D.N.; Desikan, R.S.; Busa, E.; Morris, J.C.; Dale, A.M.; Fischl, B. Thinning of the Cerebral Cortex in Aging. *Cereb. Cortex* **2004**, *14*, 721–730. [CrossRef]
30. Good, C.D.; Johnsrudeb, I.; Ashburner, J.; Henson, R.N.; Friston, K.J.; Frackowiak, R. Cerebral Asymmetry and the Effects of Sex and Handedness on Brain Structure: A Voxel-Based Morphometric Analysis of 465 Normal Adult Human Brains. *NeuroImage* **2001**, *14*, 685–700. [CrossRef]
31. Chen, X.; Sachdev, P.S.; Wen, W.; Anstey, K. Sex differences in regional gray matter in healthy individuals aged 44–48 years: A voxel-based morphometric study. *NeuroImage* **2007**, *36*, 691–699. [CrossRef]
32. Fjell, A.M.; Westlye, L.T.; Amlien, I.K.; Espeseth, T.; Reinvang, I.; Raz, N.; Agartz, I.; Salat, D.H.; Greve, U.N.; Fischl, B.; et al. Minute Effects of Sex on the Aging Brain: A Multisample Magnetic Resonance Imaging Study of Healthy Aging and Alzheimer's Disease. *J. Neurosci.* **2009**, *29*, 8774–8783. [CrossRef] [PubMed]
33. Smith, C.D.; Chebrolu, H.; Wekstein, D.R.; Schmitt, F.A.; Markesbery, W.R. Age and gender effects on human brain anatomy: A voxel-based morphometric study in healthy elderly. *Neurobiol. Aging* **2007**, *28*, 1075–1087. [CrossRef] [PubMed]
34. Sanchis-Segura, C.; Ibanez-Gual, M.V.; Adrian-Ventura, J.; Aguirre, N.; Gomez-Cruz, A.J.; Avila, C.; Forn, C. Sex differences in gray matter volume: How many and how large are they really? *Biol. Sex Differ.* **2019**, *10*, 1–19. [CrossRef] [PubMed]
35. Dong, Y.; Holly, L.T.; Albistegui-DuBois, R.; Yan, X.; Marehbian, J.; Newton, J.M.; Dobkin, B.H. Compensatory cerebral adaptations before and evolving changes after surgical decompression in cervical spondylotic myelopathy. *J. Neurosurg. Spine* **2008**, *9*, 538–551. [CrossRef] [PubMed]
36. Bernabéu-Sanz, A.; Mollá-Torró, J.V.; López-Celada, S.; López, P.M.; Fernández-Jover, E. MRI evidence of brain atrophy, white matter damage, and functional adaptive changes in patients with cervical spondylosis and prolonged spinal cord compression. *Eur. Radiol.* **2019**, *30*, 357–369. [CrossRef]
37. Durga, A.; Sepahpanah, F.; Regozzi, M.; Hastings, J.; Crane, D.A. Prevalence of Testosterone Deficiency After Spinal Cord Injury. *PM&R* **2011**, *3*, 929–932. [CrossRef]
38. Bauman, W.A.; La Fountaine, M.F.; Spungen, A.M. Age-related prevalence of low testosterone in men with spinal cord injury. *J. Spinal Cord Med.* **2013**, *37*, 32–39. [CrossRef]
39. Fomberstein, K.; Qadri, S.; Ramani, R. Functional MRI and pain. *Curr. Opin. Anaesthesiol.* **2013**, *26*, 588–593. [CrossRef] [PubMed]

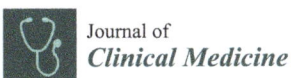
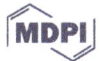

Article

Spinal Cord Motion in Degenerative Cervical Myelopathy: The Level of the Stenotic Segment and Gender Cause Altered Pathodynamics

Katharina Wolf [1,*], Marco Reisert [2], Saúl Felipe Beltrán [1], Jan-Helge Klingler [3], Ulrich Hubbe [3], Axel J. Krafft [2], Nico Kremers [4], Karl Egger [4,5] and Marc Hohenhaus [3]

1. Medical Center, Department of Neurology and Neurophysiology, Faculty of Medicine, University of Freiburg, 79106 Freiburg im Breisgau, Germany; saul.beltran@uniklinik-freiburg.de
2. Medical Center, Department of Radiology, Medical Physics, Faculty of Medicine, University of Freiburg, 79106 Freiburg im Breisgau, Germany; marco.reisert@uniklinik-freiburg.de (M.R.); axeljoachim.krafft@siemens-healthineers.com (A.J.K.)
3. Medical Center, Department of Neurosurgery, Faculty of Medicine, University of Freiburg, 79106 Freiburg im Breisgau, Germany; jan-helge.klingler@uniklinik-freiburg.de (J.-H.K.); ulrich.hubbe@uniklinik-freiburg.de (U.H.); marc.hohenhaus@uniklinik-freiburg.de (M.H.)
4. Medical Center, Department of Neuroradiology, Faculty of Medicine, University of Freiburg, 79106 Freiburg im Breisgau, Germany; nico.kremers@uniklinik-freiburg.de (N.K.); karl.egger@uniklinik-freiburg.de (K.E.)
5. Department of Radiology, Tauernklinikum Zell am See/Mittersill, 5700 Salzburg, Austria
* Correspondence: katharina.wolf@uniklinik-freiburg.de

Abstract: In degenerative cervical myelopathy (DCM), focally increased spinal cord motion has been observed for C5/C6, but whether stenoses at other cervical segments lead to similar pathodynamics and how severity of stenosis, age, and gender affect them is still unclear. We report a prospective matched-pair controlled trial on 65 DCM patients. A high-resolution 3D T2 sampling perfection with application-optimized contrasts using different flip angle evolution (SPACE) and a phase-contrast magnetic resonance imaging (MRI) sequence were performed and automatically segmented. Anatomical and spinal cord motion data were assessed per segment from C2/C3 to C7/T1. Spinal cord motion was focally increased at a level of stenosis among patients with stenosis at C4/C5 ($n = 14$), C5/C6 ($n = 33$), and C6/C7 ($n = 10$) ($p < 0.033$). Patients with stenosis at C2/C3 ($n = 2$) and C3/C4 ($n = 6$) presented a similar pattern, not reaching significance. Gender was a significant predictor of higher spinal cord dynamics among men with stenosis at C5/C6 ($p = 0.048$) and C6/C7 ($p = 0.033$). Age and severity of stenosis did not relate to spinal cord motion. Thus, the data demonstrates focally increased spinal cord motion depending on the specific level of stenosis. Gender-related effects lead to dynamic alterations among men with stenosis at C5/C6 and C6/C7. The missing relation of motion to severity of stenosis underlines a possible additive diagnostic value of spinal cord motion analysis in DCM.

Keywords: degenerative cervical myelopathy; phase-contrast MRI; automated segmentation; gender; convolutional neural network

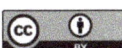

1. Introduction

The anatomical degenerations of the cervical spine, which may lead to the syndrome of degenerative cervical myelopathy (DCM) are well established (e.g., disc protrusions, ossification of ligaments, etc.) [1–4]. While relevant spinal canal degeneration may occur without any objective clinical signs or symptoms [1,5–7], further parameters may help to identify those at risk in developing cervical myelopathy.

Recent findings based on phase-contrast MRI (PC-MRI) have demonstrated significantly increased craniocaudal spinal cord motion among patients with degenerative cervical myelopathy (DCM) at the most commonly affected segment C5/C6 [8–12]. The increase of motion was demonstrated to be a focal phenomenon specifically at the stenotic segment C5/C6 [10,12], and also at the stenotic segment C4/C5 in a small group of four patients [13]. The spinal cord motion at more cranial segments remained unaffected [10,12].

Clinical impairment correlated to increased spinal cord motion within a small cohort [10]. Dynamic strain on spinal cord tissue was demonstrated and supports the conclusion of possible pathodynamic relevance [12]. To date and in contrast to the expected dynamic behavior, the extent of spinal cord motion cannot yet be associated to measurements of the severity of spinal stenosis at C5/C6 reflected by the compression ratio ($n = 12$) [10], or the adapted maximum canal compromise (aMCC; $n = 29$) [12]. This missing relationship indicates the need of either further refinements of anatomical assessments or the existence of influencing factors beyond local anatomy. Thus, MRI-based measurements of spinal cord dynamics may provide additive diagnostic information.

As there are many uncertainties regarding the spontaneous course, and consecutively, the treatment decision of mildly affected or multimorbid DCM patients, these new quantitative, non-invasively, and reliably assessable PC-MRI parameters [10–13] may be of future interest in the clinical decision-making process. Still, at the current state of basic research, there are many unanswered questions concerning the dynamic behavior of the cervical spinal cord and its influencing factors.

Based on known segmental differences of spinal cord motion across the cervical spine in healthy controls [11], it remains unclear whether spinal cord motion pattern in DCM differ from one stenotic cervical segment to another and how segmental spinal cord motion is affected by age, gender, and extent of stenosis.

We hypothesized that we could reproduce similar patterns of spinal cord motion at the different levels of cervical stenosis among DCM patients presenting with monosegmental stenosis. We assumed non-significant effects of age and gender on spinal cord motion. Also, we hypothesized to find interactions of spinal cord motion to automated assessments of spinal canal compression.

2. Methods

2.1. Study Design

We report a monocentric, prospective, matched-pair-controlled study. The first consecutive eighty patients from our ongoing longitudinal trial on DCM were analyzed (German registry of clinical trials, number: DRKS00012962). Patients were grouped according to the level of relevant cervical stenosis (C2/C3, C3/C4, C4/C5, C5/C6, and C6/C7). Relevant stenosis was defined as depleted cerebrospinal fluid (CSF)-space anterior and posterior or marked compression of the spinal cord visually diagnosed in T2-weighted MRI; mild to moderate degeneration at other segments not fulfilling these criteria were accepted.

Per group, each patient was matched one to one by age and gender to a healthy control, which we extracted from our database (German registry of clinical trials, number: DRKS00017351). Recruitment procedures as well as in- and exclusion criteria have been reported previously [12,14]. In short, patients were required to present at least mild symptoms (e.g., clumsy hands, bilateral non-radicular paresthesia, and hyperreflexia) due to monosegmental relevant cervical spinal stenosis. Clinical severity was scored via the modified Japanese Orthopedic Association (mJOA) score [15], and number of patients entering decompressive surgery was recorded. A maximum mJOA score of 18 points was accepted, as certain signs of spinal cord affection do not necessarily lead to a reduced score (e.g., hyperreflexia or intermittent hypesthesia). Controls were required to have no history or signs or symptoms of DCM and no incidental relevant cervical stenosis within the following MRI.

Patients with conflicting neurological symptoms, due to e.g., carpal tunnel syndrome, and controls volunteering with unaware neurological symptoms, were prospectively excluded by an interview, a neurological exam, and, if needed, by electrophysiological measurements before admission to the study.

Data was collected between June 2018 and February 2021. Data acquisition and analysis was performed in compliance with protocols approved by the Ethical Committee of the Albert-Ludwigs-University Freiburg (ethical approval numbers: 261/17, 338/17). Written informed consent was obtained from all participants prior to study.

2.2. Imaging Protocol

Each participant received one MRI scan (3T, SIEMENS MAGNETOM Prisma, SIEMENS Erlangen, Germany). This included a 3D T2 SPACE sequence for analysis of anatomical parameters (spatial resolution 0.64×0.64 mm^2 $\times$ 1.0 mm, TR 1500 ms, TE 134 ms, Flip angle 105°, GRAPPA factor: 3, acquisition time 3:53 min) and a prospectively ECG-triggered PC-MRI sequence for detection of craniocaudal motion in sagittal orientation covering vertebra C1 to T1 (spatial resolution 0.62×0.62 mm^2 $\times$ 3 mm, FoV 200×200 mm^2, TR = 31.8 ms, TE = 7.75 ms, flip angle 15°, bandwidth 488 Hz/Pixel, velocity encoding parameter 5 cm/s, PEAK-GRAPPA, acquisition time: approximately 2 min depending on the heart rate.). An average of 40 timepoints per heartbeat and individual was gained. During the execution of the PC-MRI, the average duration of the heartbeat (HB) per individual was automatically recorded. Thus, individual data curves of velocity (cm/s) over time (s) can be resolved and used for further derivatives.

2.3. MRI Data Processing

Automated segmentation was performed by trained hierarchical, deep convolutional neural networks (CNN) implemented within an automated data processing pipeline using the medical imaging platform Nora [16]. The details on the trainings of the CNNs, and the data processing pipeline including segmentation, phase-drift correction method, and setting of the regions of interest (ROI) has been described previously [12]. The implementation of the CNNs was similar as reported by Zhao et al. [17]. In short, different CNNs were trained for segmentation of anatomic data (CSF-space and spinal cord cross sectional area (CSA)) based on the 3D T2-weighted sequence, and for segmentation of the spinal cord for analysis of dynamic data based on the phase-contrast sequence (example Figure 1). ROIs were generated covering the central 1/3 of the spinal cord / CSF-space between two cervical vertebra bodies (Figure 1). In total, six ROIs were analyzed per individual: C2/C3, C3/C4, C4/C5, C5/C6, C6/C7, and C7/T1 (Figure 1).

All phase–contrast images were inspected visually upon artifacts (e.g., movement, metal, infoldings, and flow-artifacts by vessels) before entering further analysis. Nine patients were excluded because of overall MRI artifact due to movement or infoldings. Six patients were excluded due to drop out during the MRI scan ($n = 1$), withdrawal of consent ($n = 1$), and detection of multisegmental relevant stenosis in the study scan ($n = 4$). In three cases, dynamic parameters at C2/C3 were excluded due to a flow-artifact (one per group with stenosis at C3/C4, C5/C6, C6/C7, respectively); dynamic parameters at segment C2/C3 and C3/C4 were excluded due to an artifact within one case with stenosis at C4/C5.

2.4. PC-MRI Parameters

The following parameters of the spinal cord motion curve per heartbeat were generated per ROI: maximum velocity (cm/s), peak-to-peak (ptp)-amplitude (mm/s; maximum velocity–minimum velocity), total displacement (mm) (~area under the curve (AUC), but addition of inversed negative AUC values instead of subtraction) (Figure 2). Due to known moderate test–retest–reliability of the total displacement at segment C2, this single parameter was not considered [12].

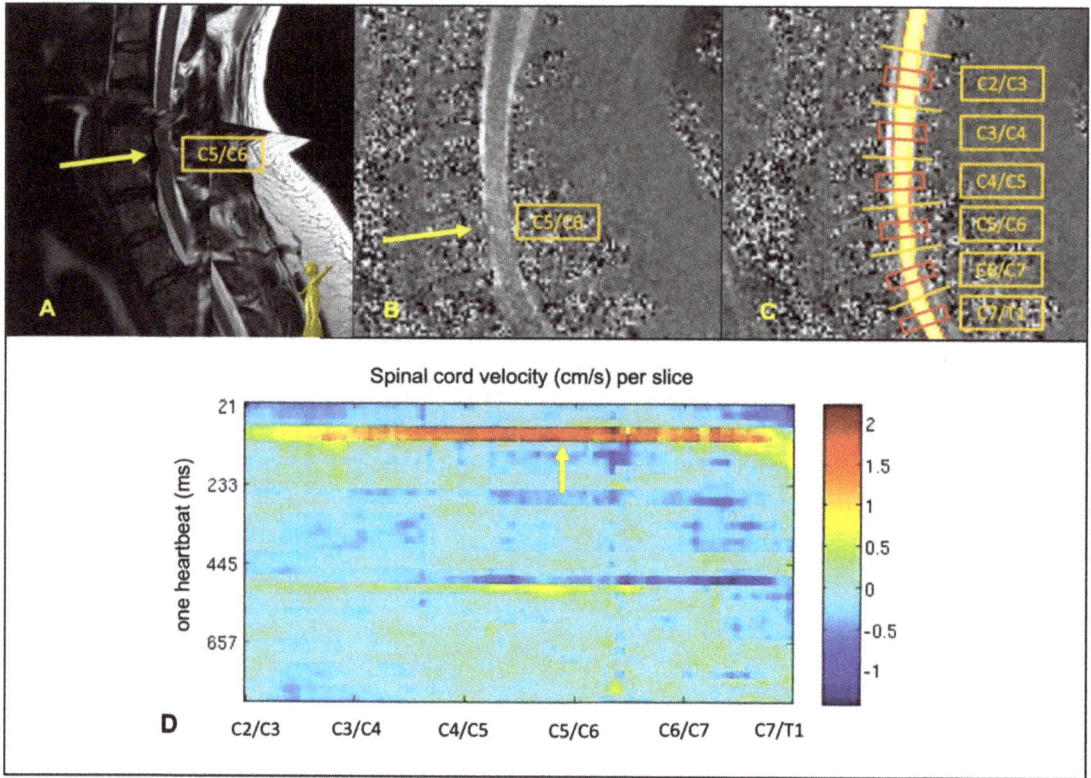

Figure 1. Example of spinal cord motion assessments within the current data processing pipeline. Top row (**A**): 3D T2w SPACE sagittal image of a patient with stenosis at C5/C6 (yellow arrow). (**B**): one exemplary phase-contrast image of the same patient within one heartbeat; the yellow arrow points onto the light grey colored spinal cord that reflects the focally increased craniocaudal spinal cord motion compared to the darker grey colored spinal cord motion at the surrounding segments. (**C**): segmentation of the phase-contrast image of the same patient, red squares demonstrate the ROIs per cervical segment covering 1/3 of the intervertebral space. (**D**): example of the spinal cord velocity plot of the same patient demonstrating color-coded spinal cord velocities (cm/s) (right side) per slice (x-axis) and per assessed time point (y-axis) during one heartbeat (ms).

In order to minimize effects of individual confounder on spinal cord motion (e.g., body size) and to analyze mechanical effects such as compression or stretching of interjacent spinal cord tissue, two indices were calculated: the C2-ptp-amplitude index (C2-pAI: [ptp-amplitude$_{(C3/4 - C7/T1)}$ ÷ ptp-amplitude$_{C2/3}$]) [12] and correspondingly, the C7-ptp-amplitude index (C7-pAI: [ptp-amplitude$_{(C2/3 - C6/C7)}$ ÷ ptp-amplitude$_{C7/T1}$]). The segments C2/C3 and C7/T1 are both suitable as references, as both have been reported to represent similar dynamics in healthy controls [11,12]. A cranio-caudal increase between two segments would indicate a mechanical stretch of the interjacent spinal cord tissue, whereas a cranio-caudal decrease would indicate a compression (Figure 2). As dynamics at adjacent segments to the stenosis were described to be altered as well [11,12], referencing was performed on the least affected, most remote segment. Thus, the C2-pAI (reference segment C2/C3) is suitable to gain information on strain mechanisms in case of caudal cervical stenosis, the C7-pAI (reference segment C7/T1), and vice versa. Indices provide a more sensitive inter-subject comparability.

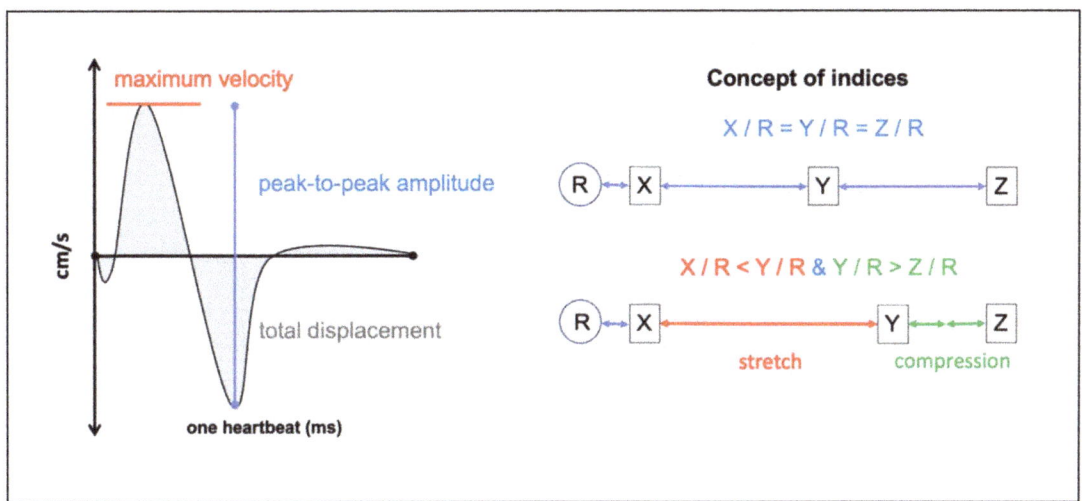

Figure 2. Schematic illustration of the dynamic spinal cord motion parameter based on the approximated 40 velocity values per individual plotted over one heartbeat (left side). Maximum velocity (red) refers to the highest positive (craniocaudal) velocity within the curve. Peak-to-peak-amplitude (blue) addresses the maximum positive (caudal) and negative (cranial) velocity within the curve and therefor adds further information on the extent of the motion. The total displacement (grey) comprises information of the entire curve (addition of the area under the curve irrespective of algebraic signs). Indices allow information beyond general group effects by intra-individual referencing. It minimizes possible general biodynamic confounders and gives information on possible strains (right side). If a point Y in relation to the reference R moves faster than a point X in relation to the reference R, the interjacent material (red arrow) becomes stretched. In case of higher motion of Y in relation to R compared to Z in relation to R, the interjacent material becomes compressed (green arrows).

2.5. Anatomical MRI-Parameters

The following anatomical parameters were automatically computed within the post-processing pipeline per segment: spinal cord CSA (mm^2), spinal canal CSA (mm^2), and the adapted maximum canal compromise (aMCC: [(spinal canal CSA one segment above + spinal canal CSA one segment below) ÷ (2 × spinal canal CSA at level)]) reflecting the severity of the individual's spinal stenosis unrelated to body size [12,18]. In addition, we calculated an adapted spinal cord occupation ratio (aSCOR) in % per segment adapted to Nouri et al. [19] using the automatically generated CSAs of the spinal cord and the spinal canal per segment (spinal cord CSA × 100 ÷ spinal canal CSA). Thus, the aSCOR adds information on the segmental relationship of occupied spinal cord CSA to remaining cerebrospinal fluid (CSF)-space, which is not reflected by the aMCC.

2.6. Data Validity

Excellent data validity of the applied data processing and test-retest-reliability of all anatomical and dynamic data assessments (ICC > 0.9 [20]) has been reported before [12].

2.7. Statistics

Statistical analysis was conducted by SPSS Statistics®(IBM Corporation, Released 2020. IBM SPSS Statistics for Macintosh, Version 27.0. Armonk, New York, USA). Data is given as mean and standard deviation (SD). Quantitative data of patients and controls were compared segment by segment. Comparison of two groups, unrelated values, was conducted upon data distribution analysis (Shapiro-Wilk): normally distributed data was compared via t-test, non-normally distributed data via Mann–Whitney U-test. Comparison of multiple related variables was calculated via bonferroni-adjusted analysis of variance (ANOVA) with repeated measurements upon validation of distribution and sphericity;

outliers were not excluded. Comparison of multiple unrelated variables was performed via Kruskal–Wallis Test. Prediction models were rated by multiple linear regressions upon validation of standard premises. Outliers were excluded if identified by two methods (Cook's distance [21], leverage [22]). p was required to be <0.05 to assume significance.

3. Results

3.1. Study Population

Sixty-five patients were included in the final analysis (Table 1). Two presented with levels of stenosis at C2/C3 (50% men), six at C3/C4 (100% men), 14 at C4/C5 (64.3% men), 33 at C5/C6 (42.4% men), and 10 with levels of stenosis at C6/C7 (60% men). Therefore, due to the small number of participants, the majority of statistical analyses was not performed among patients with stenosis at C2/C3. A total of forty healthy age- and gender-matched controls were included in the study.

Table 1. Study-population.

	Level of Stenosis	C2/C3	C3/C4	C4/C5	C5/C6	C6/C7
Patients	n	2	6	14	33	10
	Male (%)	1 (50)	6 (100)	9 (64.3)	14 (42.4)	6 (60)
	age (years) (mean ± SD)	57 ± 8	64 ± 10	65 ± 9	53 ± 12	54 ± 12
	mJOA (mean ± SD)	18	14.50 ± 3.2	15.85 ± 2.2	16.47 ± 1.8 *	15.4 ± 2.1
	mJOA 18 (%)	1 (50)	1 (16.7)	5 (35.7)	10 (31.3)	1 (10)
	mJOA 15–17 (%)	1 (50)	3 (50)	7 (50)	14 (43.8)	5 (50)
	mJOA < 15 (%)		2 (33.3)	2 (14.4)	7 (21.9)	4 (40)
	Surgical treatment (%)	0	3 (50)	8 (57.1)	18 (54.5)	6 (60)
	aMCC (mean ± SD)	2.24 ± 0.3	1.96 ± 0.7	2.97 ± 1.2 **	2.28 ± 0.9	2.20 ± 0.6
	aSCOR % (mean ± SD)	60 ± 20	74 ± 18	84 ± 9	83 ± 14	79 ± 10
Controls age- & gender-matched pairs	n	2	6	14	33	10
	Male (%)	1 (50)	6 (100)	9 (64.3)	13 (39.4)	6 (60)
	age (years, mean ± SD)	58 ± 8	64 ± 8	66 ± 9	54 ± 12	55 ± 12
	p	0.909	0.937	0.874	0.934	0.796
	aMCC (mean ± SD)	0.95 ± 0.1	1.12 ± 0.1	1.13 ± 0.1	1.21 ± 0.1	1.15 ± 0.1
	p	0.026	0.022	<0.001	<0.001	<0.001
	aSCOR % (mean ± SD)	30 ± 2	36 ± 5	37 ± 5	41 ± 7	37 ± 8
	p	0.158	0.001	<0.001	<0.001	<0.001

mJOA, modified Japanese Orthopedic Association (score); aMCC, adapted maximum cord compression; aSCOR, adapted spinal cord occupation ratio; SD, standard deviation; * incomplete data mJOA in two patients, total of $n = 31$; ** significantly higher compared to patients with stenosis at C3/C4 ($p = 0.002$) and compared to patients with stenosis at C5/C6 ($p = 0.012$).

Age, mJOA score, number of patients receiving decompressive surgery, aSCOR, and aMCC per group are listed in Table 1. Patients with stenosis at C5/C6 (53 ± 12 years) and C6/C7 (54 ± 12 years) were significantly younger than patients with stenosis at C4/C5 (65 ± 9 years, $p = 0.002$, $p = 0.021$, respectively). Age did not differ between any other group of patients. Comparison of gender between groups showed no significant difference ($p = 0.18$–0.84), with exception of patients with stenosis at C3/C4 (100% men). Duration of the heartbeat was comparable between all groups of patients ($p = 0.85$) and between patients and controls ($p = 0.25$–0.78). The comparison of the mJOA score between groups of patients was not significant (C2/C3 vs. C6/C7, $p = 0.078$, any other comparison $p > 0.5$).

As expected, the aMCC at the stenotic level was significantly higher per group compared to controls (C2/C3 $p = 0.026$, C3/C4 $p = 0.022$, C4/C5, C5/C6, C6/C7 $p < 0.001$, respectively). The aMCC among patients with stenosis at C4/C5 (2.97 ± 0.2) was significantly higher compared to patients with stenosis at C3/C4 (1.96 ± 0.7, $p = 0.002$) and at C5/C6 (2.28 ± 0.9, $p = 0.012$). The aMCC between other groups did not differ.

aSCOR was expectedly significantly higher among patients ($p \leq 0.001$, each), but within patients with stenosis at C2/C3 ($p = 0.16$).

3.2. Focal Increase of Spinal Cord Motion within All Groups of Patients

Compared to controls, patients with stenosis at C2/C3 and C3/C4 showed a trend toward higher spinal cord dynamics at stenosis and at the adjacent segments, but comparison did not reach significance ($p > 0.5$) (Figure 3, complete data sets in Table S1).

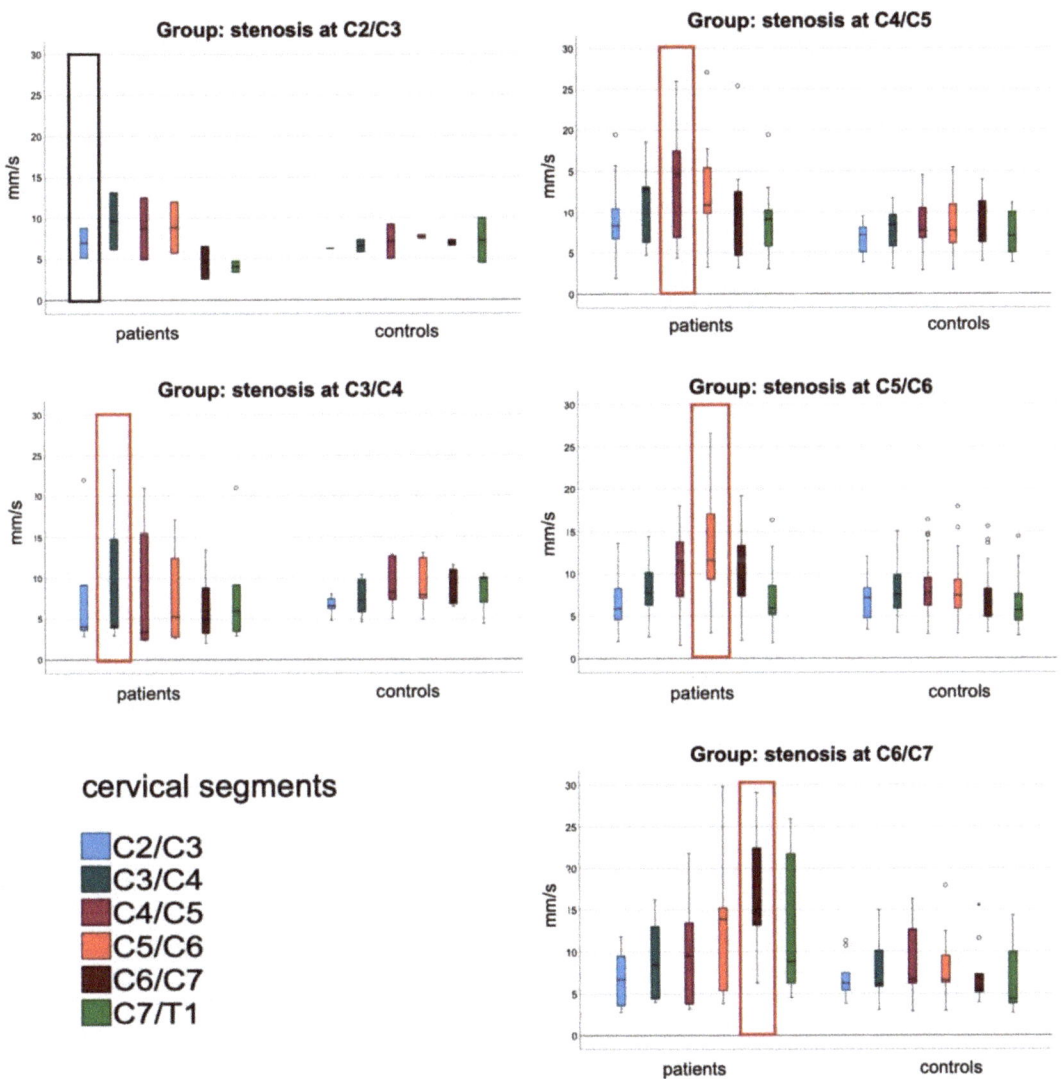

Figure 3. Boxplots per group of patients with level of stenosis at C2/C3, C3/C4, C4/C5, C5/C6, and C6/C7 compared to matched controls; the peak-to-peak amplitude of spinal cord motion is given in mm/s per cervical segment C2/C3 to C7/T1. Increase of spinal cord motion toward each level of stenosis (red rectangle) can be observed. Mild outliers are indicated by ° (1.5 to 3.0 × interquartile range), extreme outliers by * (>3.0 × interquartile range).

Spinal cord motion at level of stenosis was significantly higher among patients with stenosis at C4/C5, C5/C6, and C6/C7 (Figure 3, Table S1; e.g., ptp-amplitude (mm/s) − group C4/C5: 13.80 ± 6.7 mm/s vs. 7.94 ± 3.3 mm/s, $p = 0.007$; group C5/C6: 13.44 ± 6.4 mm/s vs. 7.89 ± 3.3 mm/s, $p < 0.001$; group C6/C7: 17.69 ± 7.5 mm/s vs. 7.31 ± 3.7 mm/s, $p = 0.001$). Similarly, the cranial and caudal adjacent segments showed significantly, or borderline significantly increased spinal cord dynamics (Figure 2, Table S1, e.g., ptp-amplitude (mm/s) one segment caudal to the stenosis: group C4/C5: 12.46 ± 6.1 vs. 8.07 ± 3.5, $p = 0.02$; group C5/C6: 9.95 ± 3.9 vs. 7.16 ± 3.1, $p = 0.002$; group C6/C7: 12.88 ± 7.9 vs. 6.57 ± 4.1, $p = 0.038$).

3.3. Mechanical Stretching and Compression of Interjacent Spinal Cord Tissue

Compared to controls, indices (pAI) at stenosis were significantly increased among patients with stenosis at C4/C5, C5/C6, and C6/C7 (Figure 4).

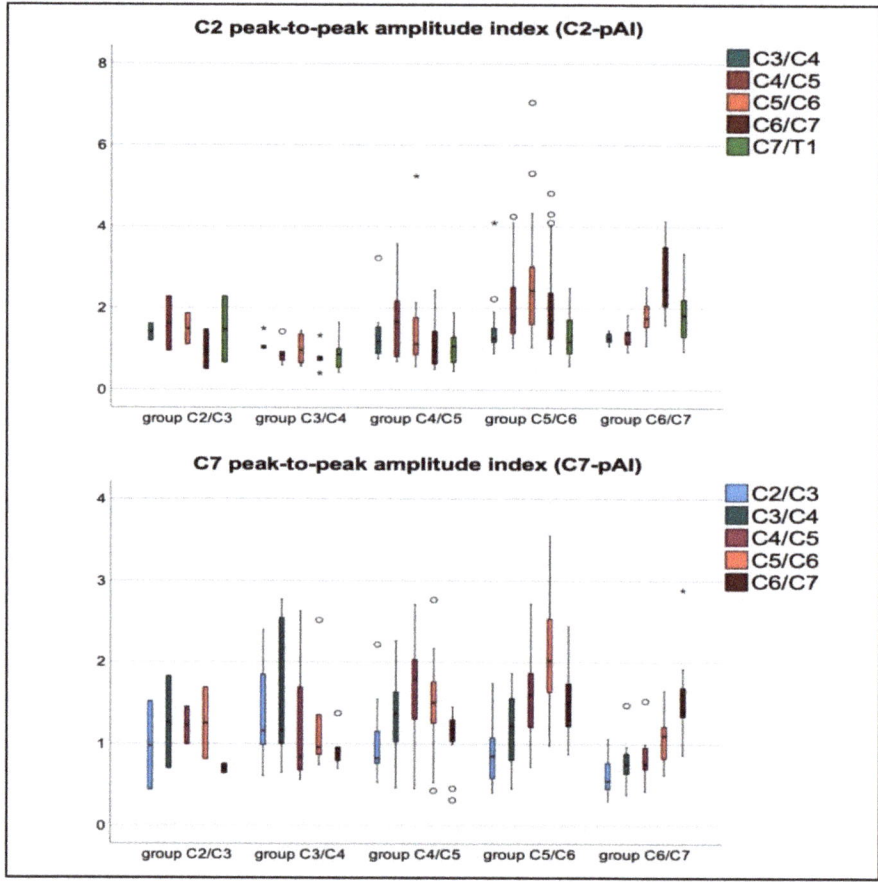

Figure 4. Boxplots of the C2-peak-to-peak amplitude index (C2-pAI, top row) and the C7-peak-to-peak amplitude index (C7-pAI, bottom row). The pAI references the spinal cord peak-to-peak amplitude per segment to the individual's spinal cord peak-to-peak amplitude at the cranial segment C2/C3, or to the caudal segment C7/T1. Cranial levels of stenosis are best reflected by the C7-pAI, caudal stenosis by the C2-pAI. An increase (y-axis) toward the stenotic level per group (x-axis) followed by a decrease is shown, indicating a stretching of the spinal cord tissue cranial of the level of stenosis followed by a mechanical compression of tissue at the caudal segments. Increase and decrease were significant among the groups of patients with stenosis at C4/C5, C5/C6, and C6/C7. Mild outliers are indicated by ° (1.5 to 3.0 × interquartile range), extreme outliers by * (>3.0 × interquartile range).

Patients with levels of stenosis at C4/C5 showed a significant decrease of the C2-pAI from C4/C5 to C6/C7 ($p = 0.011$), highlighting a primarily caudal compression of the spinal cord tissue (Table S1, Figure 4). Patients with stenosis at C5/C6 and C6/C7 showed a significant increase from C2/C3 toward stenosis, and a significant decrease from stenosis to C7/T1 (increase: $p \leq 0.001$, each, decline: $p = 0.019$–0.036, respectively; Table S1, Figure 4). Among patients with levels of stenosis at C2/C3 and C3/C4 comparison of indices showed a non-significant trend toward higher values at stenosis (Table S1).

3.4. Relations of Severity of Stenosis (aMCC/aSCOR), Age, Gender, and mJOA Score to Increased Spinal Cord Motion at Stenosis

Prediction models of each spinal cord motion parameter at stenosis by (1: aMCC at stenosis, age, gender) or (2: aSCOR at stenosis, age, gender) were calculated within all suitable groups of patients with stenosis at C3/C4, C4/C5, C5/C6, and C6/C7. Gender as a predictor could not be analyzed among patients with stenosis at C3/C4 (100% men).

aMCC, aSCOR, age, and mJOA score did not reach significance within any prediction models. One model (1: aMCC at stenosis, age, gender) significantly predicted the C2-pAI at stenosis among patients with stenosis at C6/C7 (1:$R^2 = 0.933$, $p = 0.042$), gender being the only significant predictor ($p = 0.033$).

Gender was a significant predictor of higher spinal cord motion at stenosis among men in group C5/C6 (1: $p = 0.048$; higher ptp-amplitude), and of higher spinal cord strain among men in group C6/C7 (1: $p = 0.033$, 2: $p = 0.024$; higher C2-pAI).

The comparison of spinal cord motion between men and women per group revealed increased maximum velocity and/or ptp-amplitudes at stenosis among patients with stenosis at C4/C5 and C5/C6 ($p = 0.03$, $p = 0.064$, and $p = 0.03$, $p = 0.028$, respectively; Figure 5). Total displacement did not differ between men and women in these groups ($p = 0.89$, $p = 0.25$, respectively; Table 2).

In contrast, men with stenosis at C6/C7 revealed atypically decreased spinal cord motion at segments cranial to the stenosis. Comparison to matched controls (all parameter, $p = 0.009$ to 0.027, Figure 5, Table 2), and to women with stenosis at C6/C7 ($p < 0.001$ to 0.02) showed significantly lower values. At the level of stenosis, spinal cord motion did not differ between genders. There was no significant difference of age, HB, mJOA score, spinal canal CSA, aSCOR, or aMCC between men and women per group with stenosis at C4/C5, C5/C6, or C6/C7, nor between men or women with stenosis at C5/C6 and men with stenosis at C6/C7.

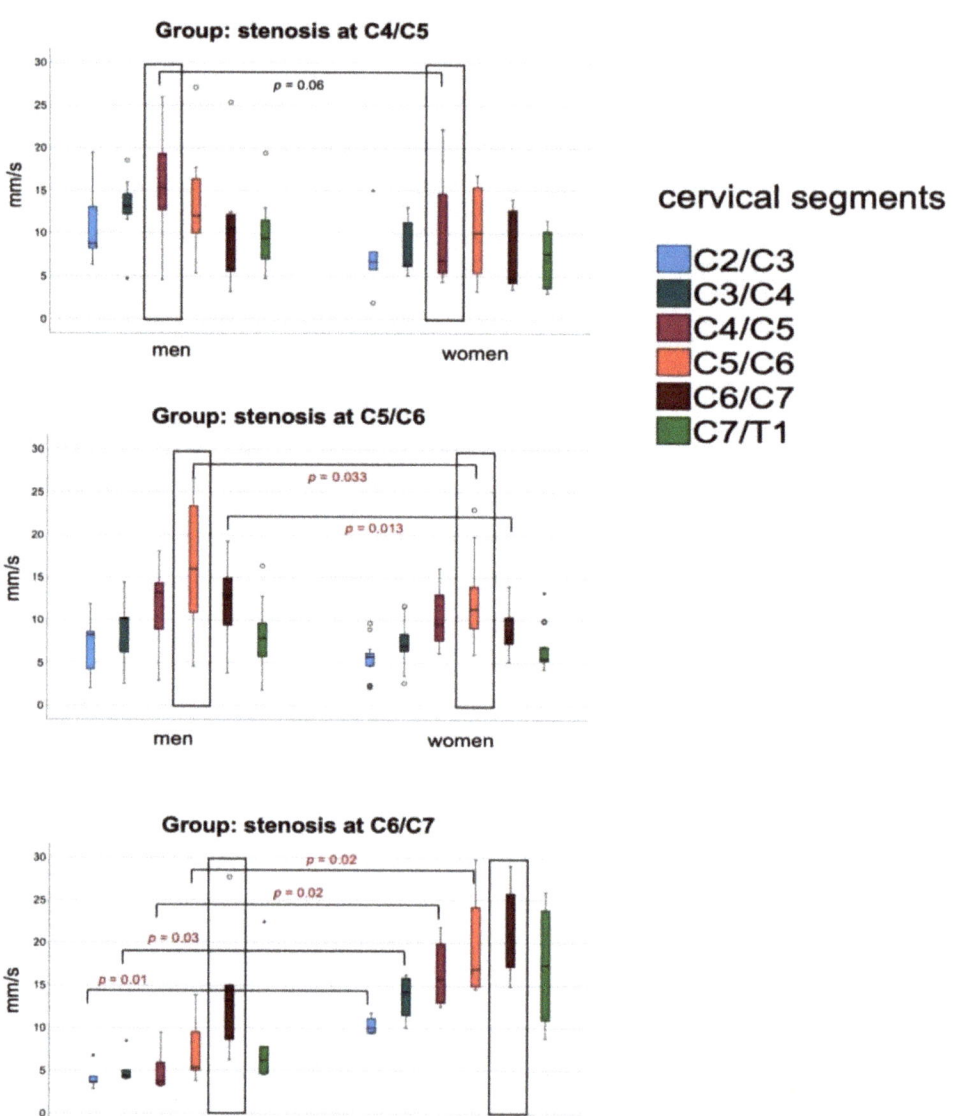

Figure 5. Boxplots demonstrating differences of peak-to-peak amplitudes (mm/s) between men and women. Level of significance is provided in brackets, borderline significance in black lettering, and significant difference in red lettering. The typical increase toward levels of stenosis followed by a decrease can be observed among all groups (black rectangle). Men with stenosis at C6/C7 show a significant decrease of spinal cord motion prior to the stenotic segment. Mild outliers are indicated by ° (1.5 to 3.0 × interquartile range), extreme outliers by * (>3.0 × interquartile range).

Table 2. Clinical, anatomical, and spinal cord motion data per suitable group of patients divided by gender.

		C4/C5	C5/C6	C6/C7
Age (years) (mean ± SD)	men	65 ± 8	53 ± 13	51 ±9
	women	66 ± 11	54 ± 11	59 ± 16
	p	0.819	0.875	0.345
mJOA (mean ± SD)	men	15.9 ± 1.9	16.5 ± 1.7	15.5 ± 2.1
	women	17.0 ± 0.8	16.3 ± 1.9	15.3 ± 2.4
	p	0.289	0.756	0.864
HB (ms) (mean ± SD)	men	944 ± 109	926 ± 138	857 ± 172
	women	962 ± 168	910 ± 134	934 ± 229
	p	0.827	0.732	0.761
aMCC at stenosis (mean ± SD)	men	2.8 ± 1.1	2.6 ± 1.2	2.5 ± 0.6
	women	3.3 ± 1.3	2.0 ± 0.7	1.8 ± 0.3
	p	0.468	*0.084*	*0.065*
aSCOR % at stenosis (mean ± SD)	men	83.0 ± 9	82.9 ± 11	82.6 ± 12
	women	85.0 ± 10	82.7 ± 16	73.3 ± 5
	p	0.72	0.968	0.182
Max. velocity (cm/s) at stenosis (mean ± SD)	men	1.00 ± 0.5	1.09 ± 0.6	0.94 ± 0.6
	women	0.59 ± 0.4	0.73 ± 0.4	1.49 ± 0.4
	p	**0.03**	**0.03**	0.13
ptp-amplitude (mm/s) at stenosis (mean ± SD)	men	15.5 ± 5.9	16.3 ± 7.1	15.2 ± 7.9
	women	10.7 ± 7.6	11.4 ± 5.1	21.5 ± 5.9
	p	*0.064*	**0.028**	0.211
Total displacement (mm) at stenosis (mean ± SD)	men	1.92 ± 0.9	1.92 ± 0.9	1.7 ± 0.6
	women	1.83 ± 1.5	1.49 ± 0.9	2.4 ± 0.9
	p	0.893	0.255	0.151
C2-pAI at stenosis (mean ± SD)	men	1.56 ± 0.7	2.76 ± 1.1	3.23 ± 0.9
	women	1.79 ± 1.3	2.45 ± 1.5	2.05 ± 0.4
	p	0.682	0.523	**0.046**
C7-pAI at stenosis (mean ± SD)	men	1.79 ± 0.8	2.21 ± 0.7	1.71 ± 0.6
	women	1.54 ± 0.6	1.96 ± 0.6	1.35 ± 0.4
	p	0.570	0.31	0.33

mJOA, modified Japanese Orthopedic Association (score); HB, heartbeat; aMCC, adapted maximum cord compression; aSCOR, adapted spinal cord occupation ratio; Max, maximum; ptp, peak-to-peak; pAI, peak-to-peak amplitude index. Significant differences in bold letters, borderline significance in italic letters.

4. Discussion

To date, our work represents the most extensive study on spinal cord motion demonstrating focal and long distant pathodynamic patterns in DCM patients while covering relevant stenoses at all cervical segments. Moreover, this is the first report on significant dynamic alterations due to gender-related effects among DCM patients. Additionally, our data suggest segmental differences of spinal cord motion behavior depending on the stenotic cervical segment and therefore underlines the importance of focal influences on spinal cord motion.

We report on 65 DCM patients presenting with monosegmental stenosis. Our study population represents a common, clinically mildly affected cohort, with C5/C6 being the most commonly stenotic segment [23]. Thus, the cohort consists of a representative sample that typically would require additional diagnostics during medical workup.

The current data replicates the dynamic alterations already observed at C5/C6 also at other stenotic cervical segments [10,12,13]. This is of interest, as the segment C5/C6 is located at the maximum of the cervical lordosis and healthy controls show a physiological increase of spinal cord motion at this segment [11,12]; Figure 3. Current results show significant differences between DCM patients and matched-paired controls specifically depending on the level of the stenotic segment: focally increased spinal cord motion appears with a maximum at stenosis and remains relatively unaffected at segments remote from stenosis. The intra-individual indices replicate an overall strain on spinal cord tissue among patients with stenoses at other cervical levels [12]. Among all larger groups of patients, a significant decrease of the indices below level of stenosis was demonstrated as well, indicating an additional compressive effect on the spinal cord tissue caudal of the stenosis. This relative decrease of spinal cord motion below the stenotic segment may be an effect of higher pressure within the spinal canal caudal of the stenosis, following the law of Bernoulli.

Consistent with earlier findings [10,12], automated measurements of the severity of the stenosis (aMCC, aSCOR) did not predict the extent of spinal cord motion, emphasizing a focal disarrangement of spinal cord dynamics and anatomy. The generally suspected origin of spinal cord motion has been extensively discussed previously [10–13]. In summary, known influences on intraspinal dynamics can be divided in global (e.g., heartbeat [24–26]), breathing [27], and pulsatile CSF-flow [28]) and focal effects, such as loss of compensatory buffer zone for the expansion of pulsatile local arteries [28]).

The demonstrated missing relationship of spinal cord motion to the severity of stenosis may possibly be due to differences of the capacity to compensate for alterations of pulsatile subarachnoid CSF-pressure changes within the spinal canal-analogous to the Windkessel effect. Thus, as there exists a well-known variance between clinical impairment and severity of spinal canal compression [1,5–7], spinal cord motion may be a possible predictor of the clinical course in case of spinal canal stenoses.

Although current data show similar spinal cord motion patterns across all groups of patients with different levels of stenosis, current data may imply differences between men and women.

While the velocity peaks of the spinal cord motion curve over one heartbeat were significantly increased among men compared to women with stenosis at C4/C5 and C5/C6 (maximum velocity, peak-to-peak amplitude), the total displacement—a parameter comprising information of the entire velocity curve—remained similar between genders. As the mean duration of the heartbeat was not different between men and women, a lower peak but with similar total displacement indicated a flattened peak and a prolonged sinusoidal spinal cord motion curve over one heartbeat among women. This finding is complementary to the recently described spinal cord motion curve pattern among DCM patients by Hupp et al. In contrast to controls with a short, singular spinal cord oscillation within the heart cycle, DCM patients showed an ongoing spinal cord motion during the entire heart cycle [13]. Among women, this effect seems to be intensified.

As an unexpected, possibly gender-related effect, a uniquely altered spinal cord motion pattern was observed among men with stenosis at C6/C7: Spinal cord motion was significantly slower at segments cranial to the stenosis followed by a vast acceleration at stenosis. Sufficient explanation for this observation cannot be concluded based on the currently assessed data (age, spinal canal CSA, aSCOR, etc.), that did not differ between genders or groups. As the assessed parameters on spinal canal anatomy and age did not significantly differ between genders, possible compensatory mechanisms as elasticity of meninges leading toward differences of volume–compensation within the subarachnoid CSF-space may play a role. The possibility of gender effects within DCM is underlined by significantly worse functional outcome of men undergoing decompressive surgery, which has been recently reported [29].

The only other trial on spinal cord motion across all cervical segments in 55 DCM patients with mono- ($n = 19$) and multisegmental ($n = 36$) stenoses based on validated analysis procedures was recently published by Hupp et al. [13]. Due to combined analysis of spinal cord motion pattern at different segments and non-matched cohorts, a point-to-point comparison is difficult. As a topic of inter-scanner and inter-protocol comparability, the currently reported velocity values among patients and controls based on different PC-MRI settings are at a higher level (approximately $\times$ 2) [12,13]. Further investigations should evaluate the inter-scanner reliability. As common ground, both studies underline pathological alterations of spinal cord motion pattern among DCM patients and its possible contributing value in DCM diagnostics. The currently presented data offers more refined results and depicts relevant differences of the pathodynamics per cervical segment between men and women. Thus, further studies should aim to investigate multicentric data and the clinical value of spinal cord motion based on segmental analysis.

Limits of the study are in part small cohorts (group C2/C3, C3/C4) and sub-cohorts. This is mostly due to the known contribution of most to least affected segments in DCM, but also to the exclusion of multisegmental relevant stenoses. At the current state of basic research and the general aim of an understanding of intrathecal dynamics, we chose to limit the possible confounding effect of multisegmental stenosis.

Effects on (yet) non-symptomatic spinal stenosis were not a topic of this study and should be investigated in further longitudinal trials. Differences in spinal canal degeneration, e.g., rather soft disc herniation vs. solid ossification of ligaments, and their possible influence on spinal cord dynamics were not systematically addressed. The study does not include a full analysis of physiological relations (e.g., body mass indices and height), nor associations to clinical function due to primary aims on pathophysiological ground research. Due to small group size, we cannot sufficiently analyze the association of clinical impairment to spinal cord motion based on the current data. The mJOA score reflects the range of patients included within the presented data, but it does not comprise details on mild spinal cord affection. First, more refined and reliable clinical and electrophysiological assessments are needed to assess the many aspects of DCM (e.g., reliable light-touch, pin-prick testing as part of the International Standards for Neurological Classification of Spinal Cord Injury [30] evoked potentials [31], the graded redefined assessment of strength, sensibility, and prehension version myelopathy [32], etc.). Second, more knowledge of the influencing factors is required in respect to gender and level of the cervical segment in order to establish reliable and comparable cut-off values.

5. Conclusions

The presented data presents focally increased spinal cord motion depending on the affected cervical stenotic segment among DCM patients. There is proof of an overall disarranged dynamic behavior resulting in mechanical strains on spinal cord tissue across the cervical spine. Men and women show significantly different spinal cord motion patterns depending on the affected cervical segment, thus indicating gender-related differences in DCM.

Supplementary Materials: The following are available online at https://www.mdpi.com/article/10.3390/jcm10173788/s1, Table S1: Table of all means, standard deviations, and *p* values of all dynamic parameters per segment and group.

Author Contributions: Conceptualization, K.W., J.-H.K., U.H., A.J.K., K.E. and M.H.; data curation, K.W., M.R., J.-H.K., A.J.K. and M.H.; formal analysis, K.W. and S.F.B.; funding acquisition, K.W., U.H., A.J.K., K.E. and M.H.; investigation, K.W., S.F.B., J.-H.K., U.H., N.K., K.E. and M.H.; methodology, K.W., M.R., A.J.K., K.E. and M.H.; project administration, K.W., K.E. and M.H.; resources, M.R. and U.H.; software, M.R. and A.J.K.; validation, K.W., J.-H.K. and M.H.; visualization, K.W. and M.R.; writing—original draft, K.W.; Writing—review and editing, M.R., S.F.B., J.-H.K., U.H., A.J.K., N.K., K.E. and M.H. All authors have read and agreed to the published version of the manuscript.

Funding: Our study received funding from the German Spine Foundation (number 12/2017) and the program "Clinical Studies 2019" of the Faculty of Medicine, University of Freiburg, Germany (number: 3091331904). The article processing charge was funded by the Baden-Württemberg Ministry of Science, Research and Art and the University of Freiburg in the funding program Open Access Publishing.

Institutional Review Board Statement: The study was conducted according to the guidelines of the Declaration of Helsinki, and approved by the Institutional Ethics Committee of the Albert-Ludwigs-University Freiburg (ethical approval number: 261/17, date of approval 9 August 2017, and number 338/17, date of approval 6 September 2017).

Informed Consent Statement: Informed consent was obtained from all subjects involved in the study. Written informed consent has been obtained from the patients to publish this paper.

Data Availability Statement: The data presented in this study are openly available in Table S1, and Tables 1 and 2.

Acknowledgments: We thank D. Gruninger (Department of Neurosurgery) and Hansjörg Mast (Department of Neuroradiology) for their constant support in study administration.

Conflicts of Interest: Axel J. Krafft is currently employed at Siemens Healthcare GmbH, Erlangen, Germany; he contributed to the study while being employed at the Department of Neuroradiology, Medical Center–University of Freiburg, Faculty of Medicine, University of Freiburg, Germany. All other authors confirm that there are no conflicts of interest. The funders had no role in the design of the study; in the collection, analyses, or interpretation of data; in the writing of the manuscript, or in the decision to publish the results.

Abbreviations

aMCC	adapted maximum canal compromise
aSCOR	adapted spinal cord occupation ratio
CNN	convolutional neural network
CSA	cross-sectional area
CSF	cerebrospinal fluid
DCM	degenerative cervical myelopathy
ICC	intra-class correlation coefficient
MRI	magnetic resonance imaging
pAI	peak-to-peak-amplitude index
PC-MRI	phase-contrast MRI
ptp	peak-to-peak
SPACE	sampling perfection with application-optimized contrasts using different flip angle evolution

References

1. Kalsi-Ryan, S.; Karadimas, S.K.; Fehlings, M.G. Cervical spondylotic myelopathy: The clinical phenomenon and the current pathobiology of an increasingly prevalent and devastating disorder. *Neuroscientist* **2013**, *19*, 409–421. [CrossRef]
2. Badhiwala, J.H.; Ahuja, C.S.; Akbar, M.A.; Witiw, C.D.; Nassiri, F.; Furlan, J.C.; Curt, A.; Wilson, J.R.; Fehlings, M.G. Degenerative cervical myelopathy—Update and future directions. *Nat. Rev. Neurol.* **2020**, *16*, 108–124. [CrossRef]
3. Davies, B.; Mowforth, O.D.; Smith, E.K.; Kotter, M.R. Degenerative cervical myelopathy. *BMJ* **2018**, *360*, k186. [CrossRef]
4. Nouri, A.; Tetreault, L.; Singh, A.; Karadimas, S.K.; Fehlings, M. Degenerative Cervical Myelopathy. *Spine* **2015**, *40*, E675–E693. [CrossRef]
5. Fehlings, M.G.; Tetreault, L.A.; Riew, K.D.; Middleton, J.W.; Aarabi, B.; Arnold, P.M.; Brodke, D.S.; Burns, A.; Carette, S.; Chen, R.; et al. A Clinical Practice Guideline for the Management of Patients with Degenerative Cervical Myelopathy: Recommendations for Patients with Mild, Moderate, and Severe Disease and Nonmyelopathic Patients with Evidence of Cord Compression. *Glob. Spine J.* **2017**, *7*, 70S–83S. [CrossRef]
6. Nouri, A.; Gondar, R.; Cheng, J.S.; Kotter, M.R.; Tessitore, E. Degenerative Cervical Myelopathy and the Aging Spine: Introduction to the Special Issue. *J. Clin. Med.* **2020**, *9*, 2535. [CrossRef] [PubMed]
7. Witiw, C.D.; Mathieu, F.; Nouri, A.; Fehlings, M.G. Clinico-Radiographic Discordance: An Evidence-Based Commentary on the Management of Degenerative Cervical Spinal Cord Compression in the Absence of Symptoms or with Only Mild Symptoms of Myelopathy. *Glob. Spine J.* **2017**, *8*, 527–534. [CrossRef]
8. Vavasour, I.M.; Meyers, S.M.; Macmillan, E.L.; Mädler, B.; Li, D.K.; Rauscher, A.; Vertinsky, T.; Venu, V.; Mackay, A.L.; Curt, A. Increased spinal cord movements in cervical spondylotic myelopathy. *Spine J.* **2014**, *14*, 2344–2354. [CrossRef] [PubMed]
9. Chang, H.S.; Nejo, T.; Yoshida, S.; Oya, S.; Matsui, T. Increased flow signal in compressed segments of the spinal cord in patients with cervical spondylotic myelopathy. *Spine* **2014**, *39*, 2136–2142. [CrossRef] [PubMed]
10. Wolf, K.; Hupp, M.; Friedl, S.; Sutter, R.; Klarhöfer, M.; Grabher, P.; Freund, P.; Curt, A. In cervical spondylotic myelopathy spinal cord motion is focally increased at the level of stenosis: A controlled cross-sectional study. *Spinal Cord* **2018**, *56*, 769–776. [CrossRef] [PubMed]

11. Hupp, M.; Vallotton, K.; Brockmann, C.; Huwyler, S.; Rosner, J.; Sutter, R.; Klarhoefer, M.; Freund, P.; Farshad, M.; Curt, A. Segmental differences of cervical spinal cord motion: Advancing from confounders to a diagnostic tool. *Sci. Rep.* **2019**, *9*, 7415. [CrossRef]
12. Wolf, K.; Reisert, M.; Beltrán, S.F.; Klingler, J.-H.; Hubbe, U.; Krafft, A.J.; Egger, K.; Hohenhaus, M. Focal cervical spinal stenosis causes mechanical strain on the entire cervical spinal cord tissue—A prospective controlled, matched-pair analysis based on phase-contrast MRI. *NeuroImage Clin.* **2021**, *30*, 102580. [CrossRef] [PubMed]
13. Hupp, M.; Pfender, N.; Vallotton, K.; Rosner, J.; Friedl, S.; Zipser, C.M.; Sutter, R.; Klarhöfer, M.; Spirig, J.M.; Betz, M.; et al. The Restless Spinal Cord in Degenerative Cervical Myelopathy. *Am. J. Neuroradiol.* **2021**, *42*, 597–609. [CrossRef] [PubMed]
14. Wolf, K.; Krafft, A.J.; Egger, K.; Klingler, J.-H.; Hubbe, U.; Reisert, M.; Hohenhaus, M. Assessment of spinal cord motion as a new diagnostic MRI-parameter in cervical spinal canal stenosis: Study protocol on a prospective longitudinal trial. *J. Orthop. Surg. Res.* **2019**, *14*, 1–7. [CrossRef]
15. Kato, S.; Oshima, Y.; Oka, H.; Chikuda, H.; Takeshita, Y.; Miyoshi, K.; Kawamura, N.; Masuda, K.; Kunogi, J.; Okazaki, R.; et al. Comparison of the Japanese Orthopaedic Association (JOA) Score and Modified JOA (mJOA) Score for the Assessment of Cervical Myelopathy: A Multicenter Observational Study. *PLoS ONE* **2015**, *10*, e0123022, Erratum in **2015**, *10*, e0128392. [CrossRef] [PubMed]
16. Nora-Imaging. Available online: http://www.nora-imaging.org (accessed on 1 July 2021).
17. Zhao, B.; Zhang, X.; Li, Z.; Hu, X. A multi-scale strategy for deep semantic segmentation with convolutional neural networks. *Neurocomputing* **2019**, *365*, 273–284. [CrossRef]
18. Nouri, A.; Martin, A.R.; Mikulis, D.; Fehlings, M.G. Magnetic resonance imaging assessment of degenerative cervical myelopathy: A review of structural changes and measurement techniques. *Neurosurg. Focus* **2016**, *40*, E5. [CrossRef]
19. Nouri, A.; Montejo, J.; Sun, X.; Virojanapa, J.; Kolb, L.E.; Abbed, K.M.; Cheng, J.S. Cervical Cord-Canal Mismatch: A New Method for Identifying Predisposition to Spinal Cord Injury. *World Neurosur.* **2017**, *108*, 112–117. [CrossRef]
20. Koo, T.K.; Li, M.Y. Cracking the code: Providing insight into the fundamentals of research and evidence-based practice a guideline of selecting and reporting intraclass correlation coefficients for reliability research. *J. Chiropr. Med.* **2016**, *15*, 155–163. [CrossRef]
21. Cook, R.D. Detection of Influential Observation in Linear Regression. *Technometrics* **1977**, *19*, 15. [CrossRef]
22. Huber, P.J. *Robust Statistics*; John Wiley: New York, NY, USA, 1981; ISBN 978-0-471-72524-4.
23. Northover, J.R.; Wild, J.B.; Braybrooke, J.; Blanco, J. The epidemiology of cervical spondylotic myelopathy. *Skelet. Radiol.* **2012**, *41*, 1543–1546. [CrossRef] [PubMed]
24. Figley, C.; Stroman, P. Investigation of human cervical and upper thoracic spinal cord motion: Implications for imaging spinal cord structure and function. *Magn. Reson. Med.* **2007**, *58*, 185–189. [CrossRef] [PubMed]
25. Tanaka, H.; Sakurai, K.; Kashiwagi, N.; Fujita, N.; Hirabuki, N.; Inaba, F.; Harada, K.; Nakamura, H. Transition of the craniocaudal velocity of the spinal cord: From cervical segment to lumbar enlargement. *Invest. Radiol.* **1998**, *33*, 141–145. [CrossRef] [PubMed]
26. Mikulis, D.J.; Wood, M.L.; Zerdoner, O.A.; Poncelet, B.P. Oscillatory motion of the normal cervical spinal cord. *Radiology* **1994**, *192*, 117–121. [CrossRef]
27. Winklhofer, S.; Schoth, F.; Stolzmann, P.; Krings, T.; Mull, M.; Wiesmann, M.; Stracke, C.P. Spinal Cord Motion: Influence of Respiration and Cardiac Cycle. *RoFo* **2014**, *186*, 1016–1021. [CrossRef] [PubMed]
28. Matsuzaki, H.; Wakabayashi, K.; Ishihara, K.; Ishikawa, H.; Kawabata, H.; Onomura, T. The origin and significance of spinal cord pulsation. *Spinal Cord* **1996**, *34*, 422–426. [CrossRef]
29. Khan, O.; Badhiwala, J.H.; Akbar, M.A.; Fehlings, M.G. Prediction of Worse Functional Status After Surgery for Degenerative Cervical Myelopathy: A Machine Learning Approach. *Neurosurgery* **2020**, *88*, 584–591. [CrossRef]
30. Kirshblum, S.C.; Waring, W.; Biering-Sorensen, F.; Burns, S.P.; Johansen, M.; Schmidt-Read, M.; Donovan, W.; Graves, D.E.; Jha, A.; Jones, L.; et al. Reference for the 2011 revision of the International Standards for Neuro-logical Classification of Spinal Cord Injury. *J. Spinal Cord Med.* **2011**, *34*, 547–554. [CrossRef]
31. Holly, L.T.; Matz, P.G.; Anderson, P.A.; Groff, M.W.; Heary, R.F.; Kaiser, M.G.; Mummaneni, P.V.; Ryken, T.C.; Choudhri, T.F.; Vresilovic, E.J.; et al. Clinical prognostic indicators of surgical outcome in cervical spondylotic myelopathy. *J. Neurosurg. Spine* **2009**, *11*, 112–118. [CrossRef] [PubMed]
32. Kalsi-Ryan, S.; Riehm, L.E.; Tetreault, L.; Martin, A.R.; Teoderascu, F.; Massicotte, E.; Curt, A.; Verrier, M.C.; Velstra, I.-M.; Fehlings, M.G. Characteristics of Upper Limb Impairment Related to Degenerative Cervical Myelopathy: Development of a Sensitive Hand Assessment (Graded Redefined Assessment of Strength, Sensibility, and Prehension Version Myelopathy). *Neurosurgery* **2019**, *86*, E292–E299. [CrossRef] [PubMed]

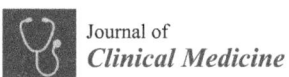

Article

Clinical Outcomes between Stand-Alone Zero-Profile Spacers and Cervical Plate with Cage Fixation for Anterior Cervical Discectomy and Fusion: A Retrospective Analysis of 166 Patients

Samuel Sommaruga [1,2,†], Joaquin Camara-Quintana [1,†], Kishan Patel [1], Aria Nouri [1,2], Enrico Tessitore [2], Granit Molliqaj [2], Shreyas Panchagnula [1], Michael Robinson [3], Justin Virojanapa [1], Xin Sun [1], Fjodor Melnikov [4], Luis Kolb [1], Karl Schaller [2], Khalid Abbed [1] and Joseph Cheng [1,3,*]

[1] Department of Neurosurgery, Yale University School of Medicine, New Haven, CT 06519, USA; samuelsommaruga@gmail.com (S.S.); jqcamara@gmail.com (J.C.-Q.); kishan.patel@yale.edu (K.P.); arianouri9@gmail.com (A.N.); shreyas.panchagnula@yale.edu (S.P.); justin.virojanapa@gmail.com (J.V.); xin.sun@yale.edu (X.S.); luis.kolb@yale.edu (L.K.); Khalid.AbbedMD@gmail.com (K.A.)
[2] Department of Neurosurgery, Geneva University Hospital, 1205 Geneva, Switzerland; enrico.tessitore@hcuge.ch (E.T.); granitmolliqaj@gmail.com (G.M.); Karl.Schaller@hcuge.ch (K.S.)
[3] Department of Neurosurgery, University of Cincinnati College of Medicine, Cincinnati, OH 45267-0515, USA; robinson.michaelw@gmail.com
[4] Yale Center for Green Chemistry and Engineering, New Haven, CT 06511, USA; fjodor.melnikov@yale.edu
* Correspondence: chengj6@ucmail.uc.edu; Tel.: +1-(513)-558-3556
† These authors contributed equally.

Abstract: Stand-alone (SA) zero-profile implants are an alternative to cervical plating (CP) in anterior cervical discectomy and fusion (ACDF). In this study, we investigate differences in surgical outcomes between SA and CP in ACDF. We conducted a retrospective analysis of 166 patients with myelopathy and/or radiculopathy who had ACDF with SA or CP from Jan 2013–Dec 2016. We measured surgical outcomes including Bazaz dysphagia score at 3 months, Nurick grade at last follow-up, and length of hospital stay. 166 patients (92F/74M) were reviewed. 92 presented with radiculopathy (55%), 37 with myelopathy (22%), and 37 with myeloradiculopathy (22%). The average operative time with CP was longer than SA (194 ± 69 vs. 126 ± 46 min) ($p < 0.001$), as was the average length of hospital stay (2.1 ± 2 vs. 1.5 ± 1 days) ($p = 0.006$). At 3 months, 82 patients (49.4%) had a follow-up for dysphagia, with 3 patients reporting mild dysphagia and none reporting moderate or severe dysphagia. Nurick grade at last follow-up for the myelopathy and myeloradiculopathy cohorts improved in 63 patients (85%). Prolonged length of stay was associated with reduced odds of having an optimal outcome by 0.50 (CI = 0.35–0.85, $p = 0.003$). Overall, we demonstrate that there is no significant difference in neurological outcome or rates of dysphagia between SA and CP, and that both lead to overall improvement of symptoms based on Nurick grading. However, we also show that the SA group has shorter length of hospital stay and operative time compared to CP.

Keywords: degenerative cervical myelopathy; radiculopathy; ACDF; dysphagia; cervical plating; stand-alone implant

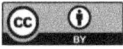

1. Introduction

Degenerative disease of the cervical spine manifests in a wide spectrum of pathologies that encompass disc degeneration, disc herniation, vertebral restructuring, osteophyte formation, and ligamentous hypertrophy [1]. Compression of the neural elements can lead to cervical radiculopathy, myelopathy, or myeloradiculopathy. In the treatment of these pathologies, an anterior, posterior, or combined anterior/posterior surgical approach can be undertaken. However, anterior approaches are often favored for patients with single level disc disease, kyphotic deformity and large focal anterior pathology [2].

Anterior cervical discectomy and fusion (ACDF) is considered the gold standard in the management of cervical disc disease [3,4]. This procedure has been improved on over time since first described by Smith and Robinson in the 1950s, mainly via technological advances. Over the past few decades, ACDF has been coupled with anterior cervical plating (CP), which is thought to reduce the risk of graft extrusion, increase the likelihood of fusion, maintain appropriate lordosis, and reduce the risk of subsidence [5]. In recent years, zero-profile, stand-alone (SA) interbody spacers have been developed as an alternative aimed at decreasing operative time, improving dysphagia complication rates, and preventing adjacent level disease [6], Figure 1. Indications for ACDF with plating or stand-alone cages are variable and are operator dependent, however, the following indications are often used, cases of instability (degenerative or post-traumatic), presence of significant degeneration, concern for fusion failure including in cases of poor bone quality (osteoporosis, rheumatoid arthritis) and tobacco use. In addition, further indication exists with significant alignment correction and increasing number of operated segments [7,8].

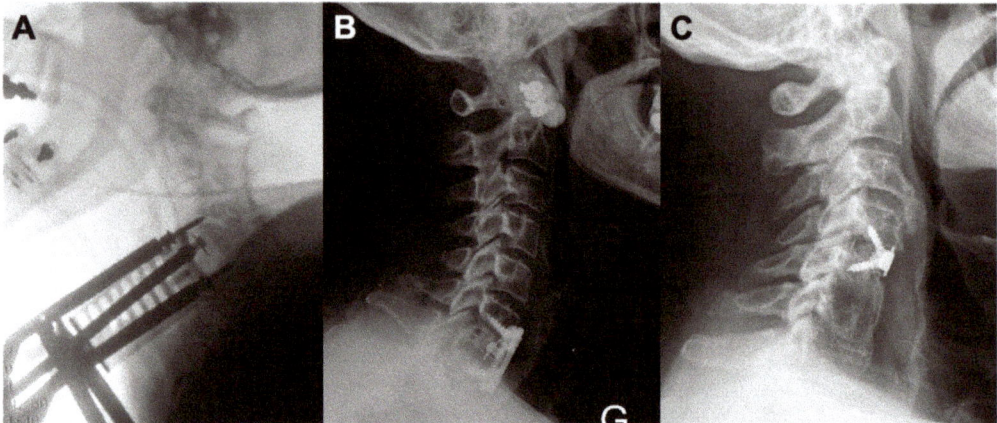

Figure 1. Anterior cervical cage placement and fixation. (**A**) Intraoperative lateral X-ray to assess ACDF cage placement. Casper pins can be seen in the vertebral bodies above and below. (**B**) Post-operative lateral X-ray showing a single level ACDF (HRCC, Eurospine) at C6-C7 secured by a plate (Venture, Medtronic). (**C**) Post-operative lateral X-ray showing a single level ACDF at C4-5 (Zero-P cage, DePuy Synthes) for the treatment of myelopathy due to adjacent segment disease after a fusion with autologous iliac crest bone at C5-6. ACDF = Anterior Cervical Discectomy and Fusion.

There is a dearth of studies in the literature comparing outcomes between SA and CP in single and multilevel ACDF for degenerative cervical disc disease. When compared, the clinical outcomes and dysphagia rates have been either equivocal or not statistically significant [5,9–13]. It remains unclear if this has been due to the limited number patients in these studies and/or the amount of follow-up time.

We sought to study a large North American patient population undergoing ACDF with SA or CP for single and multilevel degenerative disc disease. Herein, we report our experience on a retrospectively collected series of patients with follow-up of up to 24 months after surgery, and describe clinical outcomes and dysphagia rates related to these two techniques. To our knowledge, this cohort represents one of the largest that has been studied in North America.

2. Materials and Methods

Between January 2013 to December 2016, a total of 182 patients underwent single to three-level ACDF in the Department of Neurosurgery at Yale New Haven Hospital, New Haven, CT, USA. Of the 182 patients, we retrospectively reviewed 166 consecutive patients that had received ACDF (Figure 2). Yale University's IRB approved the protocol for this study (protocol number 200020713), and the study was exempt from informed consent. Inclusion criteria included: signs and symptoms of cervical radiculopathy, myelopathy, or myeloradiculopathy, unresponsiveness to conservative measures, ages between 18–85, and disc herniation identified by MRI with evidence of nerve root and/or cord compression. Exclusion criteria included: patients presenting with ossification of the posterior longitudinal ligament, a history of malignancy, evidence of systemic or local infection, history of cervical spine trauma, prior cervical spine surgery, and patients requiring simultaneous anterior and posterior surgery. Demographic information, medical comorbidities, selected medications and selected personal history were also collected.

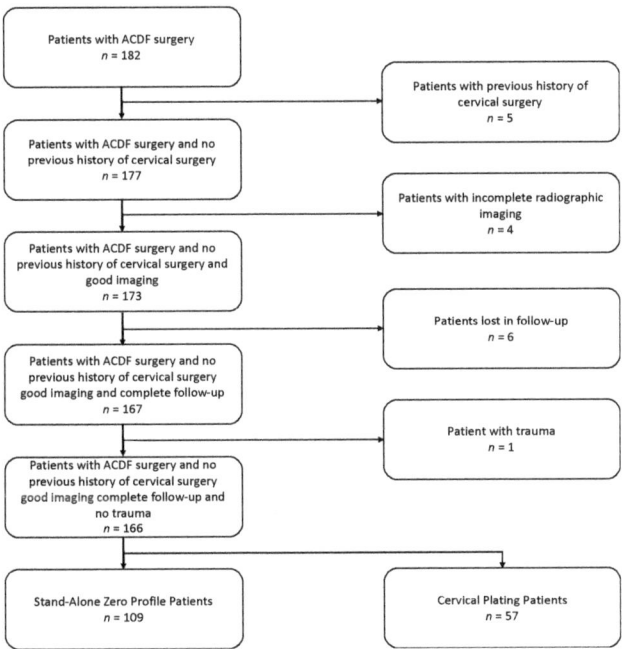

Figure 2. Flow Chart of Patient Cohort. ACDF = Anterior Cervical Discectomy and Fusion.

2.1. Surgical Procedure

All surgical procedures were performed by two senior spine surgeons using the standard Smith-Robinson approach on the patient's right side. After sterile prep and draping, a right-sided transverse incision was made with a #10 blade. The platysma was transected using bovie electrocautery. Fascial planes under the platysma were exposed cranially and caudally using Metzenbaum scissors. A corridor was then made in between the sternocleidomastoid muscle and strap muscles, preserving their respective fascial planes. Using Cloward hand-held retractors, the esophagus was protected medially and the carotid laterally. The prevertebral fascia was dissected off the ventral spine, exposing our index disc level(s) and longus colli bilaterally. Once our index disc level(s) were confirmed with a needle and fluoroscopy, bilateral colli were dissected of the lateral ventral spine using bovie electrocautery. Appropriately sized retraction blades with teeth were placed under the dissected longus colli to retract over the longus colli away from our working field. Caspar pins were then applied to the vertebral bodies above and below to help distract our disc space. Disc was removed with great care taken in removing the cartilaginous endplate to avoid disruption and damage of the bony integrity of the endplates. Posterior osteophytes were drilled using a high-speed cutting burr in combination with Kerrison rongeurs. After decompression of the spinal cord and nerve roots, the appropriate size cage was selected using trial spacers under fluoroscopic guidance to ensure good height and width as well as to not over-distract the facet joints. We used demineralized bone matrix to pack all interbody spacers. For patients undergoing SA device insertion (Globus Coalition AGX, Audubon, PA, USA), the implant was placed into the intervertebral disc space and a pilot hole was drilled at the rostral and caudal endplates under fluoroscopic guidance and this was followed by screw insertion. For patients undergoing CP devices, the spacer was inserted under fluoroscopic guidance followed by positioning of a 4-hole plate across the midline of rostral and caudal ventral vertebral bodies. Pilot holes were drilled into rostral and caudal vertebral bodies followed by screw insertion, again using fluoroscopy to ensure proper placement.

2.2. Clinical Measures

The operative procedure details such as the post-operative symptoms, the post-operative Nurick grade, the number of index levels, operating time, blood loss, presence of a CSF leak, and hospital length of stay were all collected. Nurick grade scores were collected on pre-op, 2 weeks, 3-, 6-, 12-months, and up to 24-months or last follow-up. Neurological outcome was dichotomized in the Nurick grade. Outcome measures included Bazaz dysphagia score at 3 months [14]. We defined optimal outcome as an improvement in the Nurick grade. We defined suboptimal outcome as no change or a decline in Nurick grade.

2.3. Statistical Analysis

Statistical analysis was performed with R-studio Desktop v1.1.383 (R-studio, Boston, MA, USA) programming software. Continuous variables are presented as mean (standard deviation (SD)) or median (interquartile range (IQR)), while discrete variables are presented as count (percentage (%)).

Assessments of potentially significant differences between patients with optimal and suboptimal outcomes groups were performed using the Fisher exact test for categorical variables and the Mann-Whitney U test for continuous variables.

We constructed a multivariable logistic regression model by including variables that reached a predetermined significance level of $p < 0.2$ in univariate analysis. Additionally, universal confounders and other variables selected based on expert opinion were forced into the model, including Nurick grade and number of levels of surgery. Covariates with $p > 0.1$ were removed and collinearity was assessed based on variance inflation factor. A 2-sided p value of <0.05 was used to determine which variables were independently associated with an optimal outcome.

3. Results

3.1. Demographics

Our baseline patient population characteristics are reported in Table 1. A total of 166 patients (92 females and 74 males) underwent ACDF and met our inclusion criteria, with age ranging from 23 to 85 (mean 53 years). Of the 166 patients, 92 (55%) presented with radiculopathy, 37 (22%) with myelopathy, and 37 (22%) with myeloradiculopathy. In comparing SA and CP patients, 61% and 46% suffered from radiculopathy, 14% and 39% from myelopathy, and 26% and 16% from myeloradiculopathy, respectively.

Twenty-four (14%) of our patients had diabetes, 45 (27%) were current tobacco users, 47 (28%) had a history of tobacco use longer than 1-year and 3 patients (2%) were formally diagnosed with osteoporosis. For preoperative pain management, 61 (37%) patients were currently using opioid medications, 40 (24%) were on Gabapentin or Pregabalin, 58 (35%) were using NSAIDs for over 3 months, 54 (33%) were on antidepressants, and 13 (8%) were taking steroids chronically for medical conditions. In addition, 98 (59%) patients were actively involved in physical therapy and 22 (13%) had at least one epidural steroid injection.

Among the 166 patients, 109 underwent ACDF with SA devices (66%) and 57 underwent ACDF with CP (34%). Eighty-five patients (51%) underwent 1 level ACDF; 65 patients (39%) underwent 2 levels and 16 patients (10%) had 3 levels. There was no difference in the number of levels of surgery between the SA and CP groups (Table 2). The average duration of surgery for all ACDF procedures was 150 ($\pm$64) min, with 194 ($\pm$69) and 126 ($\pm$46) min for CP and for SA respectively ($p < 0.001$). The blood loss was minimal; only 4 patients (2%) had more than 100 mL of blood loss. Only one patient had a CSF leak. The average length of hospital stay for the total population was 1.7 ± 1 days, with the SA group having a shorter length of stay compared to the CP group (1.5 ± 1 vs. 2.1 ± 2 days) ($p = 0.006$).

Table 1. Population Characteristics.

Covariate	All Patients $n = 166$	Stand Alone $n = 109$	Cervical Plate $n = 57$	p-Value
Demographics				
Age, n (SD)	53 (13)	52 (14)	54 (13)	0.50
Female, n (%)	92 (55)	66 (61)	26 (46)	0.07
Medical Comorbidities				
BMI, mean (SD)	29 (9)	28 (6)	30 (6)	0.05
Diabetes Mellitus, n (%)	24 (14)	15 (14)	9 (16)	0.73
Current Smoker, n (%)	45 (27)	30 (28)	15 (26)	0.87
Former Smoker, n (%)	47 (28)	24 (22)	23 (40)	0.03
Osteoporosis, n (%)	3 (2)	3 (3)	0	0.08
Treatments, n (%)				
Number of Medication, mean (SD)	6 (4)	6 (4)	6 (4)	0.72
1 opioid	50 (30)	32 (29)	18 (32)	0.77
2+ opioids	11 (7)	8 (7)	3 (5)	0.60
1 depression medication	44 (27)	33 (30)	11 (19)	0.11
2+ depression medications	10 (6)	7 (6)	3 (5)	0.76
Pregabalin or Gabapentin	40 (24)	30 (28)	10 (18)	0.17
Chronic NSAID	58 (35)	40 (37)	18 (32)	0.44
Chronic Steroid	13 (8)	10 (9)	3 (5)	0.60
Physical Therapy	98 (59)	67 (61)	31 (54)	0.52
Epidural Steroid Injection	22 (13)	17 (16)	5 (9)	0.25
Clinical presentation, n (%)				
Radiculopathy	92 (55)	66 (61)	26 (46)	0.07
Myelopathy	37 (22)	15 (14)	22 (39)	0.001
Myeloradiculopathy	37 (22)	28 (26)	9 (16)	0.13

NSAID = Non-steroidal anti-inflammatory drugs, SD = Standard deviation, BMI = Body mass index.

Table 2. Surgical Details.

Covariate	All Patients	Stand Alone	Cervical Plate	p-Value
Number of Levels of Surgery				
1	85 (51)	59 (54)	26 (46)	0.30
2	65 (39)	37 (34)	28 (49)	0.63
3	16 (10)	13 (12)	3 (5)	0.13

Table 2. Cont.

Covariate	All Patients	Stand Alone	Cervical Plate	p-Value
Levels of Surgery, n				
C2-C3	25	13	12	0.15
C3-C4	66	42	24	0.66
C4-C5	133	88	45	0.79
C5-C6	133	89	44	0.51
C6-C7	68	48	20	0.26
C7-T1	52	35	17	0.76
Total number of levels	477	315	162	
Length of Surgery, mean (SD)	150 min (64)	126 min (46)	194 min (69)	<0.001
Blood Loss, n (%)				
0–50 mL	132 (80)	85 (78)	47 (82)	0.49
51–100 mL	30 (18)	24 (22)	6 (10)	0.05
>100 mL	4 (2)	0	4 (7)	0.05
CSF leak, n (%)	1 (1)	0	1 (2)	0.32
Length of stay, mean (SD)	1.7 (1)	1.5 (1)	2.1 (2)	0.006
Dysphagia at 3 months, n (%)				
None	79 (96)	52 (98)	27 (93)	0.34
Mild	3 (4)	1 (2)	2 (7)	0.34
Moderate	0	0	0	N/A
Steroid use, n (%)	10 (6)	9 (8)	1 (2)	0.07

3.2. Clinical Outcomes

The mean follow-up for the SA and plate groups was 7.5 months and 10.6 months, respectively, with an overall mean follow-up of 8.6 months. Of the 166 patients, 82 (49%) had a post-surgical follow-up appointment at 3 months to assess for dysphagia. Three patients had mild dysphagia and none of them had moderate or severe dysphagia. However, all of these patients recovered with no further consequences at the last follow-up. As shown in Table 3, the mean Nurick score for the myelopathy and myeloradiculopathy groups improved regardless of the surgical technique or number of index levels. The baseline Nurick score was a score of 1 for 21 patients (28%), a score of 2 for 41 patients (55%), a score of 3 for 8 patients (11%), a score of 4 for 3 patients (4%) and a score of 6 for 1 patient (1%). The Nurick score at last follow up was 0 for 55 patients (74%), 1 for 12 patients (16%), 2 for 5 patients (7%), 3 for 1 patient (1%), and 6 for 1 patient (1%). Overall, 63 patients improved their Nurick score (defined as an optimal outcome) while 11 patients showed no change or decline in their Nurick score (defined as a suboptimal outcome).

Multivariable analysis (Table 4) revealed that length of stay is a statistically significant independent predictor of suboptimal outcome. Prolonged length of stay was associated with reduced odds of having an optimal outcome by 0.50 (95% CI = 0.35–0.85, $p = 0.003$). Moreover, the SA technique was not found to be an independent predictor of better outcomes.

Table 3. Surgery Outcomes for Myelopathy and Myeloradiculopathy Cohorts.

Patient Group	All Patients (n = 74)		Stand Alone (n = 43)		Cervical Plate (n = 31)	
Nurick Score	Baseline	Last Follow-Up	Baseline	Last Follow-Up	Baseline	Last Follow-Up
0	0	55 (74)	0	36 (84)	0	19 (61)
1	21 (28)	12 (16)	11 (26)	3 (7)	10 (32)	9 (29)
2	41 (55)	5 (7)	25 (58)	4 (9)	16 (52)	1 (3)
3	8 (11)	1 (1)	6 (14)	0	2 (7)	1 (3)
4	3 (4)	0	1 (2)	0	2 (7)	0
5	0	0	0	0	0	0
6	1 (1)	1 (1)	0	0	1 (3)	1 (3)

Table 4. Multivariable Analysis.

Covariates	OR (95% CI)	p-Value
Patient Characteristics		
Age	0.99 (0.97–1.04)	0.79
Sex (Female)	1.21 (0.27–2.30)	0.71
Diabetes	0.44 (0.12–1.23)	0.14
Surgery Characteristics		
Stand-Alone Zero Profile	0.67 (0.14–1.61)	0.49
Length of Stay	0.5 (0.35–0.85)	0.003
Number of levels of Surgery		
1 level	1	NA
2 levels	1.99 (0.15–1.70)	0.22
3 levels	3.56 (0.77–21)	0.25

OR = Odds Ratio, CI = Confidence Interval.

4. Discussion

ACDF is a well-established surgical treatment for anterior degenerative cervical pathology. ACDF is often done with the use of an anterior vertebral body plate, with the goal of maintaining stability, promoting fusion, preventing graft extrusion, preventing graft subsidence, and maintaining desired cervical lordosis. Potential instability in both degenerative and traumatic cases is a common reason for the addition of additional structural support via plate fixation. However, a known morbidity of ACDF with cervical plating is post-operative dysphagia, ranging from 2 to 67% in the post-operative period [15]. With the goal of reducing dysphagia and other perioperative morbidities, stand-alone (SA) ACDF systems were developed. Additional potential benefits of SA devices include that they can provide lordotic correction and are anchored with screw fixation. The latter aspect may be relevant in patients with segmental degenerative instability.

Despite the introduction of stand-alone cages as an alternative to cervical plating, clinical outcomes appear to be similar between the two groups. A systematic review by Cheung et al. of 19 studies comparing ACDF with a cage-only technique and conventional cage-plate technique found that stand-alone cage was associated with less dysphagia, intraoperative blood loss, and adjacent segment disease. However, the stand-alone cage was also shown to have increased rates of subsidence and less restoration of cervical lordosis [5]. Similarly, a recent meta-analysis by Gabr et al. demonstrated that stand-alone anchored spacers were associated with less dysphagia compared to the plate-screw construct [16]. Lastly, a systematic review by Boer et al. showed that there was no difference in clinical (visual analog scale, neck disability index) or radiological (cervical lordosis and fusion) outcomes between the two groups, but stand-alone devices were associated with shorter operative time [17].

The pathogenesis of dysphagia in ACDF has not been clearly elucidated. Previous studies have implicated that injury to the esophagus, soft tissue edema, localized bleeding, and adhesions surrounding the CP may contribute to post-operative dysphagia [15]. Indeed, removal of the anterior plate and lysis of associated adhesions has been shown to clinically improve patients' experience of dysphagia both immediately after surgery and at later timepoints [18]. A study by Lee et al. also noted a correlation between the thickness of the cervical plate and post-operative dysphagia, suggesting that physical obstruction may also play a role [19].

In addition to demonstrating no statistically significant difference in morbidity of SA and CP with respect to post-operative dysphagia, our study also found no significant difference in intraoperative blood loss. This data differs slightly from the results described in Cheung et al., which suggest that a cage-only technique is associated with less intraoperative bleeding. However, it is important to note that the average blood loss of ACDF is quite low, so the difference that was noted between SA and CP is not likely to be clinically significant [5]. We also found a significant reduction in operative time with cage-only implants, as well as a decrease in hospital length of stay. Consistent with other studies comparing SA to CP, our data support that either intervention confers optimal outcomes in patients with degenerative cervical myelopathy or radiculopathy. Based on Nurick scores postoperatively, 85% of patients treated in our study had improvement in neurological symptoms, social independence, walking ability, and ability to work full time, with no significant difference in outcomes between SA and CP.

Given our findings with respect to morbidity, there is no clear advantage of stand-alone cage over cervical plating. The stand-alone cage was not found to be a predictor of superior outcomes. Based on these results, it will be important in future studies to investigate the cost-effectiveness of CP vs. SA in anterior cervical discectomy and fusion; in the setting of similar surgical outcomes, as was reported in our study, the more affordable option should be pursued.

An important point to note is that while anterior approaches are indicated in patients with kyphosis, it is unclear how the choice of these 2 techniques affects surgical decision-making. Some may prefer stand-alone cages in such instances given that they can provide different degrees of lordosis. On the other hand, if the implicated disc is present adjacent to a kyphotic segment, increasing lordosis at that level may increase segmental kyphosis at the adjacent level. Further research is warranted with regards to whether these 2 techniques carry different risks and benefits with regards to patients with cervical kyphosis or malalignment.

5. Limitations

There are important limitations with our study. First, patients were not randomized to treatment modality. The two surgeons in this study had different preferences in using SA vs. CP, such that one surgeon used only SA while the other used only CP in their practice. Thus, outcomes and operative time may be biased by surgeon experience, number of years in practice, and technique. However, this also eliminates selection bias, as patients were not selected to receive SA versus CP based on any preoperative parameters or surgeon preference, as each surgeon exclusively performs ACDF with SA or CP. Second, this study does not include a power analysis to determine if the sample size in adequate. Nonetheless, it is important to note that this cohort represents one of the largest studies that examines surgical outcomes between SA and CP, and is one of few in North America. Third, our study warrants a cost analysis between the two approaches to further identify which is more favorable if no change in morbidity is observed. Moreover, if dysphagia avoidance is not an indication for SA grafts, other variables such as the relationship of operative time and blood loss, or graft extrusion, pseudoarthrosis, subsidence, and sagittal alignment should be further assessed between SA and CP techniques to further understand the advantages of the SA technique. Fourth, the Bazaz criteria were used in this study rather than other metrics, such as the EAT assessment, which have been validated as an outcome tool for dysphagia. Lastly, because this study is a retrospective analysis, we were unable to assess the presence of dysphagia in every patient included in this study, due to inconsistent reporting in the absence of symptoms.

6. Conclusions

Patients undergoing ACDF with SA had significantly decreased hospital length of stay and operative time compared to patients with CP. The type of procedure did not affect neurological outcome based on Nurick grade. Hospital length of stay was found to be a predictor of a poor outcome regardless of technique. In general, both ACDF with CP and SA are effective treatment options and provide comparable outcomes.

Author Contributions: Conceptualization, S.S., J.C.-Q. and A.N.; methodology, S.S., J.C.-Q. and A.N.; software, S.S., J.C.-Q. and A.N.; validation, S.S., J.C.-Q. and A.N.; formal analysis, S.S., J.C.-Q. and A.N.; investigation, S.S., J.C.-Q. and A.N.; resources, S.S., J.C.-Q. and A.N.; data curation, S.S., J.C.-Q. and A.N.; writing—original draft preparation, S.S., J.C.-Q., A.N., and K.P.; writing—review and editing, all authors; visualization, S.S., J.C.-Q. and A.N.; supervision, J.C.; project administration, J.C. All authors have read and agreed to the published version of the manuscript.

Funding: This research received no external funding.

Institutional Review Board Statement: The study was conducted according to the guidelines of the Declaration of Helsinki, and approved by the Institutional Review Board (or Ethics Committee) of Yale University (protocol code 200020713).

Informed Consent Statement: The study was exempt from informed consent.

Data Availability Statement: Data available on request (not publicly available for privacy protection).

Acknowledgments: We would like to acknowledge Murat Gunel and Patrick Tomak for their critical review of the manuscript.

Conflicts of Interest: The authors declare no conflict of interest.

References

1. Nouri, A.; Tetreault, L.; Singh, A.; Karadimas, S.K.; Fehlings, M. Degenerative Cervical Myelopathy. *Spine* **2015**, *40*, E675–E693. [CrossRef] [PubMed]
2. Nouri, A.; Martin, A.R.; Nater, A.; Witiw, C.D.; Kato, S.; Tetreault, L.; Reihani-Kermani, H.; Santaguida, C.; Fehlings, M.G. Influence of Magnetic Resonance Imaging Features on Surgical Decision-Making in Degenerative Cervical Myelopathy: Results from a Global Survey of AOSpine International Members. *World Neurosurg.* **2017**, *105*, 864–874. [CrossRef] [PubMed]
3. Angevine, P.D.; Arons, R.R.; McCormick, P.C. National and Regional Rates and Variation of Cervical Discectomy with and Without Anterior Fusion, 1990–1999. *Spine* **2003**, *28*, 931–939. [CrossRef] [PubMed]
4. Korinth, M.C. Treatment of Cervical Degenerative Disc Disease–Current Status and Trends. *Cent. Eur. Neurosurg. Zent. Neurochir.* **2008**, *69*, 113–124. [CrossRef] [PubMed]
5. Cheung, Z.B.; Gidumal, S.; White, S.; Shin, J.; Phan, K.; Osman, N.; Bronheim, R.; Vargas, L.; Kim, J.; Cho, S.K. Comparison of Anterior Cervical Discectomy and Fusion with a Stand-Alone Interbody Cage Versus a Conventional Cage-Plate Technique: A Systematic Review and Meta-Analysis. *Glob. Spine J.* **2018**, *9*, 446–455. [CrossRef] [PubMed]
6. Barbagallo, G.M.V.; Romano, D.; Certo, F.; Milone, P.; Albanese, V. Zero-P: A new zero-profile cage-plate device for single and multilevel ACDF. A single Institution series with four years maximum follow-up and review of the literature on zero-profile devices. *Eur. Spine J.* **2013**, *22*, 868–878. [CrossRef] [PubMed]
7. Matz, P.G.; Pritchard, P.R.; Hadley, M.N. Anterior cervical approach for the treatment of cervical myelopathy. *Neurosurgery* **2007**, *60*, S1–S64. [CrossRef] [PubMed]
8. Bible, J.E.; Kang, J.D. Anterior cervical discectomy and fusion: Surgical indications and outcomes. *Semin. Spine Surg.* **2016**, *28*, 80–83. [CrossRef]
9. Chen, Y.; Chen, H.; Wu, X.; Wang, X.; Lin, W.; Yuan, W. Comparative analysis of clinical outcomes between zero-profile implant and cages with plate fixation in treating multilevel cervical spondilotic myelopathy: A three-year follow-up. *Clin. Neurol. Neurosurg.* **2016**, *144*, 72–76. [CrossRef] [PubMed]
10. Song, K.-J.; Taghavi, C.E.; Lee, K.-B.; Song, J.-H.; Eun, J.-P. The Efficacy of Plate Construct Augmentation Versus Cage Alone in Anterior Cervical Fusion. *Spine* **2009**, *34*, 2886–2892. [CrossRef] [PubMed]

11. Yun, D.-J.; Lee, S.-J.; Park, S.-J.; Oh, H.S.; Lee, Y.J.; Oh, H.M. Use of a Zero-Profile Device for Contiguous 2-Level Anterior Cervical Diskectomy and Fusion: Comparison with Cage with Plate Construct. *World Neurosurg.* **2017**, *97*, 189–198. [CrossRef] [PubMed]
12. Shi, S.; Liu, Z.-D.; Li, X.-F.; Qian, L.; Zhong, G.-B.; Chen, F.-J. Comparison of plate-cage construct and stand-alone anchored spacer in the surgical treatment of three-level cervical spondylotic myelopathy: A preliminary clinical study. *Spine J.* **2015**, *15*, 1973–1980. [CrossRef] [PubMed]
13. Vaněk, P.; Bradáč, O.; DeLacy, P.; Lacman, J.; Beneš, V. Anterior Interbody Fusion of the Cervical Spine with Zero-P Spacer. *Spine* **2013**, *38*, E792–E797. [CrossRef] [PubMed]
14. Bazaz, R.; Lee, M.J.; Yoo, J.U. Incidence of Dysphagia after Anterior Cervical Spine Surgery. *Spine* **2002**, *27*, 2453–2458. [CrossRef] [PubMed]
15. Fountas, K.N.; Kapsalaki, E.Z.; Nikolakakos, L.G.; Smisson, H.F.; Johnston, K.W.; Grigorian, A.A.; Lee, G.P.; Robinson, J.S. Anterior Cervical Discectomy and Fusion Associated Complications. *Spine* **2007**, *32*, 2310–2317. [CrossRef] [PubMed]
16. Gabr, M.A.; Touko, E.; Yadav, A.P.; Karikari, I.; Goodwin, C.R.; Groff, M.W.; Ramirez, L.; Abd-El-Barr, M.M. Improved Dysphagia Outcomes in Anchored Spacers Versus Plate-Screw Systems in Anterior Cervical Discectomy and Fusion: A Systematic Review. *Glob. Spine J.* **2020**, *10*, 1057–1065. [CrossRef] [PubMed]
17. Boer, L.F.R.; Zorzetto, E.; Yeh, F.; Wajchenberg, M.; Martins, D.E. Degenerative Cervical Disorder—Stand-alone Cage Versus Cage and Cervical Plate: A Systematic Review. *Glob. Spine J.* **2021**, *11*, 249–255. [CrossRef] [PubMed]
18. Fogel, G.R.; McDonnell, M.F. Surgical treatment of dysphagia after anterior cervical interbody fusion. *Spine J.* **2005**, *5*, 140–144. [CrossRef] [PubMed]
19. Lee, C.-H.; Hyun, S.-J.; Kim, M.J.; Yeom, J.S.; Kim, W.H.; Kim, K.-J.; Jahng, T.-A.; Kim, H.-J.; Yoon, S.H. Comparative Analysis of 3 Different Construct Systems for Single-level Anterior Cervical Discectomy and Fusion. *J. Spinal Disord. Tech.* **2013**, *26*, 112–118. [CrossRef] [PubMed]

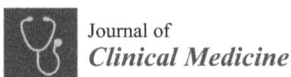

Article

The Long-Term Effect of Treatment Using the Transcranial Magnetic Stimulation rTMS in Patients after Incomplete Cervical or Thoracic Spinal Cord Injury

Agnieszka Wincek [1], Juliusz Huber [1,*], Katarzyna Leszczyńska [1], Wojciech Fortuna [2,3], Stefan Okurowski [4], Krzysztof Chmielak [2] and Paweł Tabakow [2]

1. Department of Pathophysiology of Locomotor Organs, Poznan University of Medical Sciences, 28 Czerwca 1956 nr 135/147, 60-545 Poznań, Poland; awincek@ump.edu.pl (A.W.); kat.leszczynska@gmail.com (K.L.)
2. Department of Neurosurgery, Wroclaw Medical University, Borowska 213, 50-556 Wrocław, Poland; wfortuna@onet.pl (W.F.); kchmielak@wp.pl (K.C.); p.tabakov@wp.pl (P.T.)
3. Bacteriophage Laboratory, Ludwik Hirszfeld Institute of Immunology and Experimental Therapy, Polish Academy of Sciences, Rudolfa Weigla 12, 53-114 Wrocław, Poland
4. Neurorehabilitation Center for Treatment of Spinal Cord Injuries AKSON, ul. Bierutowska 23, 51-317 Wroclaw, Poland; sokurowski@wp.pl
* Correspondence: juliusz.huber@ump.edu.pl; Tel.: +48-50-404-1843

Abstract: Repetitive transcranial magnetic stimulation (rTMS) may support motor function recovery in patients with incomplete spinal cord injury (iSCI). Its effectiveness mainly depends on the applied algorithm. This clinical and neurophysiological study aimed to assess the effectiveness of high-frequency rTMS in iSCI patients at the C2–Th12 levels. rTMS sessions (lasting 3–5 per month, from 2 to 11 months, 5 months on average) were applied to 26 iSCI subjects. The motor cortex was bilaterally stimulated with a frequency at 20–25 Hz and a stimulus strength that was 70–80% of the resting motor threshold (15.4–45.5% maximal output) during one therapeutic session. Surface electromyography (sEMG) recordings at rest and during maximal contractions and motor evoked potential (MEP) recordings were performed from the abductor pollicis brevis (APB) and the tibialis anterior (TA) muscles. The same neurophysiological studies were also performed in patients treated with kinesiotherapy only (K group, $n = 25$) and compared with patients treated with both kinesiotherapy and rTMS (K + rTMS). A decrease in sEMG amplitudes recorded at rest from the APB muscles ($p = 0.001$) and an increase in sEMG amplitudes during the maximal contraction of the APB ($p = 0.001$) and TA ($p = 0.009$) muscles were found in the K + rTMS group. A comparison of data from MEP studies recorded from both APB and TA muscles showed significant changes in the mean amplitudes but not in latencies, suggesting a slight improvement in the transmission of spinal efferent pathways from the motor cortex to the lower spinal centers. The application of rTMS at 20–25 Hz reduced spasticity in the upper extremity muscles, improved the recruitment of motor units in the upper and lower extremity muscles, and slightly improved the transmission of efferent neural impulses within the spinal pathways in patients with C2–Th12 iSCI. Neurophysiological recordings produced significantly better parameters in the K + rTMS group of patients after therapy. These results may support the hypothesis about the importance of rTMS therapy and possible involvement of the residual efferent pathways including propriospinal neurons in the recovery of the motor control of iSCI patients.

Keywords: incomplete spinal cord injury; repetitive transcranial magnetic stimulation; cervical and thoracic spinal cord injury; rehabilitation

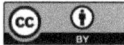

1. Introduction

An increasing number of studies provide evidence that transcranial magnetic stimulation (rTMS), together with the other classical rehabilitation methods, such as physical therapy and kinesiotherapy, may bring benefits for the recovery of sensory and motor function in patients with an incomplete spinal cord injury (iSCI) [1]. rTMS is known to evoke the long-term potentiation or depression of neuronal circuits' activity (on the supraspinal and/or spinal levels) depending on the accepted protocol, including the widely applied stimuli algorithm [2–7]. Low-frequency rTMS (less than 20 Hz) decreases cortical excitability, whereas a higher frequency (more than 30 Hz) increases activity in the corticospinal pathway axons and reduces corticospinal inhibition. Therefore, paresis and spasticity, two main clinical symptoms in patients with an iSCI, should change following rTMS therapy [8]. Both the mechanism and structures within the central nervous system responsible for positive treatment results remain unknown. Many of the studies on the treatment of iSCI patients describe this phenomenon as "functional recovery" [9–11].

Our previous study on the short-term results from rTMS in patients with a C4–Th2 iSCI provided evidence of its positive effects; however, it was conducted on a limited number of participants [10]. Thus, it is crucial to ascertain the long-lasting impacts, e.g., on thoracic spinal levels, of rTMS therapy in a larger population of iSCI patients. It is also necessary to understand how rTMS therapy can be optimized in clinical practice. One of the most promising features of rTMS is the cumulative effect of several therapeutic sessions, which according to the previous descriptions appeared differently from 2 weeks to 5 months [5,7,10]. Therefore, this study aims to investigate the long-term effects of rTMS application.

Results of experimental and clinical studies indicate a group of long axonal projections of spinal neurons from cervical to lumbosacral centers, which are called propriospinal neurons (PNs). They are responsible, among other residual efferent pathways, for the coordination of locomotor mechanisms in the spinal cord and are engaged in the recovery of motor and sensory deficits in iSCI patients [1,9,12]. They are known to have primarily crossed, rather than uncrossed, projections of long descending axons in the spinal funiculi at low thoracic and upper lumbar spinal cord neuromeres, interconnecting cervical and lumbosacral centers [13]. If studies in patients with both cervical and thoracic iSCI reveal a greater improvement in motor function following rTMS and kinesiotherapy than those previously studied in patients with a C4–Th2 iSCI, the involvement of the PN system will be indicated for the recovery in spinal interconnections. Moreover, the results of the study may contribute to wider rTMS clinical applications in the treatment of iSCI patients, which was highlighted in previous studies [2–8].

In this study, we investigated the long-term effect of the rTMS protocol at frequencies ranging from 20 to 25 Hz and a stimulus strength that was 70–80% of the resting motor threshold in patients with C2–Th12 iSCI. The rTMS efficacy was evaluated by surface electromyography (sEMG) and motor-evoked potential (MEP) recordings. We have also compared neurophysiological data in iSCI patients treated only with kinesiotherapy and those treated with kinesiotherapy and rTMS to prove the effect of repetitive magnetic stimulation included in the current standard of care. We hypothesized that such excitation of motor cortex centers may decrease spasticity and improve motor function in iSCI patients.

2. Materials and Methods

The study was performed in accordance with the Declaration of Helsinki and was approved by the Bioethics Committee from the University of Medical Sciences (including studies on healthy subjects; decision no. 559/2018). Before the clinical and neurophysiological studies, 55 participants and 50 healthy volunteers declared their stable psychological and social status and signed written informed consent prior to further participation in the study.

2.1. Participants

The preliminary sample included 70 patients with iSCI at the cervical and thoracic levels (Figure 1) that was treated surgically for spine stabilization. Fifteen were excluded because they did not meet the inclusion criteria ($n = 8$), declined to participate in the project (*n* = 6), or had died (*n* = 1). Finally, 55 patients participated in the study from February 2018 to February 2020; 26 of them with injuries at the C2–Th12 levels (C2–C7 = 15, Th1–Th12 = 11) received the kinesiotherapeutic and rTMS treatment described in Sections 2.2.1 and 2.2.2 (K + rTMS group). The timeline between the allocation and follow-up ranged from 2 to 4 months. Eighteen men (aged between 25 and 45 years) and eight women (aged between 37 and 41 years) with similar weights and heights (59 kg and 165 cm on average, respectively) were included in this group. Another sample of 25 patients with an iSCI at cervical and thoracic levels C3–Th12 (C2–C7 = 14, Th1–Th12 = 11) was treated with kinesiotherapy only (K group, therapy described in Section 2.2.1), and was included in the study to compare the results of the applied therapies. The timelines between allocation and follow-up ranged from 1 to 4 months in the K group. This group included fourteen men (aged between 23 and 46 years) and eleven women (aged between 36 and 43 years) with similar weights and heights (62 kg and 175.3 cm on average, respectively).

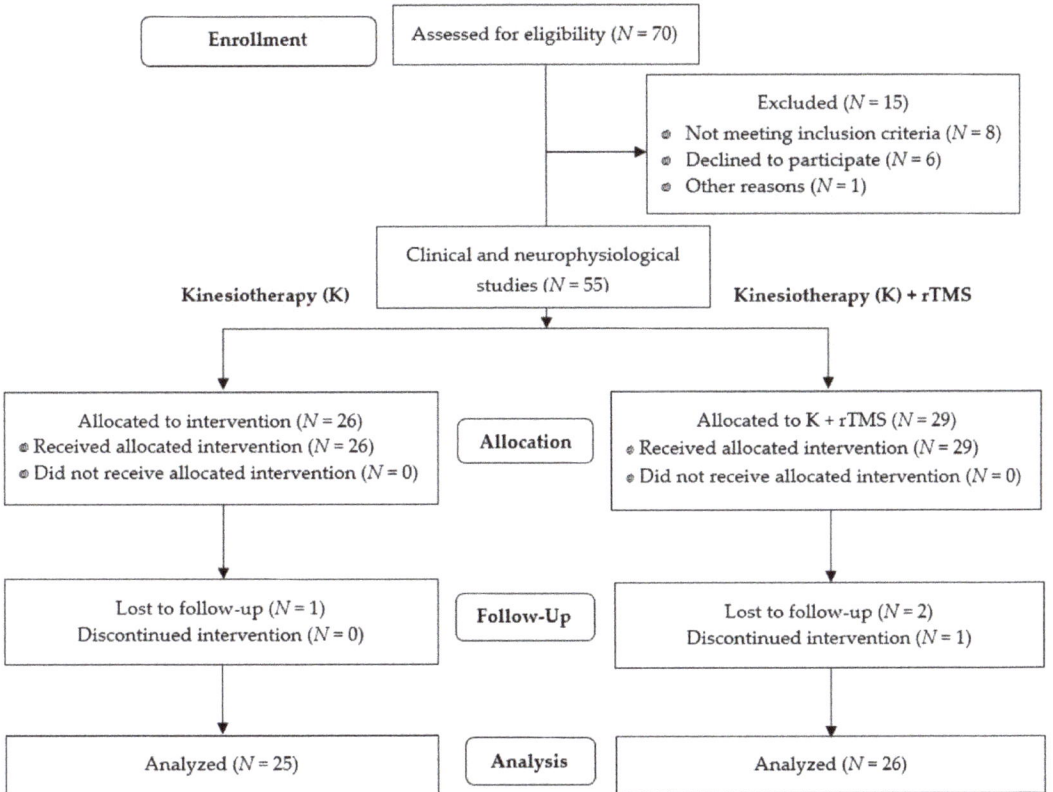

Figure 1. Flow chart of the study.

Clinical studies were conducted according to the American Spinal Injury Association (ASIA) impairment scale and the tests revealed AIS C in 20 patients and D in 6 patients in the K + rTMS group and AIS C in 19 patients and D in 6 patients in the K group. Data in Table 1 summarizes the characteristics of the patients. Patients were mainly victims of car, industrial, or sports accidents. The main inclusion criteria for both groups of patients were the preservation of one-third to one-quarter of the spinal structures within fibers and neurons in the white and gray matter based on the results of MRI studies, as well as from the results of direct MEP recordings performed before treatment that confirmed the range of the iSCI. The other inclusion criteria were: first observation not less than a year since the spinal injury, agreement to participate in the project for not less than three months, no head injuries, no epilepsy episodes, no cardiovascular diseases, no psychical disorders, no pregnancy, no oncological episodes, no pacemaker or cochlear implants, no strokes nor plexopathies episodes during treatment, no inflammatory diseases nor myelopathies before the incident, written informed consent for participation in the rTMS procedures (understanding the risk), subsequent neurophysiological examinations on demand, and a stable psychological and social status. The patients who could not be treated with rTMS because of the exclusion criteria mentioned hereinabove were included in the K group.

Table 1. Characteristics of the subjects studied in two groups before treatment.

	K Group		K + rTMS Group	
	Mean ± SD	Min–Max	Mean ± SD	Min–Max
Age	36.7 ± 5.3	23–46	37.3 ± 4.7	25–45
Height (cm)	175.3 ± 4.3	165–181	165.0 ± 4.3	158–172
Weight (kg)	62.0 ± 6.1	51–79	59.0 ± 5.5	51–83
	n		n	
AIS scale	C = 19		C = 20	
	D = 6		D = 6	
Spinal injury	C2–C7 = 14		C2–C7 = 15	
level	Th1–Th12 = 11		Th2–Th12 = 11	

K group—iSCI patients treated with kinesiotherapy, K + rTMS—iSCI patients treated with kinesiotherapy and repetitive transcranial magnetic stimulation.

The group of healthy volunteers (n = 50, 26 men and 24 women) was examined to obtain the reference values of neurophysiological recordings. The mean age of the healthy group was 38.2 ± 4.3 years (range from 26 to 45) and their heights were 155–178 cm with a mean of 168.3 ± 3.7 cm. The subjects of both patients and healthy volunteer sets did not differ significantly in age or height (p = 0.7). A general practitioner, neurologist, and neurosurgeon evaluated their health statuses.

2.2. Procedures and Intervention

2.2.1. Kinesiotherapy

Kinesiotherapy is a part of physiotherapy; it includes the application of exercises that are supervised by a physiotherapist and are focused on improving motor and sensory function. The algorithm in this study included the same intensive programs applied in all 55 patients between the rTMS sessions, which were the only physicotherapeutic interventions. A physiotherapist carried out the programs following consultations with a neurosurgeon and neurologist in the Akson Neurorehabilitation Center in Wrocław, Poland. Sets of training were included in the rehabilitation program, as shown in Figure 2; the rehabilitation program did not differ between both study groups. One rehabilitation set lasted three months; the break between sets was longer than one month. A physiotherapist supervised patient treatment 4–5 h per day, five days a week. One session of daily training consisted of a range of motion and stretching exercises with loadings for 1 h (the magnitude of loading exercises depended on the spasticity or hypertonia level, and the minimal loading was 100 g), and was adjusted individually for certain groups of partially paralyzed muscles showing activation improvement. Depending on the spasticity or hypotonia, verticalization training was performed. The use of a verticalization bed was denied when minor neurological symptoms, such as tingling or a decrease in muscle strength or function of the autonomic nervous system, were detected. Locomotor training for 3 h on a runway with handrails with support first and later without physiotherapist assistance, as well as sensory training of posture and balance for 1 h on a specially designed vibration platform, were performed. Walking exercises were administered when the Walking Index scores increased [14]. The number of repetitions in one trial (exercise) ranged from 6 to 15, depending on the patient's condition, five days per week.

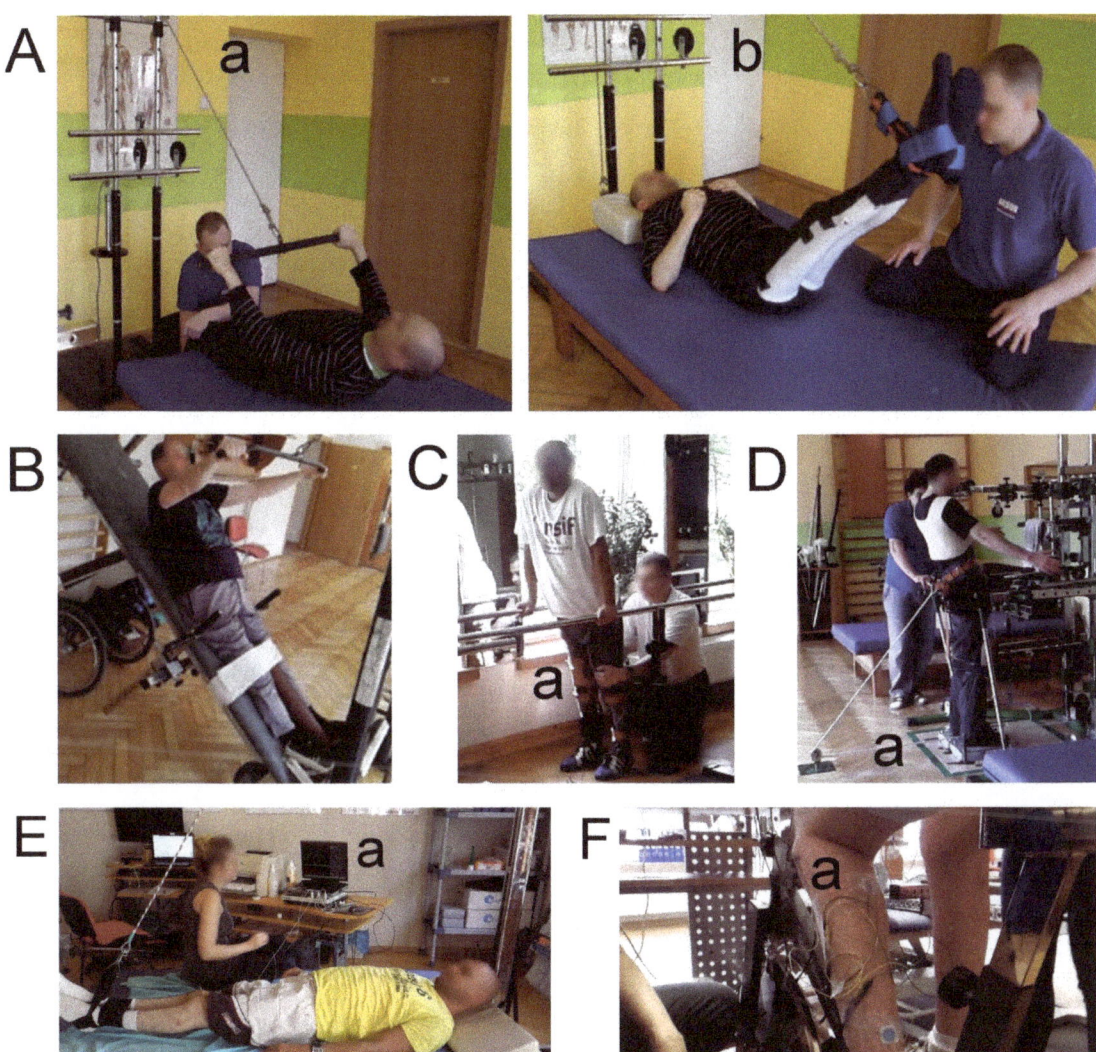

Figure 2. Photographs illustrating the principles of physiotherapeutic treatment and neurophysiological tests applied to the K group in this study: (**A**) a range of motion (**a**) and stretching exercises (**b**), (**B**) verticalization training, (**C**) training of locomotion on a runway with handrails with a support (**a**), (**D**) posture and balance exercises on a vibration platform (**a**), (**E**) bilateral recordings of surface electromyography (sEMG) from upper and lower extremity muscles with the visual feedback of a subject who observed the monitor with recordings (**a**), and (**F**) sEMG recordings with surface electrodes (**a**) during exercise on a stationary bicycle.

2.2.2. Repetitive Transcranial Magnetic Stimulation (rTMS)

Patients received rTMS therapy in the Department of Pathophysiology of the Locomotor Organs of the Poznan University of Medical Sciences, Poland, and the Neurorehabilitation Center for Treatment of Spinal Cord Injuries AKSON in Wroclaw, Poland. Both facilities applied the same rTMS algorithm. A maximum of 15 sessions of rTMS was applied within five months on average (±1 month). The MagPro R30 and MagPro X100 magnetic stimulator with MagOption Medtronic (Medtronic A/S, Skovlunde, Denmark) were used for the rTMS therapy and for performing the motor evoked potentials (MEPs) diagnostic studies (Figure 3). Treatment was induced with a circular coil (C-100, 12 cm in diameter) that was placed over the scalp in the area of the M1 motor cortex, targeted with an angle for the corona radiata excitation, where the fibers of the corticospinal tract for the upper and lower extremities originated (Figure 3B(b)). A train of stimuli with a maximum limit of 2–4 tesla (T) on the surface of a patient's head was induced from the magnetic field generator (Figure 3B(a)). The magnetic field stream delivered from the coil had a strength that was 70–80% of the resting motor threshold (RMT; 0.84–0.96 T); this field excited all neural structures up to 3–5 cm deep. It is possible that the cells of origin of the rubrospinal tract in the midbrain were also excited [1,10]. The RMT test performed as a single stimulus that was 50% of the maximal stimulus output (MSO) was used before and at the end of each course. Afterward, the individual RMT, as the minimum magnetic stimulus intensity required to elicit an MEP > 50 µV peak-to-peak amplitude above the background electromyographic activity in the relaxed key muscles, was determined. sEMG was performed on the abductor pollicis brevis (APB) and tibialis anterior (TA) muscles (Figure 3A). A single stimulus with a lower intensity (usually 38–40% of the MSO) was used before the rTMS therapeutic sessions. It evoked minimal muscle twitch for both the APB and TA. The maximal stimulus intensity that was used for diagnostic purposes was not more than 70–80% of the RMT. Diagnostic stimulations had the same locations bilaterally over the scalp as they did during the therapies. The stimuli had individually designed algorithms based on repetitive sets of neurophysiological tests and the patient's current clinical state at a subsequent stage of observation. Although the main schedule was kept the same for all patients, the frequency of the applied stimuli was adjusted higher (from 15 up to 25 Hz), depending on the severity of the spinal injury (worse MEP results) and neurogenic dysfunction detected in muscles (low-frequency and low-amplitude sEMG recordings). For example, when the amplitudes of the MEP and sEMG (during the attempt of maximal contraction) recordings were about 100 µV and the frequency index was 1, the algorithm required the application of higher frequency rTMS trains up to 25 Hz. If results were observed to be better (an increase in the amplitude and the frequency index was recorded), the frequency of rTMS was decreased toward 15 Hz. One session of therapy consisted of 3–5 rTMS sessions in a month, and one session per day was conducted; the motor cortex's bilateral stimulation was performed for about 10 min with 10 min intervals. Patients whose values in the MEP and sEMG recordings improved in the second observation, and did not report the symptoms of muscle fatigue or general tiredness, received a greater number of rTMS sessions. In general, patients received 1600 biphasic pulses, 800 pulses for each hemisphere during each session. The parameters were as follows: 15–25 Hz—frequency of the applied stimuli, 2 s trains of 40 pulses, 28 s—the interval between trains of stimuli, and a strength of about 70–80% of the RMT. The whole observation period of rTMS application was from 2 to 11 months, 5 months on average. None of the patients reported the rTMS as being painful, though they felt a slight spread of current to the upper and lower extremities; they were always awake and cooperating. None of the patients received antispastic drugs when the rTMS therapy was applied. The neurologist advised not to take antispastic drugs after the statement of participation was signed up at the beginning of the project.

2.3. Neurophysiological Studies

Patients were examined using neurophysiological methods in the Department of Pathophysiology of the Locomotor Organs of the Poznan University of Medical Sciences, Poland, except for the set of clinical studies included in the ASIA scale evaluation. Studies of efferent spinal transmission and muscle motor unit activity were performed in three periods of observations, before and after each rTMS session in K + rTMS group and separately in the K group of patients. The KeyPoint Diagnostic System (Medtronic A/S, Skovlunde, Denmark) was used for MEP and sEMG recordings in the iSCI patients and healthy volunteers ($n = 50$, control group) to obtain the reference values of neurophysiological recordings for comparison (Table 2).

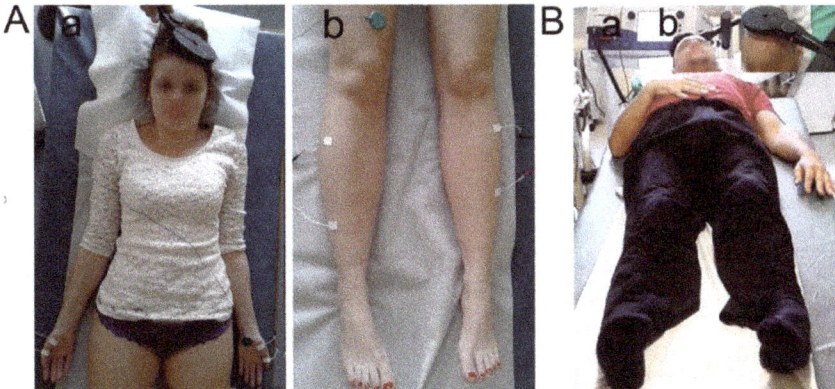

Figure 3. Photographs illustrating the principles of (**A**) electromyography (EMG) recorded from the upper (**a**) and lower (**b**) extremities and motor evoked potentials (MEPs) recordings and (**B**) repetitive transcranial magnetic stimulation (rTMS) treatment with a MagPro device ((**a**)—magnetic field generator; (**b**)—coil over the scalp) performed on the K + rTMS patients.

Table 2. Reference values of surface electromyography (sEMG) parameters that were recorded at rest and during an attempt of maximal contraction, and MEP parameters that were recorded following transcranial magnetic stimulation in a group of healthy volunteers (n = 50). Ranges and mean or median values are presented.

Recording	Measured Parameter	Healthy Volunteers
sEMG APB	Amplitude at rest (μV)	15–30 25.3 ± 2.6
	Amplitude during maximal contraction (μV)	900–1800 1025 ± 105
	Frequency index	3-3 3.0
sEMG TA	Amplitude at rest (μV)	15–30 25.6 ± 2.2
	Amplitude during maximal contraction (μV)	600–1450 725 ± 110
	Frequency index	3-3 3.0
MEP APB	Amplitude (μV)	1125–3650 1662.5 ± 472.8
	Latency (ms)	18.6–22.7 20.65 ± 2.05
MEP TA	Amplitude (μV)	1200–2975 1656 ± 370.7
	Latency (ms)	25.9–31.75 28.8 ± 1.7

Modified frequency index (3-0)—frequency of motor unit action potentials recruitment during maximal contraction sEMG recording: (3 = 95–70 Hz—normal; 2 = 65–40 Hz—moderate abnormality; 1 = 35–10 Hz—severe abnormality; 0 = no contraction); sEMG—surface electromyography; MEP—motor evoked potential; APB—abductor pollicis brevis muscle; TA—tibialis anterior muscle.

2.3.1. Surface Electromyography Recordings (sEMG)

sEMG activity was recorded from the bilateral abductor pollicis brevis (APB) and tibialis anterior (TA) muscles with surface electrodes that measured the amplitudes and frequencies at rest and during maximal contraction attempts lasting 5 s. Standard disposable Ag/AgCl recording surface electrodes that had an active surface of 5 mm^2 were used.

sEMG recordings were performed with an active electrode placed on the muscle belly, while the referencing electrode was placed on its distal tendon, according to the Guidelines of the European Federation of Clinical Neurophysiology. The ground electrode was located on the distal part of the leg. As is commonly done, the upper 10 kHz and lower 20 Hz filters of the recorder were set. Recordings were made at the time base of 80 ms/D and an amplification of 20–1000 µV. The amplitude of the sEMG recordings below 20–25 µV at rest identified proper muscle tension [15]. The average amplitude parameters (minimum–maximum, i.e., the peak-to-peak of recruiting motor unit action potential deflection with reference to the isoelectric line measured in µV), and motor unit firing frequencies (the number of recruited motor unit action potentials (in Hz)) were analyzed in recording during maximal contraction. The amplitudes below 900 and 600 µV suggested the pathological recruitment of motor unit activity during the maximal contraction of APB and TA muscles, respectively (Figure 4). In the sEMG studies, the neurophysiologist verbally encouraged the patients with iSCI to make three attempts of maximal contraction. Participants were instructed to contract the tested muscle as hard and as fast as possible until the neurophysiologist requested them to finish the attempt. The recruitment of the muscle motor units heard by the patients in the loudspeaker of the recorder motivated the subjects in a biofeedback way. The test was conducted three times, with a 1 min resting period between each set of muscle contractions; the recording with the highest amplitude (in µV) and frequency (in Hz) parameters was selected for analysis. In some patients with worse sEMG results in a supine position due to muscle fatigue, dynamic exercises (tests) on stationary bicycles were applied to increase their motivation during simultaneous sEMG recordings. The frequency index from 3 to 0 (3 = 95–70 Hz—normal; 2 = 65–40 Hz—moderate abnormality; 1 = 35–10 Hz—severe abnormality; 0 = no contraction) was used according to the description elsewhere [11,15,16], with the use of automatic analyzing software included in the KeyPoint System, which were compared to the online readings of sEMG recordings.

2.3.2. Motor Evoked Potentials (MEPs) Recordings

Motor evoked potentials were elicited via a transcranial magnetic single stimulus using the same magnetic coil as for rTMS purposes and recorded with surface electrodes from the APB and TA muscles. The latency and amplitude parameters were analyzed as the primary outcome measures for assessing the primary motor cortex's output and evaluating the efferent transmission of neural impulses to effectors via spinal cord descending tracts. Consecutive tracking attempts were made to find the optimal stimulation location (a hot spot in the area where the rTMS elicited the largest MEP amplitude), distanced 5 mm each other. The amplitudes below 1125 µV and 1200 µV for the MEPs recorded from APB and TA muscles in response to an applied single magnetic pulse indicated pathological transmission in descending spinal cord pathways of the axonal type, respectively. The methodology of MEP recordings was described in detail elsewhere [10,11].

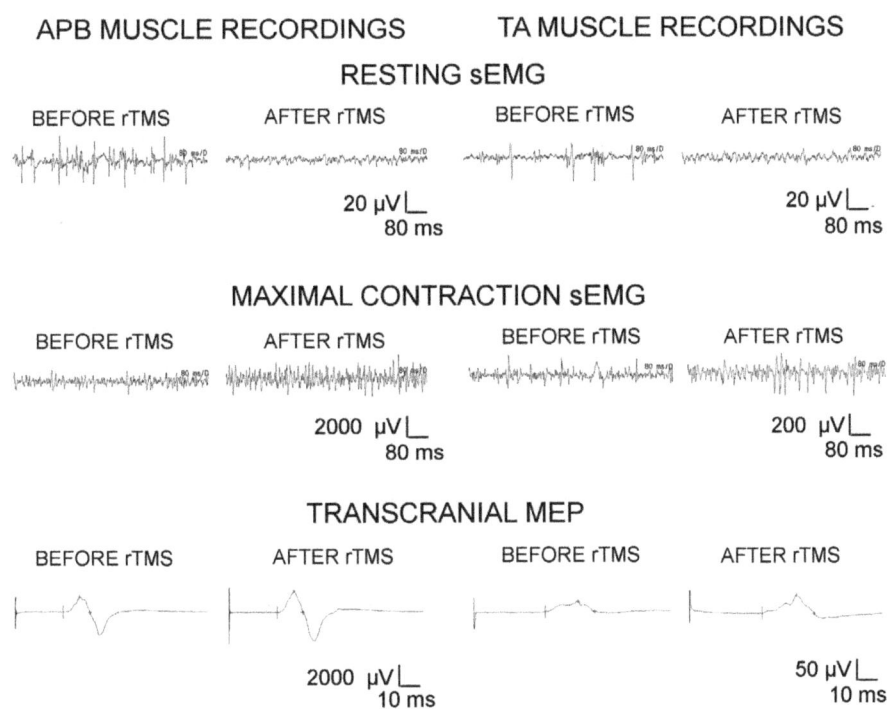

Figure 4. Examples of sEMG and MEP recordings from one iSCI patient before the first rTMS session and after the last therapeutic session. Calibration bars for different amplifications and time bases are presented.

2.4. Data Analysis and Statistics

Data were analyzed with Statistica, version 13.1 (StatSoft, Kraków, Poland). Descriptive statistics were reported as minimal and maximal values (range), with mean or median and standard deviation (SD). The normality distributions were studied with Shapiro–Wilk tests and the homogeneity of variances were studied with Levene's tests. Frequency index data were of the ordinal scale type, while amplitudes and latencies were of the interval scale type. However, they did not represent a normal distribution; therefore, the non-parametric tests had to be used. None of the collected data represented a normal distribution or were of the ordinal scale type (frequency index data); therefore, the Wilcoxon's signed-rank tests were conducted to compare the differences between results obtained before and after treatment, as well as to compare results at the beginning of the treatment using rTMS (first observation—before treatment) and at the end (third observation—after treatment). Any p-values ≤ 0.05 were considered statistically significant. The statistical software was used to determine the required sample size using the primary outcome variable of the sEMG amplitude recorded from the APB and TA muscles at rest before and after treatment with a power of 80% and a significance level of 0.05 (two-tailed). The mean and standard deviation (SD) were calculated using the data from the first seven patients, and the sample size software estimated that more than 21 patients were needed for the purposes of this study.

3. Results

Figure 4 presents examples of the sEMG and MEPs recorded in one patient with iSCI at Th11–Th12. The rTMS therapy evoked a decrease in sEMG amplitudes in both the APB and TA muscles at rest and a greater increase in amplitude than the frequency in the sEMG recordings from the APB muscles than the TA muscles. The above phenomena can be interpreted as a decrease in spasticity and an improvement in muscle motor unit activity in this patient. Similar changes induced by the rTMS were statistically shown to be significant in the entire patient population when comparing results recorded before and after therapy (Table 3).

The comparison of the data from the first and last observations shown in Figure 5A provides evidence for a significant decrease in the mean sEMG amplitude parameter recorded at rest from ABP muscles (at $p = 0.001$) in the whole population of iSCI patients following the applied therapy. However, such a phenomenon of reaching the lower physiological limit of no more than 20 µV was also observed in the sEMG recordings at rest in the TA muscles (Figure 5B).

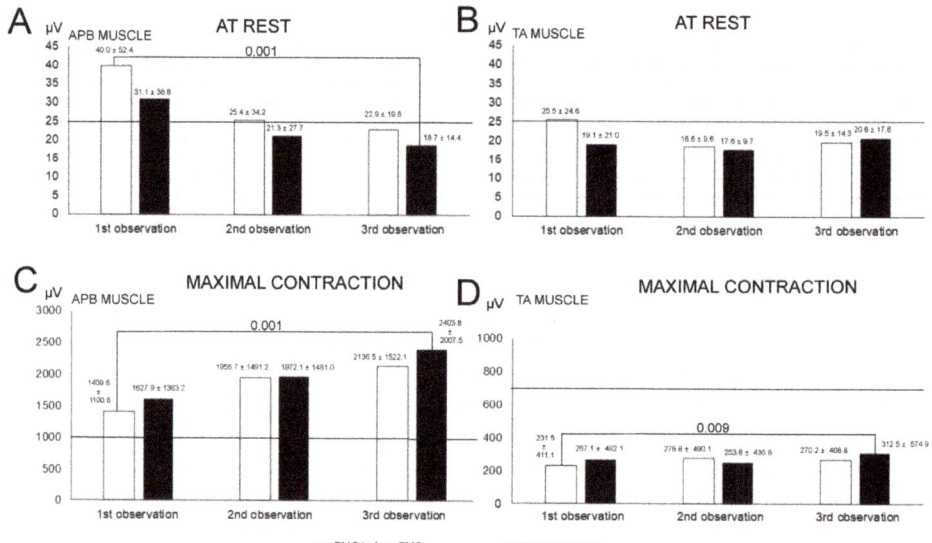

Figure 5. Comparison of mean amplitudes (expressed in µV) of the sEMG performed on the APB (**A,C**) and TA (**B,D**) muscles at rest (**A,B**) and during the attempt of maximal contraction (**C,D**) before and after each therapeutic session. Horizontal lines refer to mean values recorded in healthy subjects (control group).

The studied group of iSCI patients did not present the pathology of APB muscle motor units during maximal contractions before treatment, but the data in Figure 5C that indicates the improvement in their activity after the rTMS therapy, which was significant at $p = 0.001$, is convincing (sEMG amplitude parameter more than 1000 µV). All the iSCI patients showed TA muscle activity below the lower physiological limit (average value of amplitude = 725 µV), and rTMS therapy provided a slight but statistically significant ($p = 0.009$) increase in the sEMG amplitude parameter recorded during a maximal contraction (Figure 5D).

A comparison of the data from MEP studies recorded from both APB and TA muscles presented in Table 3 shows significant changes in the mean amplitudes but not in latencies, suggesting a slight improvement in the transmission of spinal efferent pathways from the motor cortex to the lower spinal centers. However, it should be remembered that abnormalities were not recorded before therapy in the MEP from the upper extremity muscles; those from lower extremity muscles were only residually recorded (Figure 4).

Data in Table 4 indicate the highest percentage of improvement in parameters of the sEMG (both at rest and during maximal contraction) and MEP recordings in the K + rTMS group than in the K group. This refers not only to recordings performed from muscles of the upper but also lower extremities. The neurophysiological parameters recorded in both groups of iSCI patients did not differ significantly before the therapy. However, they were significantly different in the final observation, with p-values ranging from 0.04 to 0.05.

Table 3. Comparison of results from neurophysiological studies in patients ($n = 26$) at certain periods of observation. Ranges, mean or median values, and standard deviations are presented.

Recording	Measured Parameter	1st Observation (Before Treatment)			2nd Observation (After 2–3 Months of Treatment)				3rd Observation (After 5 Months of Treatment)			Difference 1st vs. 3rd
		Before rTMS Sessions	After rTMS Sessions	p	Before rTMS Sessions	After rTMS Sessions	p		Before rTMS Sessions	After rTMS Sessions	p	p
sEMG APB	Amplitude at rest (µV)	5–200 40.0 ± 52.4	5–200 31.1 ± 38.8	0.011 *	5–200 25.4 ± 34.2	5–200 21.3 ± 27.7	0.007 *		10–100 22.9 ± 19.8	10–100 18.7 ± 14.4	0.004 *	<0.001 *
	Amplitude during maximal contraction (µV)	100–4000 1409.6 ± 1100.6	100–7000 1627.9 ± 1363.2	0.002 *	100–6000 1491.2 ± 1491.2	100–7000 1972.1 ± 1481.0	0.334		100–6000 2136.5 ± 1522.1	100–10500 2403.8 ± 2007.5	0.030 *	<0.001 *
	Frequency index	1–3 2.2 ± 0.7	1–3 2.2 ± 0.7	0.779	1–3 2.1 ± 0.7	1–3 2.2 ± 0.7	0.128		1–3 2.5 ± 0.7	0–3 2.5 ± 0.7	0.767	0.003 *
sEMG TA	Amplitude at rest (µV)	5–200 25.5 ± 34.6	5–150 19.1 ± 21.0	0.021 *	10–50 18.6 ± 9.6	10–50 17.6 ± 9.7	0.046 *		10–100 19.5 ± 14.3	10–100 20.6 ± 17.6	0.917	0.331
	Amplitude during maximal contraction (µV)	0–2000 231.5 ± 411.1	0–2200 267.1 ± 492.1	0.064	0–2000 278.8 ± 490.1	0–1700 253.8 ± 436.8	0.069		0–2100 270.2 ± 468.8	0–3000 312.5 ± 574.9	0.05 *	0.009 *
	Frequency index	0–3 0.9 ± 1.0	0–3 0.9 ± 0.9	1.0	0–3 1 ± 1.0	0–3 1 ± 1.0	1.0		0–3 0.9 ± 1.0	0–3 1.0 ± 1.1	0.109	0.320
MEP APB	Amplitude (µV)	50–12500 2052.9 ± 2511.0	0–10000 1960.6 ± 2294.8	1.0	0–10000 2351.9 ± 2599.3	0–12000 2353.8 ± 2911.2	0.602		100–15000 1942.3 ± 2668.9	100–11000 2725.1 ± 2524.1	0.05 *	0.008 *
	Latency (ms)	16.8–43.5 23.4 ± 5.2	0–37.7 22.7 ± 5.4	0.373	0–38.7 22.3 ± 5.4	0–38.7 22.7 ± 5.3	0.172		15.5–33.4 22.3 ± 3.9	14.6–33.0 23.3 ± 4.5	0.655	0.081
MEP TA	Amplitude (µV)	0–1000 76.9 ± 162.8	0–1000 80.5 ± 169.4	0.530	0–2200 128.8 ± 354.7	0–1100 107.9 ± 250.7	0.683		0–800 78.8 ± 157.6	0–1100 162.1 ± 123.6	0.05 *	0.05 *
	Latency (ms)	0–49.3 29.1 ± 18.5	0–48.0 28.7 ± 18.5	0.691	0–45.1 28.5 ± 16.4	0–45.1 28.3 ± 16.6	0.687		0–45.0 28.5 ± 17.6	0–45.0 28.1 ± 15.6	0.052	0.332

* $p < 0.05$; modified frequency index (3–0)—frequency of motor units action potentials recruitment during maximal contraction sEMG recording; (3 = 95–70 Hz—normal; 2 = 65–40 Hz—moderate abnormality; 1 = 35–10 Hz—severe abnormality; 0 = no contraction); rTMS—repetitive transcranial magnetic stimulation; sEMG—surface electromyography; MEP—motor evoked potential; APB—abductor pollicis brevis muscle; TA—tibialis anterior muscle. * Significant p-values are marked bold.

Table 4. Comparison of results from neurophysiological studies in patients from the K group (treated with kinesiotherapy only) and the K + rTMS group (treated with kinesiotherapy and repetitive transcranial magnetic stimulation). Ranges, mean or median values, and standard deviations are presented.

Recording	Measured Parameter	K Group			K + rTMS Group			K vs. K + rTMS Difference before	K vs. K + rTMS Difference after
		Before	After	Change (%)	Before	After	Change (%)	p	p
sEMG APB	Amplitude at rest (µV)	5–150 45.3 ± 22.1	5–200 35.7 ± 24.3	21.1	5–200 40.0 ± 52.4	10–100 18.7 ± 14.4	53.2	0.06	**0.03 ***
	Amplitude during maximal contraction (µV)	100–4500 1443.7 ± 1241.7	100–6500 1445.1 ± 1126.8	0.09	100–4000 1409.6 ± 1100.6	100–10500 2403.8 ± 2007.5	41.3	0.13	**0.03 ***
	Frequency index	1–3 2.0 ± 0.5	1–3 2.0 ± 0.6	0	1–3 2.2 ± 0.7	0–3 2.5 ± 0.7	12.0	0.06	**0.04 ***
sEMG TA	Amplitude at rest (µV)	10–100 22.1.6 ± 6.4	10–50 22.3 ± 7.1	0.89	5–200 25.5 ± 34.6	10–100 20.6 ± 17.6	19.2	0.07	0.06
	Amplitude during maximal contraction (µV)	0–1900 245.8 ± 381.2	0–2700 246.5 ± 321.3	0.28	0–2000 231.5 ± 411.1	0–3000 312.5 ± 574.9	25.9	0.08	**0.05 ***
	Frequency index	0–3 1 ± 1.0	0–3 1 ± 1.0	0	0–3 0.9 ± 1.0	0–3 1.0 ± 1.1	10.0	0.06	0.06
MEP APB	Amplitude (µV)	50–11200 1925.3 ± 1724.3	50–1050 2105.6 ± 1855.3	9.5	50–12500 2052.9 ± 2511.0	100–11000 2725.1 ± 2524.1	24.6	0.07	**0.05 ***
	Latency (ms)	16.2–33.4 23.1 ± 4.6	17.1–34.6 23.6 ± 3.9	2.1	16.8–43.5 23.4 ± 5.2	14.6–33.0 23.3 ± 4.5	0.42	0.14	0.13
MEP TA	Amplitude (µV)	0–1200 77.1 ± 133.5	0–1000 100.9 ± 131.6	23.5	0–1000 76.9 ± 162.8	0–1100 162.1 ± 123.6	52.5	0.11	**0.05 ***
	Latency (ms)	0–50.1 30.4 ± 17.1	0–49.2 29.4 ± 13.6	3.2	0–49.3 29.1 ± 18.5	0–45.0 28.1 ± 15.6	3.4	0.13	0.12

K group—kinesiotherapy treated group of patients n = 25, K + rTMS group—kinesiotherapy and rTMS treated group of patients n = 26. * Significant p-values are marked bold.

4. Discussion

rTMS is a non-invasive technique for neuromodulation and has therapeutic potential for motor rehabilitation following an iSCI [2–8]. In our previous study, patients who suffered a C4–Th2 iSCI that were treated with 20–22 Hz rTMS showed an improvement of functional status by means of spasticity decrease and a greater increase in muscle motor unit activity in upper than in lower extremities [10]. A statistically significant improvement in the transmission of efferent neural impulses within spinal pathways to cervical centers and upper extremity muscles was observed in the MEP recordings. In this study, we chose patients with similar injuries at the cervical or thoracic spinal levels, assumed from MRI coronal and vertical planes, where one-third to one-quarter of the neural structures were preserved, as well as from the results of direct MEP recordings performed before treatment, which confirmed the range of each iSCI. Both populations of C4–Th2 and C2–Th12 patients were different regarding the duration of treatment: up to 5 months and from 2 to 11 months (5 months of average), respectively. The results of the comparative neurophysiological tests in this study on patients with C2–Th12 iSCI provide evidence of the similarity in the above-mentioned phenomena found in the C4–Th2 iSCI patients, with additional improvements in muscle motor unit activity in the lower extremities. The results of this study also provide evidence regarding the improvement of the efferent transmission of neuronal impulses to the spinal motor centers in neuromeres below the level of the injury, as shown by the better results of the MEPs recordings from the TA muscles than in the study of Leszczyńska et al. [10]. Throughout the whole population of patients, a significant improvement of the sEMG parameters recorded from the APB muscle was commonly observed in the second period of observations (see Figure 5). It is difficult to ascertain the exact time point of the applied rTMS effectiveness, but it seems to appear after 50% of the scheduled rTMS sessions in the majority of patients. Significant changes in amplitudes parameters of MEP recordings following rTMS suggest that the maintenance of the efferent spinal cord's transmission was at least at the same level as it is before therapy. If an amplitude of MEP recordings from lower extremity muscles reflects the number of axons in the white matter actively transmitting neuronal impulses, it may also indicate the therapy's protective mechanism was inhibiting degenerative changes of the spinal structures. Patients of both groups were treated with the same algorithms of physical therapy and kinesiotherapy, which implied additional factors influencing the electrophysiological parameters of the C2–Th12 iSCI patients.

The data in Table 4 showing results of neurophysiological recordings in the iSCI patients of both groups clearly provides evidence of the superiority of treatment with kinesiotherapy and rTMS (K + rTMS group) in comparison with the effects found in patients that were treated with only kinesiotherapy (K group). This part of the study appears to be necessary to confirm the importance of rTMS therapy in future clinical practice.

The transmission in the corticospinal pathway is crucial for the recovery of motor function in iSCI patients. Functional recovery is possible either due to the sprouting of new axons, the transmission of neuronal impulses via rudimentary saved corticospinal axons, or the system of intersegmental crossed projections of propriospinal fibers [1,9]. The propriospinal neurons with crossed thoracic and upper lumbar axonal projections, which were partially preserved in patients under this study, among other residual efferent pathways, could modify the functional recovery by transmitting efferent impulses from the cervical to lumbosacral levels. Their cells of origin at the cervical levels are known to be modulated by inputs from supraspinal centers, e.g., corticospinal and rubrospinal systems, which were excited with magnetic field trains of impulses during therapeutic sessions [17,18]. However, it cannot be ignored that some spared fibers in lateral funiculi belonging to these systems participate in neural transmission as well. On the other hand, propriospinal neurons are known to especially compensate for the function of injured spinal cord pathways in long-term experimental and clinical observation [12]. They play an essential role in motor control (including locomotion) and sensory processing. They are an important substrate for spinal cord "bridging" in incomplete lesions and contribute to the plastic reorganization of spinal circuits [1]. We believe that our study results prove the effectiveness of rTMS's ability to elicit one of the systems mentioned above. Previous studies have demonstrated that PNs might also be an essential substrate for recovery in iSCI patients, as they contribute to "functional recovery" [19–21]. Considering the contemporary results of studies on patients with both cervical and thoracic iSCIs, which revealed a better improvement of motor function following rTMS and kinesiotherapy compared with those previously studied in patients with a C4–Th2 iSCI, involvement of the PN system for recovery in spinal interconnections is indicated. We assume that in our iSCI patients, PNs compensated for abnormalities in the transmission of neural impulses in white matter fibers and improved the activity of synaptic connections at the motoneuronal level. The thoracic levels of injury play a significant role as a structural basis of electrophysiological improvements since axons of propriospinal neurons cross at this level and may be the additional way of motor transmission compensation to the residual fibers after iSCI.

This study used a modified rTMS algorithm of stimulation that was described by other authors to treat patients with iSCI [2–8], which evoked positive effects toward improving motor function and reducing spasticity. This may imply that 20–25 Hz rTMS that was adjusted according to each patient's needs based on consecutive neurophysiological test results enhanced the corticospinal synaptic transmission, and this effect was sustained for at least five months. Only a few of the previous studies utilized repetitive testing of sEMG [6,7] and MEP recordings [3,8,11] in the evaluation of positive treatment results in patients with an iSCI. Most of the previous works used clinical methods of functional assessments of patients with iSCI, such as gait improvement analysis; therefore, the presented study results cannot be directly compared.

Limitations

The heterogeneity of the injuries in the patients with an iSCI in this study was its main limitation, although we attempted to recruit subjects with rigorous enrollment rules, such as the ASIA scale evaluation. By contrast, the number of presented patients and performing three trials in long-lasting observations compared to previous results seem to be the main advantages, as well as the comparison of results obtained in the group treated with kinesiotherapy with the group of patients treated with both kinesiotherapy and rTMS. We are aware that having a non-treated identical control group (ideally submitted to a placebo-like intervention) in our study would broaden the scope of the functional regeneration mechanism from the point of basic neuroscience. On the other hand, it would be difficult for iSCI patients looking for any improvement in their health status following rTMS to understand the importance of a placebo approach in the project, as they need to be informed in advance. The other limitation is the uncertainty that muscle fiber atrophy in iSCI patients might be partially caused by superimposing chronic immobility, which makes positive results of any treatment applied to iSCI patients difficult to interpret.

5. Conclusions

The comparison of the results of this study regarding the influence of rTMS at 20–25 Hz in patients with C2–Th12 iSCI in a long-term observation with previous data regarding the outcomes of similar treatment in C4–Th2 iSCI patients may confirm the hypothesis about the significance of the propriospinal system and other residual efferent pathways in the recovery of motor control. The proposed rTMS algorithm reduced spasticity symptoms more in the upper extremity muscles and improved the recruitment of upper and lower extremity muscle motor units and MEPs parameters, which may imply a slight improvement in the transmission of efferent neural impulses within spinal pathways. The comparison of neurophysiological data in iSCI patients treated only with kinesiotherapy (K group) and those treated with kinesiotherapy and rTMS (K + rTMS group) may indicate the importance of including the rTMS therapy in the current standard of care. rTMS was confirmed as a novel, non-invasive, and safe therapeutic method for enhancing voluntary motor output in motor disorders affecting the descending spinal pathways. Its potential clinical application seems to be more effective in conjunction with kinesiotherapeutic treatment, which requires further extensive studies.

Author Contributions: Conceptualization, J.H., A.W., K.L., W.F., and P.T.; Investigation, J.H., A.W., W.F., S.O., and P.T.; Methodology, J.H., A.W., K.L., W.F., S.O., and P.T.; Software, J.H.; Validation, J.H., A.W., K.C., and P.T.; Formal analysis, J.H., A.W., and K.L.; Writing—original draft preparation, J.H., A.W., and K.L.; Writing—review and editing, J.H., A.W., K.L., W.F., S.O., and P.T.; Visualization, J.H. and K.L.; Supervision, J.H. and P.T. All authors have read and agreed to the published version of the manuscript.

Funding: This research received no external funding.

Institutional Review Board Statement: The study was conducted according to the guidelines of the Declaration of Helsinki and approved by the Bioethics Committee from the University of Medical Sciences (decision no. 559/2018).

Informed Consent Statement: Informed consent was obtained from all the subjects involved in the study.

Data Availability Statement: All the data generated or analyzed during this study are included in this published article.

Conflicts of Interest: The authors declare no conflict of interest.

References

1. Oudega, M.; Perez, M. Corticospinal reorganization after spinal cord injury. *J. Physiol.* **2012**, *590*, 3647–3663. [CrossRef] [PubMed]
2. Belci, M.; Catley, M.; Husain, M. Magnetic brain stimulation can improve clinical outcome in incomplete spinal cord injured patients. *Spinal Cord* **2004**, *42*, 417–419. [CrossRef]
3. Kumru, H.; Murillo, N.; Samso, J.V.; Valls-Sole, J.; Edwards, D.; Pelayo, R.; Valero-Cabre, A.; Tormos, J.M.; Pascual-Leone, A. Reduction of spasticity with repetitive transcranial magnetic stimulation in patients with spinal cord injury. *Neurorehabil. Neural Repair* **2010**, *24*, 435–441. [CrossRef]
4. Kuppuswamy, A.; Balasubramaniam, A.V.; Maksimovic, R.; Mathias, C.J.; Gall, A.; Craggs, M.D. Ellaway PHAction of 5Hz repetitive transcranial magnetic stimulation on sensory, motor and autonomic function in human spinal cord injury. *Clin. Neurophysiol.* **2011**, *122*, 2452–2461. [CrossRef] [PubMed]
5. Benito, J.; Kumru, H.; Murillo, N.; Costa, U.; Medina, J.; Tormos, J.M.; Pascual-Leone, A.; Vidal, J. Motor and gait improvement in patients with incomplete spinal cord injury induced by high-frequency repetitive transcranial magnetic stimulation. *Top. Spinal Cord Inj. Rehabil.* **2012**, *18*, 106–112. [CrossRef] [PubMed]
6. Nardone, R.; Höller, Y.; Thomschewski, A.; Brigo, F.; Orioli, A.; Höller, P.; Golaszewski, S.; Trinka, E. rTMS modulates reciprocal inhibition in patients with traumatic spinal cord injury. *Spinal Cord* **2014**, *52*, 831–835. [CrossRef] [PubMed]
7. De Araújo, A.V.L.; Barbosa, V.R.N.; Galdino, G.S.; Fregni, F.; Massetti, T.; Fontes, S.L.; de Oliveira Silva, D.; da Silva, T.D.; Monteiro, C.B.M.; Tonks, J.; et al. Effects of high-frequency transcranial magnetic stimulation on functional performance in individuals with incomplete spinal cord injury: Study protocol for a randomized controlled trial. *Trials* **2017**, *18*, 522. [CrossRef]
8. Tazoe, T.; Perez, M.A. Effects of repetitive transcranial magnetic stimulation on recovery of function after spinal cord injury. *Arch. Phys. Med. Rehabil.* **2015**, *96*, 145–155. [CrossRef]
9. Jo, H.J.; Richardson, M.S.; Oudega, M.; Perez, M. The Potential of Corticospinal-Motoneuronal Plasticity for Recovery after Spinal Cord Injury. *Curr. Phys. Med. Rehabil. Rep.* **2020**, *8*, 293–298. [CrossRef]
10. Leszczyńska, K.; Wincek, A.; Fortuna, W.; Huber, J.; Łukaszek, J.; Okurowski, S.; Chmielak, K.; Tabakow, P. Treatment of patients with cervical and upper thoracic incomplete spinal cord injury using repetitive transcranial magnetic stimulation. *Int. J. Artif. Organs* **2019**, *43*, 323–331. [CrossRef]
11. Tabakow, P.; Raisman, G.; Fortuna, W.; Czyż, M.; Huber, J.; Li, D.; Szewczyk, P.; Okurowski, S.; Międzybrodzki, R.; Czapiga, B.; et al. Functional regeneration of supraspinal connections in a patient with transected spinal cord following transplantation of bulbar olfactory ensheathing cells with peripheral nerve bridging. *Cell Transplant.* **2014**, *23*, 1631–1655. [CrossRef]
12. Flynn, J.R.; Graham, B.A.; Galea, M.P.; Callister, R.J. The role of propriospinal interneurons in recovery from spinal cord injury. *Neuropharmacology* **2011**, *60*, 809–822. [CrossRef]
13. Jankowska, E. Interneuronal relay in spinal pathways from proprioceptors. *Prog. Neurobiol.* **1992**, *38*, 335–378. [CrossRef]
14. Ditunno, J.F.; Ditunno, P.L.; Scivoletto, G.; Patrick, M.; Dijkers, M.; Barbeau, H.; Burns, A.S.; Marino, R.J.; Schmidt-Read, M. The Walking Index for Spinal Cord Injury (WISCI/WISCI II): Nature, metric properties, use and misuse. *Spinal Cord* **2013**, *51*, 346–355. [CrossRef]
15. Lisiński, P.; Huber, J. Evolution of Muscles Dysfunction from Myofascial Pain Syndrome Through Cervical Disc-Root Conflict to Degenerative Spine Disease. *Spine* **2017**, *42*, 151–159. [CrossRef] [PubMed]

16. Huber, J.; Lisiński, P. Early results of supervised versus unsupervised rehabilitation of patients with cervical pain. *Int. J. Artif. Organs* **2019**, *42*, 695–703. [CrossRef] [PubMed]
17. Nicolas, G.; Marchand-Pauvert, V.; Burke, D.; Pierrot-Deseilligny, E. Corticospinal excitation of presumed cervical propriospinal neurones and its reversal to inhibition in humans. *J. Physiol.* **2001**, *533*, 903–919. [CrossRef] [PubMed]
18. Pierrot-Deseilligny, E. Propriospinal transmission of part of the corticospinal excitation in humans. *Muscle Nerve* **2002**, *26*, 155–172. [CrossRef] [PubMed]
19. Bunday, K.L.; Perez, M.A. Motor Recovery After Spinal Cord Injury Enhanced by Strengthening Corticospinal Synaptic Transmission. *Curr. Biol.* **2012**, *22*, 2355–2361. [CrossRef]
20. Bareyre, F.M.; Kerschensteiner, M.; Raineteau, O.; Mettenleiter, T.C.; Weinmann, O.; Schwab, M.E. The injured spinal cord spontaneously forms a new intraspinal circuit in adult rats. *Nat. Neurosci.* **2004**, *7*, 269–277. [CrossRef]
21. Calancie, B.; Alexeeva, N.; Broton, J.G.; Molano, M.R. Interlimb reflex activity after spinal cord injury in man: Strengthening response patterns are consistent with ongoing synaptic plasticity. *Clin. Neurophysiol.* **2005**, *116*, 75–86. [CrossRef] [PubMed]

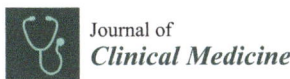

Article

Vertigo in Patients with Degenerative Cervical Myelopathy

Zdenek Kadanka, Jr. [1,2,*], Zdenek Kadanka, Sr. [1,2], Rene Jura [1,2] and Josef Bednarik [1,2]

[1] Department of Neurology, University Hospital, 625 00 Brno, Czech Republic; Kadanka.Zdenek@fnbrno.cz (Z.K.S.); Jura.Rene@fnbrno.cz (R.J.); Bednarik.Josef@fnbrno.cz (J.B.)
[2] Faculty of Medicine, Masaryk University, 625 00 Brno, Czech Republic
* Correspondence: Kadanka.Zdenek2@fnbrno.cz; Tel.: +420-532232354

Abstract: (1) Background: Cervical vertigo (CV) represents a controversial entity, with a prevalence ranging from reported high frequency to negation of CV existence. (2) Objectives: To assess the prevalence and cause of vertigo in patients with a manifest form of severe cervical spondylosis–degenerative cervical myelopathy (DCM) with special focus on CV. (3) Methods: The study included 38 DCM patients. The presence and character of vertigo were explored with a dedicated questionnaire. The cervical torsion test was used to verify the role of neck proprioceptors, and ultrasound examinations of vertebral arteries to assess the role of arteriosclerotic stenotic changes as hypothetical mechanisms of CV. All patients with vertigo underwent a detailed diagnostic work-up to investigate the cause of vertigo. (4) Results: Symptoms of vertigo were described by 18 patients (47%). Causes of vertigo included: orthostatic dizziness in eight (22%), hypertension in five (14%), benign paroxysmal positional vertigo in four (11%) and psychogenic dizziness in one patient (3%). No patient responded positively to the cervical torsion test or showed significant stenosis of vertebral arteries. (5) Conclusions: Despite the high prevalence of vertigo in patients with DCM, the aetiology in all cases could be attributed to causes outside cervical spine and related nerve structures, thus confirming the assumption that CV is over-diagnosed.

Keywords: cervical vertigo; cervical dizziness; degenerative cervical myelopathy; degenerative cervical spinal cord compression; cervical torsion test

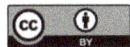

1. Introduction

Dizziness and vertigo are among the most common complaints that lead patients to visit a physician. The lifetime prevalence in adults is around 20%, reaching 40% in older adults [1]. Vertigo is not a single disease entity but a symptom of a wide range of diseases of varying aetiology. These may arise from the inner ear, the brainstem, and the cerebellum, or they may be of internal, vestibular, or psychosomatic origin.

"Cervical (or cervicogenic) vertigo" (CV) is a term often used in a clinical practice, but physicians lack sufficient data to form definite opinions and to give clinical guidelines for its diagnosis and treatment [2]. The overall prevalence of CV is not known because there are no generally accepted clinical or paraclinical tests for CV, and therefore it is predominantly a diagnosis by exclusion [3]. Colledge et al., in a community-based sample of subjects over 65 years of age, found that cervical spondylosis is the second most frequent cause of dizziness [4]. Takahashi, in an out-patient sample of 1000 patients visiting a general hospital in Japan with a chief complaint of dizziness, estimated a prevalence of CV as high as 90% [5]. These data are in striking contrast to the opinion of several leading experts in the field who doubt the diagnosis of CV entirely [6].

Based on these findings and discrepancies, we hypothesised that CV is over-diagnosed due to the absence of detailed diagnostic theory and practice in papers that reported a high prevalence of CV. As degenerative cervical myelopathy (DCM) is the most severe symptomatic form of cervical spondylosis [7], we used a well-defined cohort of DCM patients to verify our hypothesis. The aim of this paper was to assess the prevalence and cause of vertigo in these patients with special focus on CV.

2. Materials and Methods

2.1. Design

This study was designed as a cross-sectional, cohort, observational, non-interventional study.

2.2. Participants

The study sample consisted of a cohort of consecutive subjects referred to a large tertiary university hospital between March 2018 and December 2019 in whom a clinical diagnosis of DCM was established, based on the presence of at least one clinical sign and one clinical symptom of myelopathy and magnetic resonance imaging (MRI) signs of degenerative discogenic and/or spondylogenic cervical spinal cord compression [8,9].

Excluded were:
- Patients with previous surgery on the cervical spine (possibly limiting the rotation of the spine);
- Patients with other than degenerative cervical cord compressions or other non-compressive myelopathies.

All subjects gave their written, informed consent to participate in the study.

2.3. Clinical Evaluation

Clinical neurological evaluation was focused on the assessment of clinical signs and symptoms of symptomatic myelopathy (with other possible causes excluded) and possible causes of vertigo. This included a detailed history of the illness, presence of comorbidities (cardiovascular including arterial hypertension, otorhinolaryngological and psychiatric abnormalities, etc.), history of significant head or cervical spine trauma, Hallpike manoeuvre and a dedicated vertigo questionnaire (see below).

The following symptoms and signs were sought and/or determined as markers of DCM:

Symptoms
- Gait disturbance;
- Numb and/or clumsy hands;
- Lhermitte's phenomenon;
- Bilateral arm paresthesias;
- Weakness of lower or upper extremities;
- Urinary urgency, or incontinence.

Signs
- Corticospinal tract signs;
- Hyperreflexia/clonus;
- Spasticity;
- Pyramidal signs (Babinski reflex or Hoffman's sign);
- Spastic paresis of any of the extremities (most frequently, lower spastic paraparesis);
- Flaccid paresis of one or two upper extremities;
- Atrophy of the hand muscles;
- Sensory involvement in various distributions in upper or lower extremities;
- Gait ataxia.

The following clinical and demographic data were also noted:
- Age;
- Sex.

Degree of disability was assessed by the modified Japanese Orthopaedic Association (mJOA) score [10].

2.4. Imaging

All subjects underwent examination of the cervical spine on a 1.5 Tesla MRI device with a 16-channel head and neck coil. The standardised imaging protocol included conventional pulse sequences in sagittal-T1, -T2 and STIR (short-tau inversion recovery) and axial planes (gradient-echo T2). The imaging criterion for cervical cord compression was defined as a change in spinal cord contour at the level of an intervertebral disc on axial or sagittal MRI scan compared with that at midpoint level of neighbouring vertebrae [11]. Compression ratio (CR) was calculated by taking the anterior–posterior diameter of the spinal cord divided by the transverse diameter of the cord on the axial image [11]. Lower CR values indicate worse cord deformation. This measurement was taken at the level of maximum spinal cord compression identified as maximum reduction in antero/posterior spinal canal diameter in comparison with other segments. The level of maximal spinal cord compression and signs of myelopathy (signal changes of the spinal cord on T1- and T2-weighted imaging) were also established (Figure 1).

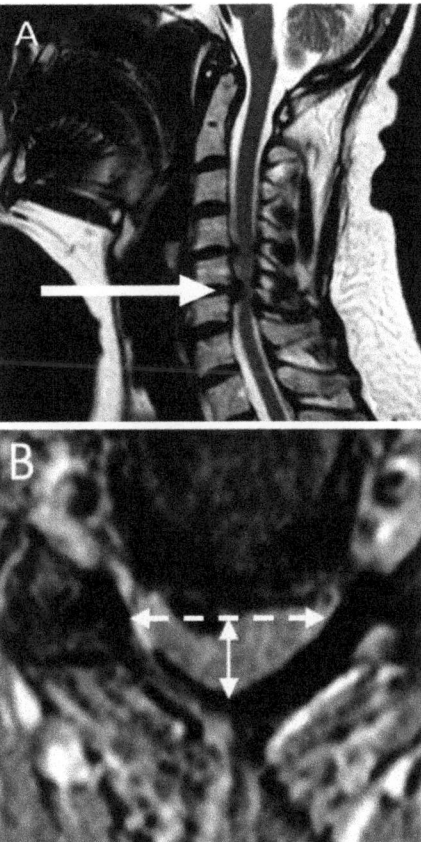

Figure 1. Patient with severe cervical spinal cord compression. (**A**) Sagittal T2-MRI sequence shows a level of maximal compression—C5/6 (arrow); (**B**) Compression ratio: anterior–posterior diameter (solid line double arrow) divided by the transverse diameter (dashed line double arrow) of the spinal cord on the axial T2 MRI image (taken at the level of maximum spinal cord compression; the result is 0.37 in this patient).

2.5. Vertigo Questionnaire

Vertigo/dizziness was defined as an unpleasant disturbance of spatial orientation or to the erroneous perception of movement [12]. An investigator-administered questionnaire originally published by Filippopoulos was administered verbally to all patients [13]. The prevalence, the type of vertigo and the body positions and movements related to the different vertigo types were assessed by a series of questions. The questionnaire is shown in Supplementary Figure S1.

2.6. Uncontrolled Blood Pressure

Patients reporting any dizziness/vertigo were asked to measure their blood pressure at home under basal conditions 3 times daily for 3 consecutive days and the average value was then calculated. Uncontrolled blood pressure was defined as an average value $\geq$140 (systolic)/90 (diastolic) mm Hg. In borderline values 24-h monitoring of blood pressure was performed and the same definition was used for uncontrolled blood pressure.

2.7. Orthostatic Hypotension

Orthostatic hypotension was evaluated in patients reporting dizziness/vertigo by measuring blood pressure after lying flat for 5 min, then 1 min and 3 min after standing. For determination of orthostatic hypotension, we used an updated definition of the American Autonomic Society as a systolic blood pressure decrease of at least 20 mm Hg or a diastolic blood pressure decrease of at least 10 mm Hg within three minutes of standing when compared with blood pressure from the sitting or supine position [14].

2.8. Benign Paroxysmal Positional Vertigo

Diagnostic criteria for benign paroxysmal positional vertigo (BPPV) consisted of vertical–torsional positional nystagmus evoked by the Dix–Hallpike manoeuvre or a predominantly horizontal positional nystagmus after rolling the head sideways from the supine position [15].

2.9. Ultrasound of Carotid and Vertebral Arteries

All ultrasound examinations were performed by an experienced neurosonologist using advanced ultrasound equipment (Philips PureWave HD 15; Massachusetts, USA) with a 3–12 MHz multi-frequency ultrasound probe. Patients were examined in a supine position with the neck slightly extended. Arterial wall thickness was evaluated and any extracranial atherosclerosis and/or occlusive disease was detected, with particular attention to the carotid bifurcation. In the event of carotid stenosis, its severity was measured in B mode and colour mode, with complementary measurements of peak systolic flow velocity and diastolic velocity gauged by Doppler ultrasound, based on the European Carotid Surgery Trial criteria (70–99% stenosis was considered significant) [16]. Vertebral arteries (VAs) were visualised in a longitudinal plane at the sixth cervical vertebra, where the vertebral artery usually enters the transverse foramina. For analysis, the course of the VA was divided into two segments: Vertebral (V1) (from the origin of the vertebral artery until the point where it enters the fifth or sixth cervical vertebra) and V2 (the part of the vertebral artery that courses cranially to the transverse foramina until it emerges besides the lateral mass of the atlas) [17]. Each segment of the VA was studied in B mode and colour-code mode. Any stenotic lesions of the VAs were evaluated according to B mode and flow pattern. Criteria used for grading $\geq$50% stenosis were focal elevated blood flow velocity with a PSV cut-off point at the V1 segment of the vertebral artery of 140 cm/s, and 125 cm/s at the V2 segment [18].

2.10. Cervical Torsion Test

A cervical torsion test was performed in all patients. The procedure was adapted after the work of L'Hereux-Lebeau [19]. Subjects were seated in a rigid but fully rotatable chair that provided support to the entire body. Their legs were flexed with a slight bend at the knees. They were securely held in the chair with shoulder- and lap-belts. It was requested that their eyes should be closed during the procedure. First, the subject´s trunk was passively turned 70 degrees to the right, with the head still, then returned to centre, followed by turning the trunk 70 degrees to the left, and returning to centre. Each position was held for 30 s with the head stabilised by the observer for all positions. Nystagmus was evaluated with Frenzel goggles. The test was considered positive when nystagmus was found in any of the four positions, or vertigo provoked or increased (Figure 2).

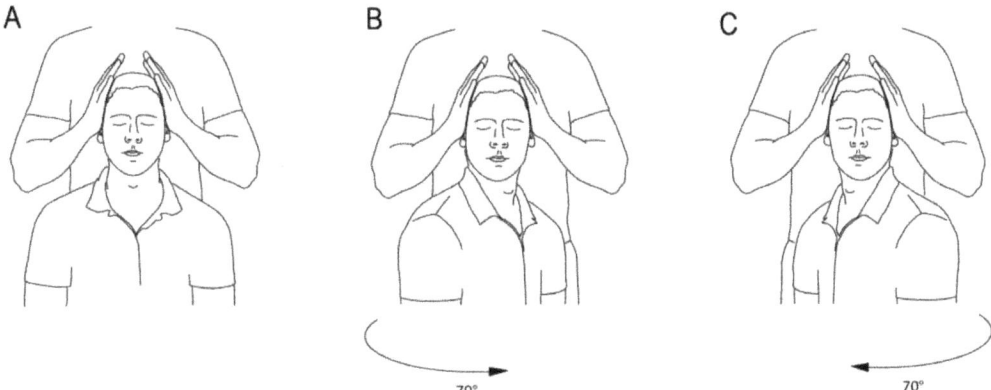

Figure 2. Cervical torsion test. (**A**) Subject seated in a rigid but fully rotatable chair, head fixed. (**B**) The subject´s trunk passively turned 70 degrees to the right, with the head still, then returned to centre. (**C**) Turning the trunk 70 degrees to the left, then returned to centre.

The final diagnosis of DCM, together with the diagnosis of possible causes of vertigo, was defined by a neurologist (ZKJ) and then reviewed and confirmed by two other researchers (ZK and JB). Finally, detailed internal, otorhino-laryngological, neuro-otological or psychiatric examinations were performed according to suspected aetiology and the definite cause of vertigo was additionally verified by a highly qualified specialist. In case of discordance with the cause suspected by a neurologist, the final cause was established by consensus. We always cooperated with the same specialist.

3. Results

3.1. Study Cohort

We screened 51 patients in whom a diagnosis of DCM was established. Eight of them were excluded because of previous cervical spine surgery and five of them were not willing to participate in the study and did not sign informed consent. Thirty-eight patients complied with the DCM diagnosis and exclusion criteria, signed informed consent and completed the study protocol. The study cohort included 17 females (44.7%) with a median age (range) of 59 (41–85) years. The average mJOA score of the evaluated cohort was 16 (median), 9–17 (range). None of them reported significant injury of the head or cervical spine during the last year before inclusion in the study. Detailed demographic and imaging characteristics are summarised in Table 1.

Table 1. Demographic and imaging characteristics.

Patients No	Gender	Age	mJOA Score	Maximum Cervical Cord Compression Level	Signs of Myelopathy on MRI	CR	ICA Stenosis	VA Stenosis
1	F	46	17	C5/6	no	0.31	no	none
2	M	44	17	C4/5	no	0.3	no	none
3	F	60	17	C6/7	yes	0.32	no	none
4	F	60	16	C6/7	no	0.37	no	none
5	F	51	17	C4/5	no	0.44	no	none
6	M	43	16	C4/5	no	0.45	no	none
7	M	71	15	C5/6	yes	0.35	yes	none
8	M	60	17	C4/5	no	0.3	no	none
9	M	65	16	C3/4	yes	0.4	no	none
10	M	51	16	C5/6	yes	0.43	no	none
11	M	65	17	C5/6	no	0.36	no	none
12	F	50	17	C5/6	no	0.36	no	none
13	F	63	11	C5/6	yes	0.36	yes	none
14	F	71	16	C5/6	no	0.41	no	none
15	M	58	16	C4/5	no	0.43	no	none
16	F	69	12	C4/5	yes	0.39	no	none
17	M	60	15	C6/7	yes	0.42	no	none
18	F	59	16	C6/7	no	0.40	no	none
19	M	63	17	C5/6	yes	0.42	no	none
20	M	52	16	C5/6	no	0.28	no	none
21	M	69	15	C5/6	no	0.3	no	none
22	F	57	16	C5/6	yes	0.38	no	none
23	M	82	17	C6/7	no	0.36	no	none
24	F	59	15	C5/6	yes	0.36	no	none
25	M	67	13	C5/6	yes	0.49	yes	none
26	M	64	15	C5/6	no	0.41	no	none
27	M	45	17	C3/4	no	0.37	no	none
28	M	77	9	C4/5	yes	0.41	no	none
29	F	40	17	C5/6	no	0.43	no	none
30	M	59	17	C5/6	yes	0.44	no	none
31	F	51	17	C5/6	no	0.39	no	none
32	M	48	15	C5/6	yes	0.21	no	none
33	F	48	17	C5/6	no	0.23	no	none
34	F	59	17	C5/6	no	0.33	no	none
35	F	48	17	C4/5	yes	0.23	no	none
36	F	52	17	C4/5	no	0.44	no	none
37	M	58	16	C5/6	yes	0.38	no	none
38	M	68	17	C5/6	no	0.39	no	none

mJOA: modified Japanese Orthopaedic Association score; CR: compression ratio; ICA: internal carotid artery; VA: vertebral artery; MRI: magnetic resonance imaging; F: female; M: male.

3.2. Dizziness/Vertigo

Subjective feelings of dizziness/vertigo in the previous six months were reported by 18 patients (47%). Patients characterised dizziness/vertigo as a feeling of impending blackout when rapidly standing up (eight patients), as a spinning vertigo (like in a carrousel) (five patients), as a swaying vertigo (like on a small boat) (four patients) and one patient was not able to specify it. Detailed characteristics of dizziness/vertigo and its aetiology in DCM patients are summarised in Table 2.

Table 2. Detailed characteristics of dizziness/vertigo and its aetiology in DCM patients.

Patients No	Type of Vertigo	Vertigo According to Body Movement	Cervical Torsion Test	Hallpike Test	Drop in BP ≥ 20/10 mmHg after at Least 3 min of Standing	Upright Tilt Table Test	Uncontrolled AH Detection	Final Aetiology of Dizziness
1	none	none	negative	negative	No	NA		NA
2	none	none	negative	negative	No	NA		NA
3	none	none	negative	negative	No	NA		NA
4	none	none	negative	negative	No	NA		NA
5	unspecified dizziness	also present when sitting or lying down	negative	negative	No	NA	24 h monitoring	uncontrolled AH
6	none	none	negative	negative	No	NA		NA
7	spinning	also present when sitting or lying down	negative	negative	No	NA	self-measurement	uncontrolled AH
8	none	none	negative	negative	No	NA		NA
9	none	none	negative	negative	No	NA		NA
10	blackout when standing	triggered by a change of position	negative	negative	Yes	NA		orthostatic vertigo
11	none	none	negative	negative	No	NA		NA
12	blackout when standing	triggered by a change of position	negative	negative	No	positive		orthostatic vertigo
13	swaying	only present when standing or walking	negative	negative	No	NA	24 h monitoring	uncontrolled AH
14	blackout when standing	triggered by a change of position	negative	negative	Yes	NA		orthostatic vertigo
15	none	none	negative	negative	No	NA		NA
16	swaying	also present when sitting or lying down	negative	negative	No	NA		psychogenic vertigo
17	none	none	negative	negative	No	NA		NA
18	swaying	only present when standing or walking	negative	negative	No	NA	self-measurement	uncontrolled AH
19	none	none	negative	negative	No	NA		NA
20	none	none	negative	negative	No	NA		NA
21	blackout when standing	triggered by a change of position	negative	negative	Yes	NA		orthostatic vertigo
22	none	none	negative	positive	No	NA		NA
23	blackout when standing	triggered by a change of position	negative	negative	Yes	NA		orthostatic vertigo
24	spinning	triggered by head movement	negative	positive	No	NA		BPPV
25	blackout when standing	triggered by a change of position	negative	negative	Yes	NA		orthostatic vertigo
26	blackout when standing	triggered by a change of position	negative	negative	Yes	NA		orthostatic vertigo
27	none	none	negative	negative	No	NA		NA

Table 2. Cont.

Patients No	Type of Vertigo	Vertigo According to Body Movement	Cervical Torsion Test	Hallpike Test	Drop in BP ≥ 20/10 mmHg after at Least 3 min of Standing	Upright Tilt Table Test	Uncontrolled AH Detection	Final Aetiology of Dizziness
28	spinning	trigered by head movement	negative	positive	No	NA		BPPV
29	none	none	negative	negative	No	NA		NA
30	none	none	negative	negative	No	NA		NA
31	spinning	triggered by head movement	negative	positive	No	NA		BPPV
32	blackout when standing	trigered by a change of position	negative	negative	No	positive		orthostatic vertigo
33	spinning	triggered by head movement	negative	positive	No	NA		BPPV
34	swaying	only present when standing or walking	negative	negative	No	NA	self-measurement	uncompensated AH
35	none	none	negative	negative	No	NA		NA
36	none	none	negative	negative	No	NA		NA
37	none	none	negative	negative	No	NA		NA
38	none	none	negative	negative	No	NA		NA

NA: not attributable; BPPV: benign paroxysmal positional vertigo; AH: arterial hypertension; BP: blood pressure.

The following causes of vertigo were found in these patients: orthostatic dizziness in eight patients (44% of patients with vertigo, 22% of all patients), uncontrolled arterial hypertension in five (28% and 14%, respectively), BPPV in four (22% and 11%, respectively) and psychogenic dizziness in one (6% and 3%, respectively). The presence of uncontrolled arterial hypertension had to be confirmed by 24-h monitoring in two out of five patients (Table 2).

None of the 38 patients studied displayed a positive response to the cervical torsion test, irrespective of the presence or absence of subjectively described vertigo in the previous six months.

Three patients (0.8%) exhibited haemodynamically significant stenosis of the internal carotid arteries (two of them suffered from recently diagnosed, uncontrolled hypertension, while one had orthostatic dizziness). None of the patients studied had significant stenosis of the vertebral arteries (Table 1).

4. Discussion

Our study demonstrated a high prevalence of dizziness/vertigo in a cohort of patients with severe cervical spondylosis. Dizziness/vertigo was reported by 47% of the DCM patients. The aetiology of dizziness/vertigo in all patients in our DCM cohort, however, could be explained by mechanisms other than lesion(s) of the nervous system in the cervical region (i.e., orthostatic dizziness, uncontrolled hypertension, BPPV, psychogenic dizziness) or stenotic changes in the cervical segment of vertebral arteries. We thus have not been able to present any evidence in favour of the high prevalence of cervical dizziness/vertigo attributed either to advanced symptomatic spondylosis of the cervical spine and/or stenotic changes of vertebral arteries reported by other authors [4,5,20].

Vertigo, in general, is a common condition, yet definitions vary and management guidelines are often contradictory [21]. Patients with intrinsic problems (cardiovascular, pulmonary, etc.) are unlikely to suffer from pure rotational vertigo and the severity of this condition is often overrated by their clinicians [6]. Orthostatic dizziness in the adult population has accounted for 42% of all participants with vertigo and for 55% of non-vestibular dizziness diagnoses [22]. These findings correlate with the results of this study— in 44% of symptomatic (vertigo-suffering) patients, orthostatic aetiology was confirmed. Five patients were diagnosed with uncontrolled hypertension, making up 28% of the symptomatic group. In general, hypertension and dizziness are both highly prevalent and significantly associated, highlighting a pressing need for investments in preventive measures [23]. BPPV is the most common of the peripheral types of vertigo. Tan noted that 9% of elderly patients undergoing general geriatric assessment exhibited unrecognised BPPV [24]. This percentage proved even higher in a larger series of patients—approximately 34% [25]. Our study disclosed four patients with BBPV (22% of symptomatic subjects), but the group was too small to draw any definite conclusions. We decided to use the questionnaire by Filippopoulos to determine the prevalence of vertigo [13]. Unfortunately, the questionnaire cannot exactly differentiate between possible underlying pathologies, but it can lead us in a certain direction. A feeling of impending blackout when standing up rapidly is typical for orthostatic dizziness [26]. Vertigo (mostly spinning) triggered by head movements is typical for benign paroxysmal vertigo [27]. Swaying vertigo is often described as a somatoform and/or phobic vertigo [28]. In recent decades, cervical vertigo has emerged as a special category of dizziness, generating considerable controversy. The diagnosis remains debatable; there remains a lack of validated tests to confirm this entity, and exclusion clinical diagnosis appears to be the default standard [3,19]. A diagnosis of CV, however, is made too often by many physicians, largely because the simultaneous occurrence of vertigo and cervical spondylosis is very common [29]. Several explanations of the aetiology of CV have been published. Disturbed cervical proprioception is suggested by probably the most cited study [30]. Neck afferents (nerves) not only assist the coordination of eye, head, and body, but they also affect spatial orientation and control of posture. This implies the theory that stimulation of, or lesions (damage) in, these structures could produce CV [31]. In experimental studies, vertigo, ataxia, and nystagmus have been induced in animals by injecting local anaesthetics into the neck [32]. Ataxia in healthy human beings, induced by unilateral injection of local anaesthetics in the neck, has also been associated with a broad-based, staggering gait and hypotonia of the ipsilateral arm and leg [32]. According to these findings, some authors have suggested that cervical spinal cord compression is the most frequent cause of cervical vertigo [33]. The cervical torsion test is supposed to be the most useful to distinguish between cervical afferent disturbance and vestibular dysfunction in patients with dizziness/vertigo [19]. It is the reason why it was used in this study to elucidate the role of the cervical proprioceptors in DCM patients. The principle of the test is to achieve stimulation of the proprioceptors of the neck; the trunk of the body is rotated with the head kept stationary. This examination, however, was not able to evoke vertigo in any patient in this cohort. The second most common hypothesis as to the aetiology of CV is that it may arise out of impaired blood circulation in the vertebrobasilar arteries. In 1933, DeKleyn first described a syndrome of vertigo produced by head movement. In post-mortem studies, he noted compromised circulation in the VA with head rotation. Later, stroke accompanying maximum rotation of the head was described in archery [30]. However, because of the collateral blood flow through the contralateral VA and the circle of Willis, VA occlusion does not lead to symptoms in most individual cases. Thus, cases of symptomatic rotational vertebral artery occlusion are very rare [34]. Investigation of the effect of the position of the head on flow rate in the vertebral arteries, as measured by Doppler ultrasound at rotations of 30 degrees up to 60 degrees to either side, revealed no changes in blood flow in healthy subjects, which means that common rotation of the cervical spine cannot elicit vertigo [35]. Thus, in conclusion, the available literature indicates that hypoperfusion in the vertebrobasilar territory has no close correlation with clinical symptoms of cervical vertigo, and should not be raised as the sole reason in explaining CV [36,37]. This finding was also confirmed by this study. Moreover, vertebrobasilar insufficiency remains a controversial clinical entity lacking clear diagnostic criteria [38].

Limitations of the Study

This study has several limitations. The sample size is small. However, we consider a cohort of 30–40 DCM patients large enough to confirm the hypothesis of CV as a prevalent condition; we used robust inclusion/exclusion criteria and an extensive evaluation, including neurological and vestibular clinical assessments. Our results have limited importance only for patients with severe cervical spondylosis and symptomatic cervical myelopathy, not for other conditions or a general population. We used the cervical torsion test to evaluate the role of cervical proprioceptors in the pathophysiology of CV, but there are no generally accepted clinical or paraclinical tests for CV and therefore it is predominantly a diagnosis by exclusion.

5. Conclusions

In conclusion, despite a comparatively high prevalence (47%) of dizziness/vertigo in patients with severe cervical spondylosis, it is primarily necessary to be in doubt about the diagnosis of so-called "cervical vertigo" and to seek other (often treatable) aetiologies, thus avoiding the possibility of overlooking other serious neurological, otorhinolaryngological or circulatory problems.

Supplementary Materials: The following are available online at https://www.mdpi.com/article/10.3390/jcm10112496/s1, Figure S1: Structured questionnaire assessing the prevalence, the type of vertigo and the body positions and movements related to the different vertigo types.

Author Contributions: Conceptualization, Z.K.J. and J.B.; methodology, Z.K.J., Z.K.S. and J.B.; validation, Z.K.J.; formal analysis, Z.K.S. and J.B.; investigation, Z.K.J., R.J. and Z.K.S.; resources, Z.K.J. and J.B.; data processing, Z.K.J.; writing—original draft preparation, Z.K.J.; writing—review and editing, J.B. and Z.K.S.; supervision, J.B.; project administration, J.B.; funding acquisition, J.B. All authors have read and agreed to the published version of the manuscript. David Pollak (Leicester, UK) helped work up the English.

Funding: This research was funded by the Czech Health Research Council, grant ref. NV 18-04-00159, by the Ministry of Health of the Czech Republic project for conceptual development in research organizations, ref. 65269705 (University Hospital, Brno, Czech Republic), and by Specific Research project ref. MUNI/A/1600/2020 provided by Masaryk University Brno.

Institutional Review Board Statement: The study was conducted according to the guidelines of the Declaration of Helsinki and approved by the Ethics Committee of Masaryk University Brno, protocol code EKV-2017-055, 19 March 2018.

Informed Consent Statement: Informed consent was obtained from all subjects involved in the study.

Data Availability Statement: The data presented in this study are available on request from the corresponding author. The data are not publicly available.

Conflicts of Interest: The authors declare that they have no conflict of interest.

References

1. Kovacs, E.; Wang, X.; Grill, E. Economic burden of vertigo: A systematic review. *Health Econ. Rev.* **2019**, *9*, 37. [CrossRef] [PubMed]
2. Thompson-Harvey, A.; Hain, T.C. Symptoms in cervical vertigo. *Laryngoscope* **2019**, *4*, 109–115. [CrossRef] [PubMed]
3. Reiley, A.S.; Vickory, F.M.; Funderburg, S.E.; Cesario, R.A.; Clendaniel, R.A. How to diagnose cervicogenic dizziness. *Arch. Physiother.* **2017**, *7*, 12. [CrossRef]
4. Colledge, N.R.; Barr-Hamilton, R.M.; Lewis, S.J.; Sellar, R.J.; Wilson, J.A. Evaluation of investigations to diagnose the cause of dizziness in elderly people: A community based controlled study. *BMJ* **1996**, *313*, 788–792. [CrossRef] [PubMed]
5. Takahashi, S. Importance of cervicogenic general dizziness. *J. Rural Med.* **2018**, *13*, 48–56. [CrossRef] [PubMed]
6. Strupp, M.; Dlugaiczyk, J.; Ertl-Wagner, B.B.; Rujescu, D.; Westhofen, M.; Dieterich, M. Vestibular Disorders. *Dtsch. Aerzteblatt Online* **2020**, *117*, 300–310. [CrossRef] [PubMed]
7. Milligan, J.; Ryan, K.; Fehlings, M.; Bauman, C. Degenerative Cervical Myelopathy. *Can. Fam. Physician* **2019**, *65*, 619–624.
8. Kalsi-Ryan, S.; Karadimas, S.K.; Fehlings, M.G. Cervical Spondylotic Myelopathy. *Neuroscientist* **2012**, *19*, 409–421. [CrossRef]
9. Martin, A.R.; De Leener, B.; Cohen-Adad, J.; Cadotte, D.W.; Nouri, A.; Wilson, J.R.; Tetreault, L.; Crawley, A.P.; Mikulis, D.J.; Ginsberg, H.; et al. Can microstructural MRI detect subclinical tissue injury in subjects with asymptomatic cervical spinal cord compression? A prospective cohort study. *BMJ Open* **2018**, *8*, e019809. [CrossRef]
10. Tetreault, L.; Kopjar, B.; Nouri, A.; Arnold, P.; Barbagallo, G.; Bartels, R.; Qiang, Z.; Singh, A.; Zileli, M.; Vaccaro, A.; et al. The modified Japanese Orthopaedic Association scale: Establishing criteria for mild, moderate and severe impairment in patients with degenerative cervical myelopathy. *Eur. Spine J.* **2016**, *26*, 78–84. [CrossRef]
11. Kadanka, Z.; Adamova, B.; Keřkovský, M.; Dusek, L.; Jurová, B.; Vlckova, E.; Bednarik, J. Predictors of symptomatic myelopathy in degenerative cervical spinal cord compression. *Brain Behav.* **2017**, *7*, e00797. [CrossRef]
12. Strupp, M.; Dieterich, M.; Brandt, T. The Treatment and Natural Course of Peripheral and Central Vertigo. *Dtsch. Aerzteblatt Online* **2013**, *110*, 505–516. [CrossRef]
13. Filippopulos, F.M.; Albers, L.; Straube, A.; Gerstl, L.; Blum, B.; Langhagen, T.; Jahn, K.; Heinen, F.; Von Kries, R.; Landgraf, M.N. Vertigo and dizziness in adolescents: Risk factors and their population attributable risk. *PLoS ONE* **2017**, *12*, e0187819. [CrossRef]
14. Freeman, R.; Wieling, W.; Axelrod, F.B.; Benditt, D.G.; Benarroch, E.E.; Biaggioni, I.; Cheshire, W.; Chelimsky, T.C.; Cortelli, P.; Gibbons, C.H.; et al. Consensus statement on the definition of orthostatic hypotension, neurally mediated syncope and the postural tachycardia syndrome. *Clin. Auton. Res.* **2011**, *21*, 69–72. [CrossRef]
15. Bhattacharyya, N.; Gubbels, S.P.; Schwartz, S.R.; Edlow, J.A.; El-Kashlan, H.; Fife, T.; Holmberg, J.M.; Mahoney, K.; Hollingsworth, D.B.; Roberts, R.; et al. Clinical Practice Guideline: Benign Paroxysmal Positional Vertigo (Update). *Otolaryngol. Neck Surg.* **2017**, *156*, S1–S47. [CrossRef]
16. Warlow, C. MRC European Carotid Surgery Trial: Interim results for symptomatic patients with severe (70–99%) or with mild (0–29%) carotid stenosis. *Lancet* **1991**, *337*, 1235–1243. [CrossRef]
17. Cloud, G.; Markus, H. Diagnosis and management of vertebral artery stenosis. *Qjm Int. J. Med.* **2003**, *96*, 27–54. [CrossRef]
18. Koch, S.; Bustillo, A.J.; Campo, B.; Campo, N.; Campo-Bustillo, I.; McClendon, M.S.; Katsnelson, M.; Romano, J.G. Prevalence of vertebral artery origin stenosis and occlusion in outpatient extracranial ultrasonography. *J. Vasc. Interv. Neurol.* **2014**, *7*, 29–33.
19. L'Heureux-Lebeau, B.; Godbout, A.; Berbiche, D.; Saliba, I. Evaluation of Paraclinical Tests in the Diagnosis of Cervicogenic Dizziness. *Otol. Neurotol.* **2014**, *35*, 1858–1865. [CrossRef]
20. Reddy, R.S.; Tedla, J.S.; Dixit, S.; Abohashrh, M. Cervical proprioception and its relationship with neck pain intensity in subjects with cervical spondylosis. *BMC Musculoskelet. Disord.* **2019**, *20*, 447. [CrossRef]
21. Dieterich, M.; Brandt, T. Perception of Verticality and Vestibular Disorders of Balance and Falls. *Front. Neurol.* **2019**, *10*, 172. [CrossRef] [PubMed]

22. Radtke, A.; Lempert, T.; Von Brevern, M.; Feldmann, M.; Lezius, F.; Neuhauser, H. Prevalence and complications of orthostatic dizziness in the general population. *Clin. Auton. Res.* **2011**, *21*, 161–168. [CrossRef] [PubMed]
23. Moreira, M.D.; Trelha, C.S.; Marchiori, L.L.D.M.; Lopes, A.R. Association between complaints of dizziness and hypertension in non-institutionalized elders. *Int. Arch. Otorhinolaryngol.* **2014**, *17*, 157–162. [CrossRef] [PubMed]
24. Tan, J.; Deng, Y.; Zhang, T.; Wang, M. Clinical characteristics and treatment outcomes for benign paroxysmal positional vertigo comorbid with hypertension. *Acta Oto-Laryngol.* **2016**, *137*, 482–484. [CrossRef]
25. Xue, H.; Chong, Y.; Jiang, Z.D.; Liu, Z.L.; Ding, L.; Yang, S.L.; Wang, L.; Xiang, W.P. Etiological analysis on patients with vertigo or dizziness. *Chin. Med. J.* **2018**, *98*, 1227–1230.
26. Kim, H.A.; Bisdorff, A.; Bronstein, A.M.; Lempert, T.; Rossi-Izquierdo, M.; Staab, J.P.; Strupp, M.; Kim, J.-S. Hemodynamic orthostatic dizziness/vertigo: Diagnostic criteria. *J. Vestib. Res.* **2019**, *29*, 45–56. [CrossRef]
27. Britt, C.J.; Ward, B.K.; Owusu, Y.; Friedland, D.; Russell, J.O.; Weinreich, H.M. Assessment of a Statistical Algorithm for the Prediction of Benign Paroxysmal Positional Vertigo. *JAMA Otolaryngol. Neck Surg.* **2018**, *144*, 883. [CrossRef]
28. Dieterich, M.; Staab, J. Functional dizziness: From phobic postural vertigo and chronic subjective dizziness to persistent postural-perceptual dizziness. *Curr. Opin. Neurol.* **2017**, *30*, 107–113. [CrossRef]
29. Bécares-Martínez, C.; López-Llames, A.; Martín-Pagán, A.; Cores-Prieto, A.E.; Arroyo-Domingo, M.; Marco-Algarra, J.; Morales-Suárez-Varela, M. Cervical spine radiographs in patients with vertigo and dizziness. *Radiol. Med.* **2019**, *125*, 272–279. [CrossRef]
30. Judy, B.F.; Theodore, N. Bow Hunter's Syndrome. *World Neurosurg.* **2021**, *148*, 127–128. [CrossRef]
31. Chu, E.C.P.; Chin, W.L.; Bhaumik, A. Cervicogenic dizziness. *Oxf. Med Case Rep.* **2019**, *2019*, 476–478. [CrossRef]
32. De Jong, P.T.V.M.; De Jong, J.M.B.V.; Cohen, B.; Jongkees, L.B.W. Ataxia and nystagmus induced by injection of local anesthetics in the neck. *Ann. Neurol.* **1977**, *1*, 240–246. [CrossRef]
33. Liu, X.-M.; Pan, F.-M.; Yong, Z.-Y.; Ba, Z.-Y.; Wang, S.-J.; Liu, Z.; Zhao, W.-D.; Wu, D.-S. Does the longus colli have an effect on cervical vertigo? *Med.* **2017**, *96*, e6365. [CrossRef]
34. Rendon, R.; Mannoia, K.; Reiman, S.; Hitchman, L.; Shutze, W. Rotational vertebral artery occlusion secondary to completely extraosseous vertebral artery. *J. Vasc. Surg. Cases Innov. Tech.* **2019**, *5*, 14–17. [CrossRef]
35. Simon, H.; Niederkorn, K.; Horner, S.; Duft, M.; Schröckenfuchs, M. Effect of head rotation on the vertebrobasilar system. A transcranial Doppler ultrasound contribution to the physiology. *HNO* **1994**, *42*, 614–618.
36. Wang, Z.; Wang, X.; Yuan, W.; Jiang, D. Degenerative pathological irritations to cervical PLL may play a role in presenting sympathetic symptoms. *Med. Hypotheses* **2011**, *77*, 921–923. [CrossRef]
37. Bayrak, I.K.; Durmus, D.; Bayrak, A.O.; Diren, B.; Canturk, F.; Diren, H.B. Effect of cervical spondylosis on vertebral arterial flow and its association with vertigo. *Clin. Rheumatol.* **2008**, *28*, 59–64. [CrossRef]
38. Chandratheva, A.; Werring, D.; Kaski, D. Vertebrobasilar insufficiency: An insufficient term that should be retired. *Pract. Neurol.* **2020**, 2–3. [CrossRef]

Article

Walk and Run Test in Patients with Degenerative Compression of the Cervical Spinal Cord

Zdenek Kadanka Jr. [1,2,*], Zdenek Kadanka Sr. [1,2], Tomas Skutil [2], Eva Vlckova [1,2,3] and Josef Bednarik [1,2,3]

1. Department of Neurology, University Hospital, 625 00 Brno, Czech Republic; Kadanka.Zdenek@fnbrno.cz (Z.K.S.); Vlckova.Eva@fnbrno.cz (E.V.); Bednarik.Josef@fnbrno.cz (J.B.)
2. Faculty of Medicine, Masaryk University, 625 00 Brno, Czech Republic; Tomas.Skutil@gmail.com
3. Central European Institute of Technology, Masaryk University, 625 00 Brno, Czech Republic
* Correspondence: Kadanka.Zdenek2@fnbrno.cz; Tel.: +420-532232354

Abstract: Impaired gait is one of the cardinal symptoms of degenerative cervical myelopathy (DCM) and frequently its initial presentation. Quantitative gait analysis is therefore a promising objective tool in the disclosure of early cervical cord impairment in patients with degenerative cervical compression. The aim of this cross-sectional observational cohort study was to verify whether an objective and easily-used walk and run test is capable of detecting early gait impairment in a practical proportion of non-myelopathic degenerative cervical cord compression (NMDCC) patients and of revealing any correlation with severity of disability in DCM. The study group consisted of 45 DCM patients (median age 58 years), 126 NMDCC subjects (59 years), and 100 healthy controls (HC) (55.5 years), all of whom performed a standardized 10-m walk and run test. Walking/running time/velocity, number of steps and cadence of walking/running were recorded; analysis disclosed abnormalities in 66.7% of NMDCC subjects. The DCM group exhibited significantly more pronounced abnormalities in all walk/run parameters when compared with the NMDCC group. These were apparent in 84.4% of the DCM group and correlated closely with disability as quantified by the modified Japanese Orthopaedic Association scale. A standardized 10-m walk/run test has the capacity to disclose locomotion abnormalities in NMDCC subjects who lack other clear myelopathic signs and may provide a means of classifying DCM patients according to their degree of disability.

Keywords: degenerative cervical myelopathy; non-myelopathic degenerative cervical cord compression; cervical spinal cord compression; 10-m walk rest; 10-m run test

1. Introduction

Degenerative cervical myelopathy (DCM) is a neurological condition resulting from spinal cord compression arising out of degenerative narrowing of the cervical spinal canal. It constitutes the leading cause of spinal cord dysfunction in adults worldwide [1,2]. Pathological changes include osteophytosis, intervertebral disc bulging, and ligament ossification and hypertrophy, all leading to static and dynamic injury to the spinal cord [3,4]. Early diagnosis and management of DCM are vital to the provision of appropriate care for those living with this condition. Accurate diagnosis requires agreement between clinical and imaging findings. When DCM is suspected, a detailed history and physical examination should be undertaken first [2]. Common presenting symptoms include: numb and/or clumsy hand(s), bilateral arm pain and/or paresthesias, gait disturbance, Lhermitte's sign, and urinary urgency, frequency, and/or incontinence. Objective physical signs of myelopathy include upper motor neuron signs in the upper and/or lower limbs (for example, hyper-reflexia/clonus, pyramidal Hoffmann's, Trömner's or Babinski's signs, spasticity or spastic paresis of any of the extremities—most frequently spastic lower paraparesis), flaccid paresis of one or both upper extremities, atrophy of intrinsic hand muscles, sensory involvement in various distributions in upper or lower extremities, and gait ataxia with positive Romberg sign [5–9].

Some of the objective signs of myelopathy required for the diagnosis of DCM, detected in the course of a detailed, although largely qualitative clinical neurological examination, may serve as comparatively late indicators of cervical cord impairment. Further, degenerative compression of the cervical cord may remain free of any of the symptoms or signs of DCM. This condition–known as "presymptomatic" or "non-myelopathic" degenerative cervical cord compression (NMDCC) is highly prevalent in those above 60 years of age, involving, on average, about 40% of this European/American subpopulation [10,11]. This lies in striking contrast to the prevalence of DCM, estimated at the far lower figure of 2.3% [10]. Quantitative electrophysiological and MRI methods, however, serve to document functional or microstructural impairment in NMDCC patients, indicating that myelopathy precedes the occurrence of commonly detected clinical signs and symptoms. Thus, a diagnosis of DCM based on standard clinical bedside examination may be too late for adequate proactive treatment to be undertaken [3,12,13].

Impaired gait is one of the cardinal symptoms of DCM. Therefore quantitative gait assessment shows promise as an accurate and objective tool in the diagnosis and classification of DCM, with considerable potential in the evaluation of the impacts of therapeutic interventions [14]. Studies utilizing objective gait assessment have largely concentrated upon comparing the gait parameters of healthy individuals with DCM patients, or analyzing the pre-operative status and post-operative outcomes in DCM patients [5,15,16]. Gait impairment has been reported as a strong indication for surgical intervention and may be used as an index in the assessment of post-operative recovery [17]. Certain studies have concluded that a subtle gait disturbance is the most common and the earliest presentation of DCM [5,18,19]. Promoting this somewhat vague observation to the realm of objective assessment thus has the potential to detect early impairment and facilitate timely diagnosis of DCM [14]. There is evidence that individuals with moderate and severe DCM demonstrate slower gait speed and reduced cadence [15,20]. Correlation between quantitative assessment of gait by means of sophisticated spatiotemporal gait parameters and the degree of disability quantified by the modified Japanese Orthopaedic Association (mJOA) score has also been reported [14]. The aim of this study was, therefore, to verify whether an objective and easy-to-use gait analysis employing a standardized 10-m walk and run test is capable of detecting early gait impairment in a practical proportion of NMDCC subjects and reflecting the severity of disability in DCM patients.

2. Materials and Methods

2.1. Design

Single center, cross-sectional observational cohort study.

2.2. Participants

The study sample consisted of three groups: a group of DCM patients, subjects with NMDCC and a control group of healthy volunteers.

All subjects met the following inclusion criteria:

age ≥18 years;
ability to walk at least 10 m without the assistance of another person.
Patients or subjects were excluded if they were affected by any of the following: severe respiratory or cardiac disease hindering walking abilities or safe mobilization;
history of any other neurological disorders with persistent deficit;
symptomatic musculoskeletal problems affecting gait, especially coxarthrosis or gonarthrosis;
symptomatic lumbar spinal stenosis (MRI of the lumbar spine performed only in patients with symptoms or signs suspected of lumbar spinal stenosis);
previous surgical decompression to alleviate DCM.

Approval was granted by the local ethics committee and informed written consent was obtained from all study participants.

DCM patients and NMDCC subjects were recruited from subjects referred between January 2018 and December 2020 to a large tertiary university hospital with a multi-disciplinary center specializing in degenerative compressive neurological syndromes.

DCM patients were considered as those exhibiting generally-accepted clinical and imaging diagnostic criteria for DCM, based on the presence of at least one clinical sign and one clinical symptom of myelopathy revealed by magnetic resonance imaging (MRI) signs of degenerative discogenic and/or spondylogenic cervical spinal cord compression [5,21]. The following symptoms and signs were considered as markers of DCM.

Symptoms: gait disturbance; numb and/or clumsy hands; Lhermitte's sign; bilateral arm paresthesias; weakness of lower or upper extremities; urinary urgency or incontinence.

Signs: corticospinal tract signs: hyperreflexia/clonus; spasticity; pyramidal signs (Babinski's, Trömner's or Hoffmann's signs); spastic paresis of any of the extremities (most frequently, lower limb spastic paraparesis); flaccid paresis of one or both upper extremities; atrophy of the hand muscles; sensory involvement in various distributions in the upper or lower extremities; gait ataxia.

NMDCC patients were considered as those with MRI signs of cervical cord compression and may have exhibited one clinical myelopathic symptom, but it was essential that they were free of clinical myelopathic signs and/or lacked the combination of one clinical symptom and one clinical sign of symptomatic myelopathy required for a diagnosis of DCM.

2.3. MRI Examination and Assessment of Cervical Cord Compression

All subjects underwent examination of the cervical spine provided by a 1.5 Tesla MRI device with a 16-channel head and neck coil. The standardized imaging protocol included conventional pulse sequences in sagittal-T1, -T2 and STIR (short-tau inversion recovery) and axial planes (gradient-echo T2). The clinical status of all patients was blinded to the neuroradiologists who examined the cervical spine MRIs. The imaging criterion for cervical cord compression was defined as a change in spinal cord contour at the level of an intervertebral disc on axial or sagittal MRI scan compared with that at the midpoint levels of neighboring vertebrae [11,12,22].

The control group was made up of healthy volunteers without symptomatic lower limb injuries, neurological disorders, or cardiovascular or respiratory impairment that would hinder gait analysis. All volunteers underwent MRI examination of the cervical spine (either as participants in another epidemiological study or for cervical pain or cervical radiculopathy) that disclosed neither signs of degenerative cervical cord compression nor any cervical cord abnormality [11].

2.4. mJOA Score

The degree of disability in DCM patients was assessed in terms of mJOA score, a generally accepted disability scale. This is an investigator-administered tool used to evaluate neurological function in patients with DCM [23]. It is defined on an 18-point scale that addresses upper (5 points) and lower extremities (7 points, JOA–LE) motor function, sensation (3 points) and micturition (3 points).

2.5. Gait Assessment

Gait assessment was performed in standardized fashion for all participants. After a back-and-forth warming-up walk, each subject was asked to walk a 10-m walkway from a standing start, following the instructions: "Once you are given the instruction to start, you should walk as quickly as possible until you are asked to stop. You are not allowed to run". At least one foot per step had always to make contact with the ground in order for the process to be considered "walking" [24]. Distance was calculated using markings on the track. Next, they were asked to run the same 10-m walkway as fast as they could, if possible. For patients who exhibited unstable gait, the supervision of another person was provided to prevent a possible fall. In the case of serious risk of falling, we omitted the running test. The times taken for the walk/run and the number of steps were counted by an observer and expressed as walking/running time(s), velocity (cm/s), number of steps and cadence (steps/min). No videorecording was performed.

2.6. Statistics

Continuous parameters were summarized as mean (X) ± standard deviation (SD) and/or median (minimum-maximum), or 5th–95th percentiles. Categorical parameters were expressed as absolute and relative frequencies. The normal distribution of continuous variables was investigated by means of graphic tools, the Kolmogorov–Smirnov and the Shapiro–Wilk tests. For assessment of correlation between gait/run parameters and mJOA and mJOA–LE scales in DCM and between gait/run parameters and age in healthy controls, the Spearman's rank sum correlation coefficient and/or the chi-square test were deployed. Differences between the sexes in HC in gait/run parameters were calculated via the Mann–Whitney U test, while differences in gait/run parameters between groups (HC, NMDCC and DCM) were calculated via the Kruskal–Wallis and post-hoc tests with Bonferroni's correction.

3. Results

3.1. Participant Demography

There were 100 healthy volunteers, aged 56.1 ± 13.1 (x ± SD); 55.5 (median); 30–82 (minimum-maximum) years; 52 (52%) were women. The NMDCC group consisted of 126 patients, aged 58.2 ± 9.9; 59; 30–79 years; 65 (51.6%) women. The mJOA score reached 18 points in all healthy volunteers and in vast majority of NMDCC subjects. Slight abnormality of mJOA at the level of 17 points was found in 13 out of 126 NMDCC subjects (10.3%) due to mild lack of stability and/or mild difficulties in attempt to button the shirt. No NMDCC subject had mJOA < 17. Some of them had signs of cervical radiculopathy but in all these 13 NMDCC subjects we found no clear myelopathic signs during routine clinical evaluation including those with subjective gait problems. The DCM group was made up of 45 patients, aged 59.3 ± 11.8; 58; 36–82 years, 20 (45.5%) women. There were no significant differences between the three groups in terms of age or sex proportions ($p > 0.05$). All healthy volunteers and NMDCC subjects were able to perform the 10-m walk and run test, while eleven participants from the DCM group were unable to run and took only the walk test.

3.2. Gait Analysis

3.2.1. Healthy Controls

The values of all parameters displayed normal Gaussian distribution. All parameters correlated highly significantly with age (higher figures with advancing age for time and number of steps, lower values for velocity and cadence for both the walk and the run). They differed between the sexes (higher values of time and number of steps for both walk and run in women, no difference in cadence) (Table 1). Thus, all parameters were assessed independently in four subgroups of healthy controls (men and women aged > 60 and ≤60 years of age) and normal limits were expressed as x + 2SD (time, number of steps) or x-2SD (velocity, cadence). As the values of all the parameters obtained in both groups of patients were distributed non-normally, the 5th and 95th percentiles of values in the HC group were calculated as alternative normal limits (Table 2A).

Table 1. Correlation of walk/run parameters with age and sex in healthy controls.

HC (N = 100)		Correlation with Age: Spearman's Rank Correlation Coefficient: r (p)	Comparison between Sexes: Chi-Square Test: p
		Age	Sex
Time/Velocity (cm/s)	Walk	0.610/−0.610 (<0.001)	0.006 ‡
	Run	0.657/−0.657 (<0.001)	0.001 ‡
Number of steps	Walk	0.497 (<0.001)	<0.001 ‡
	Run	0.353 (<0.001)	<0.001 ‡
Cadence (steps/min)	Walk	−0.268 (0.007)	0.659 †
	Run	−0.564 (<0.001)	0.707 †

HC: Healthy controls; ‡ Significantly higher values in women; † Insignificantly lower values in women.

Table 2. 10-m walking/running test: age- and sex- stratified normal limits (set in the group of healthy controls).

Healthy Controls (N = 100): Subgroups	Parameters: 10 m Walk			
	Time (s)/ Velocity (cm/s)		Number of Steps/ Cadence (Steps/min)	
	X ± SD	Normal limits Time: X+2SD/95.perc. Velocity: X−2SD/5.perc.	X ± SD	Normal Limits N.steps: X+2SD/95.perc. Cadence: X−2SD/5.perc.
Men ≤ 60 years N = 27	4.2 ± 0.5/ 238.3 ± 30.9	5.2/5.3 176.5/186.9	10.7 ± 1.2 153.6 ± 22.8	13.1/13.0 108.0/125.2
Men > 60 years N = 21	5.0 ± 0.8/ 198.8 ± 37.3	6.6/6.4 124.2/145.0	12.8 ± 2.1 158.3 ± 32.3	17.0/16.0 93.7/103.9
Women ≤ 60 years N = 31	4.5 ± 0.6/ 221.3 ± 28.6	5.7/5.6 164.1/178.5	12.2 ± 1.3 162.3 ± 25.1	14.8/14.5 112.1/129.4
Women > 60 years N = 21	6.1 ± 1.0/ 165.8 ± 30.2	8.1/8.1 105.4/110.0	14.6 ± 2.4 143.8 ± 24.4	19.4/18.0 95.0/101.5
Healthy Controls (N = 100): Subgroups	Parameters: 10 m Run			
	Time (s)/ Velocity (cm/s)		Number of Steps/ Cadence (Steps/min)	
	X ± SD	Normal Limits Time: X+2SD/95.perc. Velocity: X−2SD/5.perc.	X ± SD	Normal Limits N.steps: X+2SD/95.perc. Cadence: X−2SD/5.perc.
Men ≤ 60 years N = 27	2.6 ± 0.3/ 383.7 ± 58.7	3.2/3.3 266.3/304.0	8.7 ± 1.3 199.1 ± 27.6	11.3/11.0 143.9/151.3
Men > 60 years N = 21	3.4 ± 0.7/ 296.8 ± 55.8	4.8/4.2 185.2/237.0	9.4 ± 1.0 167.9 ± 29.5	11.4/11.2 108.9/116.9
Women ≤ 60 years N = 31	3.0 ± 0.4/ 336.2 ± 40.2	3.8/3.6 255.8/279.0	9.7 ± 1.2 193.6 ± 21.2	12.1/12.0 151.2/158.4
Women > 60 years N = 21	4.2 ± 1.0/ 238.2 ± 51.0	6.2/6.3 136.2/158.0	10.6 ± 1.0 155.9 ± 31.2	12.6/12.0 93.5/96.8

X: mean; SD: standard deviation; Perc.: percentile; N: Number.

10 m Walk—Number (Proportion) of Abnormal Values [&]			
Group Parameter	NMDCC (N = 126)	DCM (N = 45)	Comparison of the groups: chi-square test (p)
Time	57 (45.2%)/60 (47.6%)	31 (68.9%)/32 (71.1%)	0.006/0.007
Velocity	57 (45.2%)/60 (47.6%)	31 (68.9%)/32 (71.1%)	0.006/0.007
Number of steps	21 (16.7%)/22 (17.5%)	14 (31.1%)/23 (51.1%)	0.04/<0.001
Cadence	6 (4.8%)/33 (26.2%)	5 (11.1%)/20 (44.4%)	0.136/0.02
Any abnormality (walk)	59 (46.8%)/66 (52.4%)	32 (71.1%)/34 (75.5%)	0.005/0.007
10 m Run—Number (Proportion) of Abnormal Values [&]			
Group Parameter	NMDCC (N = 126)	DCM (N = 34) [#]	Comparison of the groups: chi-square test (p)
Time	53 (42.1%)/59 (46.8%)	23 (67.6%)/24 (70.6%)	0.008/0.014
Velocity	53 (42.1%)/59 (46.8%)	23 (67.6%)/24 (70.6%)	0.008/0.014
Number of steps	41 (32.5%)/41 (32.5%)	22 (64.7%)/22 (64.7%)	<0.001/<0.001
Cadence	24 (19.0%)/42 (33.3%)	8 (23.5%)/15 (44.1%)	0.562/0.244
Any abnormality (run)	72 (57.1%)/82 (65.1%)	27 (79.4%)/28 (82.4%)	0.018/0.054
Any abnormality (walk and/or run)	84 (66.7%)/91 (72.2%)	38 (84.4%)/40 (88.9%)	0.024/0.023

NMDCC: Non-myelopathic degenerative cervical cord compression; DCM: Degenerative cervical myelopathy; [&]: number (proportion) of abnormalities calculated for cut-offs set as X ± 2SD/5. or 95.perc.; [#]: eleven DCM patients were not able to run.

3.2.2. NMDCC

Summaries of gait parameters in NMDCC and DCM patients appear in Table 3 and Figure 1a–c. Significant differences were evident in all gait parameters among all the groups studied ($p < 0.001$; Table 3). In comparison with healthy controls (Table 3), NMDCC patients took longer to complete the ten meters at a run or walking, moved at lower speeds and required higher numbers of steps. Abnormality within the walking parameters appeared in 46.8% of NMDCC subjects. Time/velocity exhibited the highest sensitivity (45.2%), followed by number of steps (16.7%), and cadence (4.8%). All these abnormalities were disclosed in the course of investigation of time and number of steps (Table 2B).

Table 3. Summary statistics of walk/run test parameters in the groups studied.

Parameters Groups	HC	NMDCC	DCM	Kruskal–Wallis p Value *
	X (SD); Median (Min.–Max.)			
Walk time (s)	4.9 (1.3); 4.7 (3.3–13.6) [a]	6.2 (1.1); 6.0 (4.2–9.9) [b]	7.2 (2.5); 7.0 (5.0–18.0) [c]	<0.001
Walk velocity (cm/s)	209.0 (42.5); 212.5 (73–306) [a]	165.9 (27.2); 167 (101–238) [b]	139.6 (34.2); 150 (56–200) [c]	<0.001
Walk steps (No.)	12.4 (2.2); 12 (9–23) [a]	13.2 (1.9); 13 (8–18) [b]	14.8 (2.9); 15 (10–23) [c]	<0.001
Walk cadence (steps/min.)	155.2 (29.2); 152.9 (100.0–263.4) [a]	130.7 (20.6); 130 (53.3–228.6) [b]	120.7 (18.0); 120 (63.3–159.4) [b]	<0.001
Run time	3.3 (0.9); 3.1 (2–8) [a]	4.1 (0.9); 4.0 (2.4–6.7) [b]	4.6 (1.4); 4.8 (2.5–9.4) [c]	<0.001
Run velocity (cm/s)	320.1 (74.1); 323.5 (125–497) [a]	255.9 (56.5); 250 (149–416) [b]	219.0 (61.7); 221 (150–400) [c]	<0.001
Run steps (No.)	9.6 (1.4); 10 (6–12) [a]	11.3 (2.4); 11 (7–18) [b]	12.8 (3.0); 13 (8–22) [c]	<0.001
Run cadence (steps/min.)	181.8 (33.3); 182.6 (75.0–264.0) [a]	167.1 (25.9); 169.4 (114.3–266.7) [b]	160.2 (20.0); 161.2 (108.5–200.0) [b]	<0.001

HC: Healthy controls; NMDCC: non-myelopathic cervical cord compression; DCM: degenerative cervical myelopathy; X: mean; SD: standard deviation; * p-value represents comparison of all the groups (Kruskal–Wallis test); post hoc tests: a,b,c—same letters marking values of categories within any given row denote groups that are not mutually statistically different.

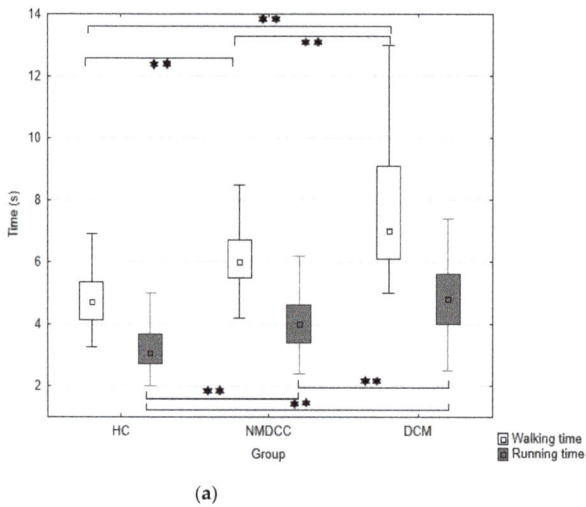

(a)

Figure 1. Cont.

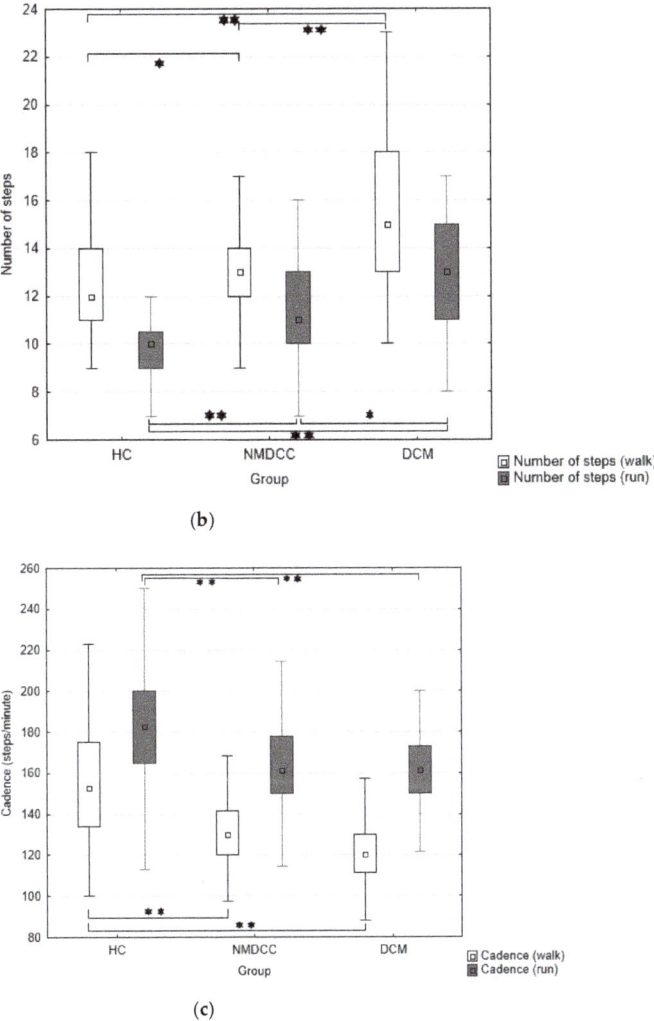

(b)

(c)

Figure 1. Box-plots and whisker-plots expressing median, lower and upper quartiles, minimum and maximum (without outliers) of walking/running time (**a**), number of steps taken during walk and run (**b**) and cadence of walk and run (**c**) in healthy controls (HC), non-myelopathic degenerative cervical compression (NMDCC) patients and those with degenerative cervical myelopathy (DCM). * $p < 0.05$; ** $p < 0.01$.

Similarly, abnormality within the run parameters appeared in 57.1% of subjects, with the highest sensitivity exhibited by time/velocity (42.1%), followed by number of steps (32.5%) and cadence (19.0%). Again, all abnormalities were disclosed in the course of investigation of time/velocity and number of steps (Table 2B).

Abnormality of walk and/or run test parameters appeared in 66.7% of NMDCC patients (Table 2B).

3.2.3. DCM

DCM patients exhibited significantly longer times/lower velocities, higher numbers of steps and lower cadence during both the walk and run tests in comparison with both healthy controls and NMDCC patients (Table 3, Figure 1a–c). Abnormality of walk parameters appeared in 71.1% of DCM patients, with the highest sensitivity for time/velocity (68.9%), followed by number of steps (31.1%) and cadence (11.1%) All abnormalities were disclosed in the course of investigation of time and number of steps (Table 2B). Similarly, abnormality of run parameters appeared in 79.4% of subjects, with the highest sensitivity for time/velocity (67.6%), followed by number of steps (64.7%) and cadence (23.5%). Again, all abnormalities were disclosed in the course of investigation of time/velocity and number of steps (Table 2B). Abnormality of walk and/or run test parameters appeared in 84.4% of DCM patients (Table 2B).

Time/velocity and number of steps as assessed from walk and run tests correlated significantly with both mJOA and mJOA–LE scales (Table 4). In addition, cadence of walk correlated with both mJOA and mJOA–LE scores, although this did not hold true for running (Table 4).

Table 4. Correlation between severity of disability and walk/run parameters in DCM patients.

DCM Patients (N = 45)		Spearman's Rank Correlation Coefficient r (p)	
		mJOA:	mJOA LE
Time (s)	Walk	−0.766 (<<0.001)	−0.790 (<<0.001)
	Run	−0.505 (0.002)	−0.568 (<0.001)
Velocity (cm/s)	Walk	0.766 (<<0.001)	0.790 (<<0.001)
	Run	0.505 (0.002)	0.568 (<0.001)
Number of steps	Walk	−0.589 (<0.001)	−0.649 (<<0.001)
	Run	−0.485 (0.004)	−0.471 (0.005)
Cadence (steps/min)	Walk	0.514 (<0.001)	0.483 (<0.001)
	Run	0.173 (0.329)	0.239 (0.173)

DCM: degenerative cervical myelopathy; mJOA: modified Japanese Orthopaedic Association scale; mJOA LE: modified Japanese Orthopaedic Association subscale for lower extremities; <<0.001: p value less than 10^{-6}.

4. Discussion

This is, to the best of our knowledge, the first study to show that gait analysis utilizing a standardized and simple 10-m walk and run test reflects gait impairment not only in DCM patients, but in a substantial proportion (66.7%) of individuals with NMDCC. Gait impairment constitutes the most prominent clinical manifestation of cervical myelopathy, and thus its amelioration may have a substantial impact on the recovery of patient functionality [25,26].

In routine clinical practice, observational gait analysis is by far the most commonly used approach to evaluating gait disturbance in DCM, including mJOA score. The accuracy and consistency of essentially subjective observation are however, questionable, particularly for subtle gait changes [27]. Timed walk tests are more sensitive to change and are known to be valid and reliable in DCM [28], but they provide no information concerning the underlying gait parameters that have contributed to the measured speed [29]. Recently, there has been a resurgence of research interest in applying quantitative and objective gait analysis to the evaluation of patients with DCM [25,26]. Gait analysis is now largely mostly performed on the basis of a specific movement protocol that includes evaluation of the range of motion of the lower extremities, of muscle strength, and of balance differences [15,25]. An assessment may also be obtained from three-dimensional computer analysis, including a number of spatiotemporal kinetic and kinematic parameters, all of which have been demonstrated as impaired in DCM patients [26,30]. Kalsi-Ryan et al. recently presented a study that found significant differences between control subjects and patients with mild, moderate, and severe DCM, and characterized specific differences in gait parameters between severity subtypes of DCM [14]. These computer analyses, however, are hardly practical in the context of clinical neurological practice. Thus, this study was based on finding an easy and reliable test, readily available to the clinical neurologist. The protocol employed was simple and easy to reproduce, based on the straightforward instruction "walk as fast as possible, but do not run", and followed by a run test (if possible). This contrasts with other protocols in which the walk has been undertaken at a subject selected pace.

The rationale to evaluate both walking and running abilities in degenerative cervical cord compression subjects is based on the fact that walking and running are generally considered as distinct gait modes, with strikingly different mechanics and energetics. Having the ability to walk does not mean that the individual has the ability to run, as running requires greater balance, muscle strength and greater joint range of movement [31,32]. As expected, 11 out of 45 DCM patients (24.4%) of DCM patients were not able to run, but running test disclosed abnormality in an additional 13% of DCM patients (and in 19.9% of NMDCC subjects) with normal walking test, justifying thus the usefulness of its use.

This study confirms that gait analysis based on a clinically practical and easily administered test is a highly sensitive approach to the disclosure of gait disturbance in DCM patients. The results were in close correlation, especially in terms of walking and running time and the number of steps taken, with the mJOA scale and mJOA–LE, its subscale for the lower extremities, the most widely-employed subjective scale for grading severity of disability. Abnormalities in gait parameters, however, were also found in a substantial proportion of NMDCC patients; further, this cohort exhibited significant differences in all the parameters assessed when compared with age-adjusted healthy controls. A number of reasons for these findings may be suggested. Firstly, DCM diagnosis is based on the presence of clinical symptoms and signs (at least one) of myelopathy, although some patients may complain of a certain degree of gait disturbance in the absence of clear, objective, physical signs of myelopathy [5,6]. In the light of current criteria, a diagnosis of DCM is critically dependent on the clinical expertise of the examining specialist; an objective approach to gait assessment may well serve as an additional clinical tool, enabling timely and reproducible establishment of a DCM diagnosis. Secondly, the approach employed herein based its test protocol of gait analysis on a fast walk and a run where feasible, rather than the usual assessment of a slow walk. The results arising out of a fast walk may be more sensitive than those of a "regular" walk. Of course, a run test is not suitable for DCM patients with moderate-to-severe disability. Nevertheless, in that part of the cohort herein capable of independent locomotion, 75.6% of DCM patients and 100% of those with NMDCC proved able to run, and the running test disclosed additional abnormalities in a quarter (25.5%) of them. Among the parameters assessed, not surprisingly, walking and running times showed the highest sensitivity, followed by number of steps, while cadence of walk/run did not disclose any abnormalities in patients returning normal times and numbers of steps and did not prove immediately useful. Thirdly, the parameters of walk and run correlated closely with age and sex, and therefore normal limits were adjusted for these two demographic parameters. This might have enhanced the sensitivity of the test.

Early recognition and treatment of DCM, before the onset of spinal cord damage, is essential for optimal outcomes. Unfortunately, despite the lack of any study showing a benefit of a prophylactic surgical decompression in NMDCC, some spondylosurgeons recommend and perform such intervention. Recommendations based on expert opinion and longitudinal studies on natural course of NMDCC and risk factors for progression to DCM [12,22,33] generally recommend consideration of surgical treatment in those patients who present with clinical or electrophysiological evidence of cervical radicular dysfunction or central conduction deficits disclosed by electrophysiological examination and are thus at higher risk for developing myelopathy [34,35]. There is also no clear agreement on the conservative treatment of both NMDCC and mild DCM patients. Intermittent immobilization in a cervical collar and "low-risk" activity modification together with close observation of both mild DCM patients and NMDCC subjects with high risk for progression into symptomatic DCM are usually recommended.

Limitations of the Study

Despite the use of age and sex-adjusted normal values and the exclusion of subjects with known tandem lumbar spinal stenosis or musculoskeletal comorbidities that might have interfered with gait, a higher tendency towards degenerative changes in the lumbar spine or hip joints in patients with degenerative cervical cord compression is to be anticipated [36]. This may lead to results indicating more severe impairment in a performance-oriented test of this nature. Moreover, such a test is prone to be influenced by the motivation of the subject tested. Exclusion of patients with symptomatic lumbar spinal stenosis or musculoskeletal comorbidities that are quite frequent in older population and especially in DCM patients eliminates significant proportion of DCM patients in particular and decreases external validity of the test. Our study was performed in the Caucasian (European) population with very low prevalence of the ossification of the posterior longitudinal ligament and the results thus may be of limited value in evaluation of other populations of patients with degenerative cervical cord compression. The methodology to measure the times taken for the walk/run and to count the number of steps manually by an observer is easy to implement in the clinical setting, but might hypothetically serve as a potential source of error.

5. Conclusions

In conclusion, the main benefit of a standardized 10-m walk/run test in comparison to already used scoring systems, such as mJOA score, is its objective and quantitative character and sensitivity to mild gait impairment due to myelopathy. It has the capacity to disclose locomotor abnormalities in the early stages of degenerative cervical cord compression that may be confirmed as another risk factor for progression into symptomatic DCM in future longitudinal studies. Furthermore, it may support clinical diagnosis of DCM in case of vague clinical myelopathic symptoms and signs and could be employed in routine clinical practice as a tool to evaluate clinical course or effect of therapy in already diagnosed DCM.

Author Contributions: Conceptualization, Z.K.J. and J.B.; methodology, J.B.; software, E.V., T.S.; validation, Z.K.J., E.V. and J.B.; formal analysis, Z.K.S. and J.B.; investigation, Z.K.J. and Z.K.S.; resources, Z.K.J. and J.B.; data processing, E.V., T.S.; writing—original draft preparation, Z.K.J.; writing—review and editing, J.B. and Z.K.S.; visualization, E.V., T.S.; supervision, J.B.; project administration, J.B.; funding acquisition, J.B. All authors have read and agreed to the published version of the manuscript.

Funding: This research was funded by the Czech Health Research Council, grant ref. NV 18-04-00159, by the Ministry of Health of the Czech Republic project for conceptual development in research organizations, ref. 65269705 (University Hospital, Brno, Czech Republic), and by Specific Research project ref. MUNI/A/1600/2020 provided by Masaryk University Brno.

Institutional Review Board Statement: The study was conducted according to the guidelines of the Declaration of Helsinki, and approved by the Ethics Committee in each institution.

Informed Consent Statement: Informed consent was obtained from all subjects involved in the study.

Data Availability Statement: The data presented in this study are available on request from the corresponding author. The data are not publicly available.

Conflicts of Interest: The authors declare that they have no conflict of interest.

References

1. Rhee, J.M.; Heflin, J.A.; Hamasaki, T.; Freedman, B. Prevalence of Physical Signs in Cervical Myelopathy: A Prospective, Controlled Study. *Spine* **2009**, *34*, 890–895. [CrossRef]
2. Badhiwala, J.H.; Ahuja, C.S.; Akbar, M.A.; Witiw, C.D.; Nassiri, F.; Furlan, J.C.; Curt, A.; Wilson, J.R.; Fehlings, M.G. Degenerative Cervical Myelopathy—Update and Future Directions. *Nat. Rev. Neurol.* **2020**, *16*, 108–124. [CrossRef]
3. Keřkovský, M.; Bednařík, J.; Jurová, B.; Dušek, L.; Kadaňka, Z.; Kadaňka, Z.; Němec, M.; Kovaľová, I.; Šprláková-Puková, A.; Mechl, M. Spinal Cord MR Diffusion Properties in Patients with Degenerative Cervical Cord Compression. *J. Neuroimaging* **2017**, *27*, 149–157. [CrossRef] [PubMed]

4. Nouri, A.; Tetreault, L.; Singh, A.; Karadimas, S.K.; Fehlings, M.G. Degenerative Cervical Myelopathy: Epidemiology, Genetics, and Pathogenesis. *Spine* **2015**, *40*, E675–E693. [CrossRef] [PubMed]
5. Kalsi-Ryan, S.; Karadimas, S.K.; Fehlings, M.G. Cervical Spondylotic Myelopathy: The Clinical Phenomenon and the Current Pathobiology of an Increasingly Prevalent and Devastating Disorder. *Neuroscientist* **2013**, *19*, 409–421. [CrossRef] [PubMed]
6. Tetreault, L.; Goldstein, C.L.; Arnold, P.; Harrop, J.; Hilibrand, A.; Nouri, A.; Fehlings, M.G. Degenerative Cervical Myelopathy: A Spectrum of Related Disorders Affecting the Aging Spine. *Neurosurgery* **2015**, *77* (Suppl. 4), S51–S67. [CrossRef]
7. Harrop, J.S.; Naroji, S.; Maltenfort, M.; Anderson, D.G.; Albert, T.; Ratliff, J.K.; Ponnappan, R.K.; Rihn, J.A.; Smith, H.E.; Hilibrand, A.; et al. Cervical Myelopathy: A Clinical and Radiographic Evaluation and Correlation to Cervical Spondylotic Myelopathy. *Spine* **2010**, *35*, 620–624. [CrossRef]
8. Tracy, J.A.; Bartleson, J.D. Cervical Spondylotic Myelopathy. *Neurologist* **2010**, *16*, 176–187. [CrossRef] [PubMed]
9. Davies, B.M.; Mowforth, O.D.; Smith, E.K.; Kotter, M.R. Degenerative Cervical Myelopathy. *BMJ* **2018**, *360*. [CrossRef] [PubMed]
10. Smith, S.S.; Stewart, M.E.; Davies, B.M.; Kotter, M.R.N. The Prevalence of Asymptomatic and Symptomatic Spinal Cord Compression on Magnetic Resonance Imaging: A Systematic Review and Meta-Analysis. *Glob. Spine J.* **2020**, 2192568220934496. [CrossRef]
11. Kovalova, I.; Kerkovsky, M.; Kadanka, Z.; Kadanka, Z.; Nemec, M.; Jurova, B.; Dusek, L.; Jarkovsky, J.; Bednarik, J. Prevalence and Imaging Characteristics of Nonmyelopathic and Myelopathic Spondylotic Cervical Cord Compression. *Spine* **2016**, *41*, 1908–1916. [CrossRef] [PubMed]
12. Bednarik, J.; Kadanka, Z.; Dusek, L.; Kerkovsky, M.; Vohanka, S.; Novotny, O.; Urbanek, I.; Kratochvilova, D. Presymptomatic Spondylotic Cervical Myelopathy: An Updated Predictive Model. *Eur. Spine J.* **2008**, *17*, 421–431. [CrossRef]
13. Labounek, R.; Valošek, J.; Horák, T.; Svátková, A.; Bednařík, P.; Vojtíšek, L.; Horáková, M.; Nestrašil, I.; Lenglet, C.; Cohen-Adad, J.; et al. HARDI-ZOOMit Protocol Improves Specificity to Microstructural Changes in Presymptomatic Myelopathy. *Sci. Rep.* **2020**, *10*, 17529. [CrossRef]
14. Kalsi-Ryan, S.; Rienmueller, A.C.; Riehm, L.; Chan, C.; Jin, D.; Martin, A.R.; Badhiwala, J.H.; Akbar, M.A.; Massicotte, E.M.; Fehlings, M.G. Quantitative Assessment of Gait Characteristics in Degenerative Cervical Myelopathy: A Prospective Clinical Study. *J. Clin. Med.* **2020**, *9*, 752. [CrossRef] [PubMed]
15. Kuhtz-Buschbeck, J.P.; Jöhnk, K.; Mäder, S.; Stolze, H.; Mehdorn, M. Analysis of Gait in Cervical Myelopathy. *Gait Posture* **1999**, *9*, 184–189. [CrossRef]
16. Singh, A.; Choi, D.; Crockard, A. Use of Walking Data in Assessing Operative Results for Cervical Spondylotic Myelopathy: Long-Term Follow-up and Comparison with Controls. *Spine* **2009**, *34*, 1296–1300. [CrossRef]
17. Zheng, C.-F.; Liu, Y.-C.; Hu, Y.-C.; Xia, Q.; Miao, J.; Zhang, J.-D.; Zhang, K. Correlations of Japanese Orthopaedic Association Scoring Systems with Gait Parameters in Patients with Degenerative Spinal Diseases. *Orthop. Surg.* **2016**, *8*, 447–453. [CrossRef]
18. Gorter, K. Influence of Laminectomy on the Course of Cervical Myelopathy. *Acta Neurochir.* **1976**, *33*, 265–281. [CrossRef] [PubMed]
19. Lunsford, L.D.; Bissonette, D.J.; Zorub, D.S. Anterior Surgery for Cervical Disc Disease. Part 2: Treatment of Cervical Spondylotic Myelopathy in 32 Cases. *J. Neurosurg.* **1980**, *53*, 12–19. [CrossRef]
20. Kim, C.R.; Yoo, J.Y.; Lee, S.H.; Lee, D.H.; Rhim, S.C. Gait Analysis for Evaluating the Relationship between Increased Signal Intensity on T2-Weighted Magnetic Resonance Imaging and Gait Function in Cervical Spondylotic Myelopathy. *Arch. Phys. Med. Rehabil.* **2010**, *91*, 1587–1592. [CrossRef]
21. Martin, A.R.; De Leener, B.; Cohen-Adad, J.; Cadotte, D.W.; Nouri, A.; Wilson, J.R.; Tetreault, L.; Crawley, A.P.; Mikulis, D.J.; Ginsberg, H.; et al. Can Microstructural MRI Detect Subclinical Tissue Injury in Subjects with Asymptomatic Cervical Spinal Cord Compression? A Prospective Cohort Study. *BMJ Open* **2018**, *8*. [CrossRef] [PubMed]
22. Kadanka, Z.; Adamova, B.; Kerkovsky, M.; Kadanka, Z.; Dusek, L.; Jurova, B.; Vlckova, E.; Bednarik, J. Predictors of Symptomatic Myelopathy in Degenerative Cervical Spinal Cord Compression. *Brain Behav.* **2017**, *7*, e00797. [CrossRef] [PubMed]
23. Benzel, E.C.; Lancon, J.; Kesterson, L.; Hadden, T. Cervical Laminectomy and Dentate Ligament Section for Cervical Spondylotic Myelopathy. *J. Spinal Disord.* **1991**, *4*, 286–295. [CrossRef] [PubMed]
24. Srinivasan, M.; Ruina, A. Computer Optimization of a Minimal Biped Model Discovers Walking and Running. *Nature* **2006**, *439*, 72–75. [CrossRef]
25. Moorthy, R.K.; Bhattacharji, S.; Thayumanasamy, G.; Rajshekhar, V. Quantitative Changes in Gait Parameters after Central Corpectomy for Cervical Spondylotic Myelopathy. *J. Neurosurg. Spine* **2005**, *2*, 418–424. [CrossRef]
26. Malone, A.; Meldrum, D.; Bolger, C. Three-Dimensional Gait Analysis Outcomes at 1 Year Following Decompressive Surgery for Cervical Spondylotic Myelopathy. *Eur. Spine J.* **2015**, *24*, 48–56. [CrossRef] [PubMed]
27. Williams, G.; Morris, M.E.; Schache, A.; McCrory, P. Observational Gait Analysis in Traumatic Brain Injury: Accuracy of Clinical Judgment. *Gait Posture* **2009**, *29*, 454–459. [CrossRef] [PubMed]
28. Singh, A.; Crockard, H.A. Quantitative Assessment of Cervical Spondylotic Myelopathy by a Simple Walking Test. *Lancet* **1999**, *354*, 370–373. [CrossRef]
29. Yavuzer, G.; Oken, O.; Elhan, A.; Stam, H.J. Repeatability of Lower Limb Three-Dimensional Kinematics in Patients with Stroke. *Gait Posture* **2008**, *27*, 31–35. [CrossRef]
30. Nishimura, H.; Endo, K.; Suzuki, H.; Tanaka, H.; Shishido, T.; Yamamoto, K. Gait Analysis in Cervical Spondylotic Myelopathy. *Asian Spine J.* **2015**, *9*, 321–326. [CrossRef]

31. Cappellini, G.; Ivanenko, Y.P.; Poppele, R.E.; Lacquaniti, F. Motor Patterns in Human Walking and Running. *J. Neurophysiol.* **2006**, *95*, 3426–3437. [CrossRef] [PubMed]
32. Novacheck, T.F. The Biomechanics of Running. *Gait Posture* **1998**, *7*, 77–95. [CrossRef]
33. Bednařík, J.; Sládková, D.; Kadaňka, Z.; Dušek, L.; Keřkovský, M.; Voháňka, S.; Novotný, O.; Urbánek, I.; Němec, M. Are Subjects with Spondylotic Cervical Cord Encroachment at Increased Risk of Cervical Spinal Cord Injury after Minor Trauma? *J. Neurol. Neurosurg. Psychiatry* **2011**, *82*, 779–781. [CrossRef]
34. Wilson, J.R.; Barry, S.; Fischer, D.J.; Skelly, A.C.; Arnold, P.M.; Riew, K.D.; Shaffrey, C.I.; Traynelis, V.C.; Fehlings, M.G. Frequency, Timing, and Predictors of Neurological Dysfunction in the Nonmyelopathic Patient with Cervical Spinal Cord Compression, Canal Stenosis, and/or Ossification of the Posterior Longitudinal Ligament. *Spine* **2013**, *38* (Suppl. 1), S37–S54. [CrossRef] [PubMed]
35. Fehlings, M.G.; Tetreault, L.A.; Riew, K.D.; Middleton, J.W.; Aarabi, B.; Arnold, P.M.; Brodke, D.S.; Burns, A.S.; Carette, S.; Chen, R.; et al. A Clinical Practice Guideline for the Management of Patients with Degenerative Cervical Myelopathy: Recommendations for Patients With Mild, Moderate, and Severe Disease and Nonmyelopathic Patients With Evidence of Cord Compression. *Global Spine J.* **2017**, *7* (Suppl. 3), 70S–83S. [CrossRef] [PubMed]
36. Adamova, B.; Bednarik, J.; Andrasinova, T.; Kovalova, I.; Kopacik, R.; Jabornik, M.; Kerkovsky, M.; Jakubcova, B.; Jarkovsky, J. Does Lumbar Spinal Stenosis Increase the Risk of Spondylotic Cervical Spinal Cord Compression? *Eur. Spine J.* **2015**, *24*, 2946–2953. [CrossRef] [PubMed]

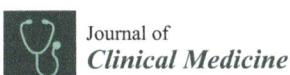

Article

Spinal Cord Morphology in Degenerative Cervical Myelopathy Patients; Assessing Key Morphological Characteristics Using Machine Vision Tools

Kalum Ost [1], W. Bradley Jacobs [2,3,†], Nathan Evaniew [3,4,†], Julien Cohen-Adad [5,6,7], David Anderson [8] and David W. Cadotte [1,3,4,8,*]

1. Hotchkiss Brain Institute, Cumming School of Medicine, University of Calgary, Calgary, AB T2N 1N4, Canada; kalum.ost@ucalgary.ca
2. Department of Clinical Neurosciences, Section of Neurosurgery, Cumming School of Medicine, University of Calgary, Calgary, AB T2N 1N4, Canada; wbjacobs@ucalgary.ca
3. Combined Orthopedic and Neurosurgery Spine Program, University of Calgary, Calgary, AB T2N 1N4, Canada; Nathan.Evaniew@albertahealthservices.ca
4. Section of Orthopaedic Surgery, Department of Surgery, University of Calgary, Calgary, AB T2N 1N4, Canada
5. NeuroPoly Lab, Institute of Biomedical Engineering, Polytechnique Montrèal, Montrèal, QC H3T 1J4, Canada; jcohen@polymtl.ca
6. Functional Neuroimaging Unit, CRIUGM, Universitè de Montrèal, Montrèal, QC H3T 1J4, Canada
7. Mila-Quebec AI Institute, Montrèal, QC T2N 1N4, Canada
8. Department of Biochemistry and Molecular Biology, Cumming School of Medicine, University of Calgary, Calgary, AB T2N 1N4, Canada; david.anderson1@ucalgary.ca
* Correspondence: david.cadotte@ucalgary.ca; Tel.: +403-944-3490
† These authors contributed equally to this work.

Abstract: Despite Degenerative Cervical Myelopathy (DCM) being the most common form of spinal cord injury, effective methods to evaluate patients for its presence and severity are only starting to appear. Evaluation of patient images, while fast, is often unreliable; the pathology of DCM is complex, and clinicians often have difficulty predicting patient prognosis. Automated tools, such as the Spinal Cord Toolbox (SCT), show promise, but remain in the early stages of development. To evaluate the current state of an SCT automated process, we applied it to MR imaging records from 328 DCM patients, using the modified Japanese Orthopedic Associate scale as a measure of DCM severity. We found that the metrics extracted from these automated methods are insufficient to reliably predict disease severity. Such automated processes showed potential, however, by highlighting trends and barriers which future analyses could, with time, overcome. This, paired with findings from other studies with similar processes, suggests that additional non-imaging metrics could be added to achieve diagnostically relevant predictions. Although modeling techniques such as these are still in their infancy, future models of DCM severity could greatly improve automated clinical diagnosis, communications with patients, and patient outcomes.

Keywords: degenerative cervical myelopathy; personalized medicine; machine learning; spinal cord

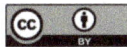

1. Introduction

Degenerative Cervical Myelopathy (DCM) is the most common form of spinal cord injury worldwide [1], and is associated with substantial impairment of patient quality of life. DCM manifests in patients as progressively worsening pain, numbness, dexterity loss, gait imbalance, and sphincter dysfunction [2], the result of degenerative compression of the cervical spinal cord. Timely diagnosis of DCM is critically important to minimize neurological deterioration, but is challenging because the symptomatology of DCM overlaps with many other common diseases [3]. DCM symptoms often do not appear until neurological damage has already occurred [4,5], and patients who receive treatment after a longer prodrome of neurological deficits may have worse long-term prognosis [6]. Surgical decompression is the mainstay of treatment, with 1.6 per 100,000 people requiring surgery to treat DCM in their lifetime [7]. In addition to a thorough history and physical examination, routine MRI of the cervical spine is an essential diagnostic test that confirms the presence and extent of spinal cord compression [8].

Once DCM has been diagnosed, patients and their care provides must decide whether to proceed with surgical treatment via surgical decompression. Predictive outcome modeling through computationally aided MRI analysis in this scenario is an attractive possibility, but is currently in its infancy. Current analysis tools include the Functional Magnetic Resonance Imaging of the Brain (FMRIB) Software Library [9], Statistical Parametric Maps [10], and the Medical Image NetCDF format [11]. These tools, however, tend to be generalized and lack the specificity required for spinal cord analyses. Although logistic regression models have been tested and have demonstrated limited success [12], there remains room for improvement. Spinal cord segmentation analysis using qMRI imaging data of patients by tools such as the Spinal Cord Toolbox (SCT) [13] has recently been shown to provide improved predictive power [14], but these tools tend to break down when analyzing damaged spinal cords [15]. Studies which did find success in predicting myelopathic outcomes opted instead to manually inspect the spinal cord [4,16] or manually correct the output of automated analyses [17], reducing the benefits these automated processes provide. To optimize their use, it is imperative to evaluate the extent and source of these limitations. To this end, we assessed the SCT software package for its analytical capabilities in predicting disease severity of DCM. We applied this software package to routinely acquired MRI images from a subset of patients who went on to receive clinical diagnoses of DCM across Alberta, Canada.

2. Methods

2.1. Computational Tools Used

The program versions for the methods used below were as follows: `Spinal Cord Toolbox, v.5.0.1` [13], `3D Slicer v.4.10.2` [18], `SciKit-Learn v.0.23.2` [19], `SciPy v.1.5.2` [20], `matplotlib v.3.3.2` [21], `seaborn v.0.11.1` [22], `numpy v.1.19.2` [23], and `pandas v.1.2.0` [24]. As *CovBat* was still in development at time of this paper's publication [25], its state at the time of this analysis can be replicated by using the GitHub commit 23a0429, available at https://github.com/andy1764/CovBat_Harmonization/commit/23a0429c2a81e7682da94ff2d0f5e634ab91b429 (accessed on 9 June 2020).

2.2. Data Preparation

We identified cervical spine MRI images that were used to diagnose 328 patients with DCM who were serially enrolled in the Canadian Spine Outcomes and Research (CSORN) longitudinal registry (initiated in 2016, ongoing [8]). Data were obtained from multiple clinics across the province of Alberta (Figure 1); each clinic had their own procedures and protocols, resulting in variation in image quality and resolution. This was accounted for, to some extent, via batch effect compensation (see Section 2.4).

Our sample set consisted of a diverse number of imaging methodologies. For example, 257 of our 328 patients records used a magnetic field strength of 1.5T, while the remaining 71 used a field strength of 3T. In general, images were also acquired at a relatively low resolution, with T2 weighted, sagittally oriented images primarily with a center-to-center slice thickness of 3 mm (318 images), 2 mm (52 images), with the remaining images (21 images) ranging from 0.9 mm to 5 mm. Axially oriented T2 weighted images were more diverse, but also relatively low resolution: they primarily consisted of images with a 2.5 mm (164 images), 4 mm (128 images), 3 mm (124 images), and 2 mm (90 images) slice thickness, with the remainder varying between 1.4 mm and 5 mm (54 images).

Digital Imaging and Communications in Medicine (DICOM) data were evaluated, anonymized, and converted into the NIfTI file format, resulting in 1335 total MRI sequences. Imaging files were then manually inspected to confirm data integrity (presence of required files and lack of substantial imaging motion or aliasing), and converted into a BIDS-compliant format [26]. This resulted in 3 patient records and 151 imaging files being excluded, leaving the dataset at 1184 imaging files across 325 patient records. The majority of files dropped were excluded due to excessive noise being present in the image or motion artifacts/patient movement between samples. Other reasons for image exclusion were mislabeling (the MRI images being of the tubular spine, rather than the cervical spine) and insufficient slice count (resulting in the inability for segmentation algorithms to make accurate estimates of spinal cord metrics). Axial images were particularly low quality, making up two thirds of the excluded set (101 of the 151 excluded images).

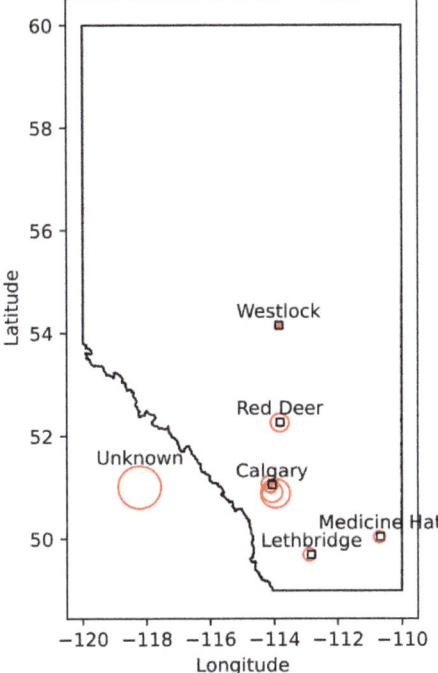

Figure 1. The distribution of clinics in Alberta, as well as their relative contribution of the dataset. Larger circles indicate larger contributions (in number of patients), with each circle representing one clinic.

2.3. Spinal Cord Segmentation

Spinal cord segmentation (masking the contents of the spinal cord vs. the other contents of the image) was done manually for a subset of 50 patients, containing a total of 195 images, as to provide a control against automated segmentation techniques (discussed below). These were done via manual inspection across all images by one person using the 3D Slicer application [18].

Automated segmentation for the full set of spinal cord images was then completed using SCT [13]. SCT was selected over its alternatives for two reasons. First, it is the only all-in-one package we are aware of that is specialized for application on the spinal cord, rather than being generalized to MR imaging in general [9,10]. Second, it is well documented and open source, making it easy to use and apply in clinical practices without major legal difficulties or financial burden. SCT provides two primary ways to initially segment the spinal cord; 'PropSeg' [27] and 'DeepSeg' [28]. PropSeg functions by initially detecting an initial slice of the spinal cord, then propagating that slice across the remainder of the spinal cord, adjusting as it goes. DeepSeg, in contrast, tries to identify the entire segmentation simultaneously, using either a Convolutional Neural Network (CNN) or Support Vector Machine (SVM) to do so. The model can also take into account only data in a given 2D slice, or the entire 3D image; we chose to test all combinations available. This resulted in 5 different automated segmentation methods being assessed in total. A segmentation method comparison, performed on a sagittal MRI image slice from a patient with severe DCM, is shown in Figure ??.

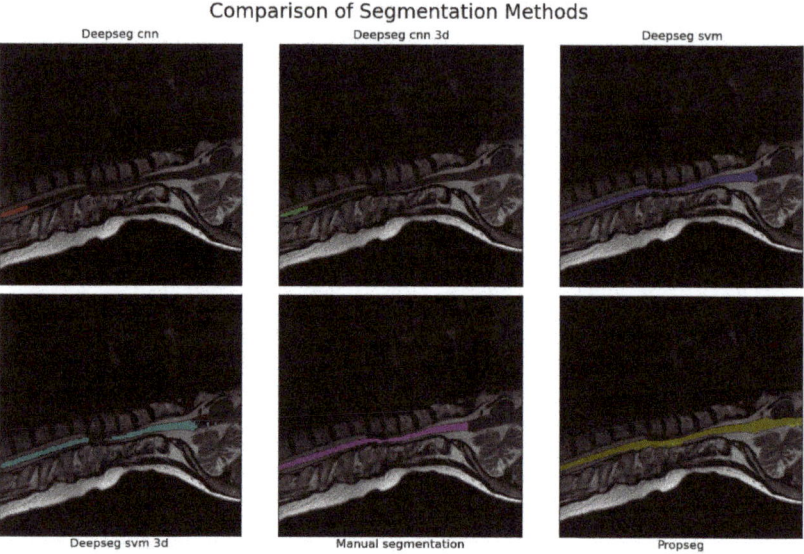

Figure 2. An example of the segmentations produced by each of the methodologies tested. The image used was that of a sagittal, T2w image from a patient with severe DCM (as evaluated by mJOA score). The manually segmented example is provided in the bottom center, with all others being produced via automated analyses using SCT [13]. The CNN kernel in particular seems to struggle when faced with spinal cord compressions, with the SVM kernel and propseg method having relatively minor issues in comparison (usually leaking or outright ignoring the compressed areas instead). This pattern appeared to hold true for all segmentations manually reviewed during the process to create Table 1.

Table 1. Total number of segmentations resulting from each algorithm which were found to be "best-of-type" for a given patient. Ties were allowed, enabling one patient image to have up to two "best" segmentations.

Orientation	Contrast	Deepseg (cnn)	Deepseg (3d svm)	Deepseg (svm)	Propseg
sagittal	T2w	2	9	51	7
sagittal	T1w	0	0	6	29
sagittal	PDw	0	0	0	1
axial	T2w	13	0	63	0
axial	T1w	0	0	1	0
axial	PDw	0	0	0	0

SCT can fail to produce a segmentation outright; there seems to be no discernible trend as to what causes this. In these cases, the segmentation method was simply skipped for the image, with subjects for which all methods failed being excluded. This resulted in

1 patient record being dropped, leaving 324 patients records containing 1066 total images for further analysis.

2.4. Metric Extraction and Standardization

Following segmentation, we used SCT's `sct_process_segmentation` script to extract metrics from each spinal cord image's segmentations (both automated and manual). All metrics were taken from the entire spinal cord volume, and included the means and standard deviations of the cross-sectional area of the spinal cord segmentation slices (mm squared), anterior/posterior angle (degrees), right/left angle (degrees), anterior/posterior diameter (mm), right/left diameter (mm), eccentricity (ratio of two prior diameter measurements), orientation (relative angle, image to spine), and solidity (ratio of true and convex-fit cross-sectional area). The total length of the spinal cord (mm) was also obtained, being produced by the same analysis pipeline; given its tenuous-at-best relation to the morphology associated with DCM, this was kept to evaluate SCT's options in full. That is to say, we did not expect length (sum) to be useful to any model, but included for the sake of being thorough.

Collected metrics from each automated segmentation were grouped by "imaging methodology" (the combination of segmentation method, MRI contrast, and MRI orientation) and joined with their respective patient's modified Japanese Orthopedic Association (mJOA) score. The mJOA is a clinician-reported instrument that measures the symptoms and disability of patients suffering from DCM, whereby lower mJOA scores indicate greater impairment and worse disease severity. It is the recommended and most commonly used metric to assess disability caused by DCM [29]. Scores can range from 18 (healthy) to 0 (inability to move hands or legs, total loss of urinary sphincter control, and complete loss of hand sensation). mJOA scores are also classified categorically as mild (a score of 15 or greater), moderate (a score of 12 to 14), or severe (a score or 11 or less) [30].

We then opted to harmonize the data to remove any effects unique to each scanner in our sample set. This was done using the *CovBat* harmonization program [25], grouping the data by scanner used to acquire it. The scanner of a given image was determined from the DICOM headers of the images, similar to the methods used in the original assessment of the *CovBat* program [25]. Specifically, images were deemed to share the same scanner if they shared the same scanner manufacturer, scanner model, and magnetic field strength. Please note that geography was *not* accounted for, unlike in Chen et al.'s [25] original presentation of the tool. This was because per clinic differences in how the scanner was operated were assumed to be minimal, given the shared health care zone all data was collected within. Not filtering by geography also has the convenient side-effect of keeping our dataset nearly completely intact, as the *CovBat* harmonization process requires that at least 3 elements exist in every group; only one methodology failed to reach this count, leading to only 2 segmentations total being lost. Thus, all patients and images remaining from prior filters remained represented in at least one methodology in the resulting set.

2.5. Model Metric Selection

External non-image derived metrics (such as age, sex, and other demographic information) were available, but were intentionally left out from both the data preparation processes prior and the data modeling below. This was to allow our models to evaluate the predictive merit of current automated image processing techniques, without external bias from said parameters. It has already been established that external metrics such as patient demographics are partially effective at predicting DCM severity in patients [31], and creating a composite model runs the risk of over-fitting the data and reducing diagnostic power.

Prior to fitting each model to their associate methodology dataset, data were grouped by the associated image's acquisition contrast (T1w, T2w, or PDw), segmentation method (options listed prior), and imaging orientation (axial, sagittal, or coronal); the resulting combination is referred to as the "assessment methodology" from this point forward. Initially, as a result of the combinations of these categories, there were potentially 45 different assessment methodologies, though only 30 of these were actually present in our data set. Assessment methodologies with fewer than 3 samples were dropped from the data set, as their lower sample size could lead to inaccurate or misleading results. This resulted in 3 further assessment methodologies being dropped, leaving 27.

Before fitting to models, each assessment methodology was then processed using False Discovery Rate Feature Selection via SciKit-Learn's `SelectFdr` function. The scoring function was set to the F-test score of the metric to the mJOA score (evaluated with SciKit-Learn's '`f_regression`' function) or DCM severity category (evaluated with SciKit-Learn's '`f_classif`' function). The F-test was selected for its ability to evaluate whether data would conform well in a regression model; as we kept to simple regression-based models for this study (see below), this fit our use case perfectly. The allowable probability of false discovery was set to $p = 0.05$. This feature selection process served both to reduce the list of spinal cord morphological metrics to only those anticipated to be correlated with our target metric (our mJOA score or the mJOA severity categories), but also to filter out assessment methodologies which are likely to be ineffective (by selecting 0 features for them). This resulted in a drastic reduction in valid assessment methodologies, with at most 3 passing this stage per severity category and model type (linear or categorical) and proceeding to the final model assessment.

2.6. mJOA Correlation and Categorization Model Assessment

The remaining assessment methodologies were then fit to either SciKit-Learn's '`LinearRegression`' model (for linear metric to mJOA score models) or '`LogisticRegression`' model (for DCM severity classification models). These simple models fit linearly to each parameter, allowing for metrics to be evaluated sans-interaction effects, and does so very quickly. This made them ideal for rapid, diverse, and simple assessments, perfect for evaluating the SCT derived metrics on their own. All groups were split into train-test groups using 5-fold shuffle split grouping, and cross-validated by fitting the modeling method to each group in turn. Each resulting model's effectiveness was then evaluated using r^2 for the linear regression models, and using receiver operating characteristic area under curve (ROC AUC) for categorical models. The effectiveness of the model type was then assessed via the mean score of all resulting models. To confirm that the somewhat experimental CovBat method worked correctly, all processes prior were run on both the standardized-only metric sets and the CovBat-harmonized metric sets as well. Categorical imbalance was also evaluated for each model type via assessing the accuracy of a "dummy" model, which simply guessed the most common category at all times.

3. Results
3.1. Spinal Cord Metrics of DCM Patients by mJOA Severity

Overall, with human-derived segmentation methods, very few metrics demonstrated significant differentiation by mJOA severity class, with only derived mean area, mean diameter (along both orientations), and anterior-posterior variance showing such distinction. A summary table of these metrics can be found in Table 2, with a visualized distribution with statistical annotations presented in Figure 3. This suggests that most metrics are not, on their own, sufficient to distinguish between the various mJOA severity classes, let alone predict the mJOA score accurately.

Table 2. Variation of metric measures across mJOA severity classes in the manually segmented subset, summarized. Please note that the 'Mean/STD' column denotes whether the metric used was the mean of the 'Metric' column or the 'Standard Deviation' of said 'Metric' column. A visualized version of this data, alongside statistical assessments, can be found in Figure 3.

Metric	Mean/STD	Severe	Moderate	Mild
MEAN(area)	mean	62.223	64.066	68.393
MEAN(area)	std	10.999	14.206	12.574
STD(area)	mean	14.710	16.319	14.879
STD(area)	std	4.599	5.341	4.587
MEAN(angle_AP)	mean	0.585	0.193	0.320
MEAN(angle_AP)	std	1.595	1.338	0.964
STD(angle_AP)	mean	8.331	8.274	7.018
STD(angle_AP)	std	4.982	4.895	4.252
MEAN(angle_RL)	mean	8.029	6.554	5.188
MEAN(angle_RL)	std	8.354	9.779	8.244
STD(angle_RL)	mean	12.848	11.755	11.153
STD(angle_RL)	std	5.536	5.816	4.706
MEAN(diameter_AP)	mean	6.679	6.957	7.038
MEAN(diameter_AP)	std	0.666	0.778	0.787
STD(diameter_AP)	mean	1.109	1.231	1.073
STD(diameter_AP)	std	0.430	0.451	0.309
MEAN(diameter_RL)	mean	12.332	12.113	13.030
MEAN(diameter_RL)	std	1.308	1.520	1.339
STD(diameter_RL)	mean	2.049	2.175	2.300
STD(diameter_RL)	std	0.644	0.609	0.818
MEAN(eccentricity)	mean	0.820	0.795	0.811
MEAN(eccentricity)	std	0.045	0.040	0.051
STD(eccentricity)	mean	0.085	0.108	0.099
STD(eccentricity)	std	0.034	0.036	0.041
MEAN(orientation)	mean	8.222	8.692	7.331
MEAN(orientation)	std	4.680	5.956	4.338
STD(orientation)	mean	9.313	12.100	9.530
STD(orientation)	std	6.215	8.879	6.452
MEAN(solidity)	mean	0.920	0.925	0.917
MEAN(solidity)	std	0.031	0.028	0.034
STD(solidity)	mean	0.046	0.043	0.049
STD(solidity)	std	0.027	0.025	0.023
SUM(length)	mean	165.963	175.729	162.561
SUM(length)	std	59.023	63.725	46.554

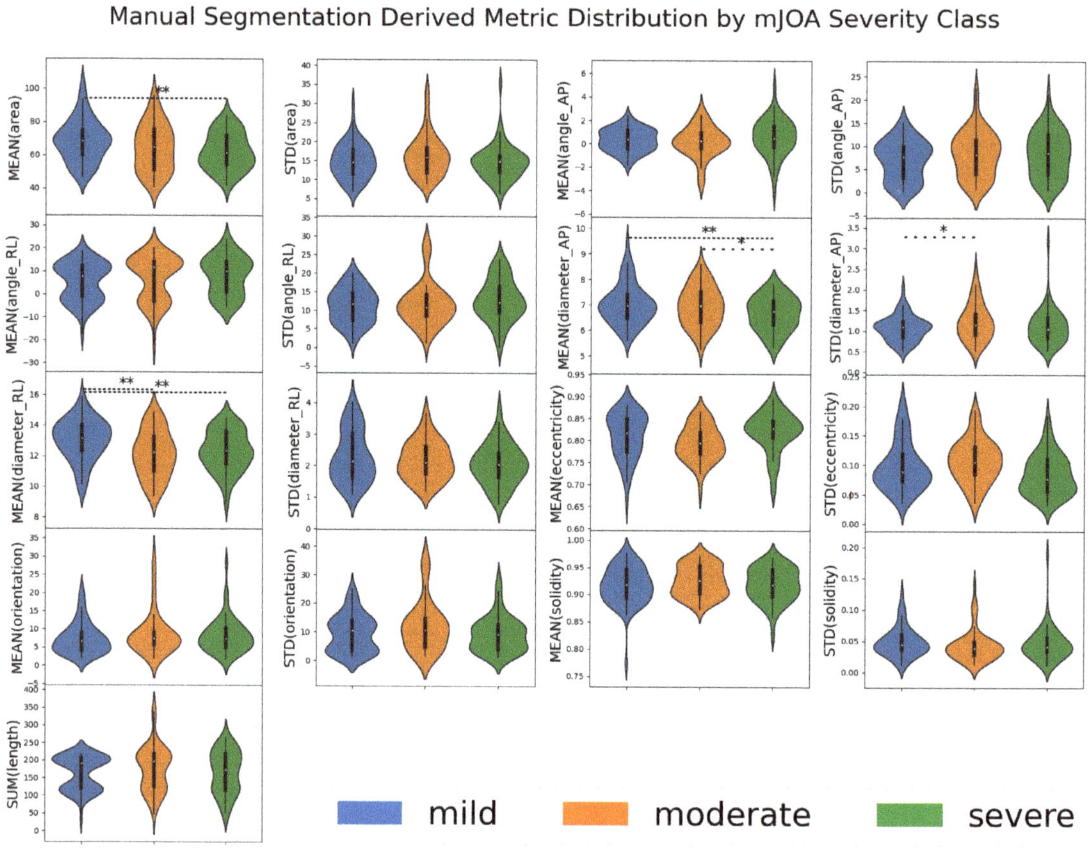

Figure 3. A violin plot of the distribution metrics extracted from manually segmented spinal cord images for 50 patients via the SCT. Each box represents one of the metrics evaluated by SCT, with the results grouped by mJOA severity classes. When the metric for one mJOA severity class was significantly different from another mJOA severity class (as determined by one-way ANOVA using SciPy's `f_oneway` function returning a p-value less than 0.05), a line denoting such is present. A single * with a sparse dotted line denotes $p < 0.05$, ** with a tightly dotted line denotes $p < 0.01$. Metrics were taken from automated SCT analysis [13] of segmentations from 195 spinal cord MRI images.

3.2. Manual vs. Automated Segmentation Metrics

All the automated segmentation methods were then compared to the manual method to determine whether significant differences existed via one-way ANOVA. This allows us to assess whether statistically significant differences in data distribution existed between our automation derived and manually derived imaging metrics. If such a difference is found to exist, it suggests that the automated process differs in some meaningful way, which may in turn become useful for predicting DCM score and/or mJOA severity. A summary of these metrics can be found in Table 3, with the distributions of said metrics shown and statistically assessed in Figure 4. In summary, the majority of metrics were found to be functionally distinct when measured automatically compared to manually, with the exceptions being eccentricity (both mean and standard deviation) and solidity (both mean and standard deviation). No automated segmentation method appeared to replicate the measures observed with manual methods for all metrics; these deviations could potentially prove useful, however, if how they differ from the manual segmentation method is diagnostically predictive.

Table 3. Variation of metric measures across automated segmentation methods. A visualized version of this data, alongside statistical assessments, can be found in Figure 4.

		Deepseg (cnn)		Deepseg (svm)			
Metric	Mean/Deviation	2d	3d	2d	3d	Manual	Propseg
MEAN(area)	mean	47.140	56.110	46.721	31.736	65.567	54.437
MEAN(area)	std	11.938	71.798	16.471	18.332	12.525	13.785
STD(area)	mean	13.528	24.376	14.993	16.562	15.366	13.336
STD(area)	std	5.627	37.167	5.033	7.937	4.841	4.717
MEAN(angle_AP)	mean	−0.099	−0.045	−0.173	0.273	0.374	0.039
MEAN(angle_AP)	std	4.842	8.273	3.535	3.917	1.283	1.381
STD(angle_AP)	mean	16.065	16.594	20.933	20.005	7.820	5.138
STD(angle_AP)	std	12.614	12.492	15.748	10.252	4.704	2.664
MEAN(angle_RL)	mean	5.600	4.448	5.036	5.475	6.639	5.166
MEAN(angle_RL)	std	10.255	12.174	7.908	8.534	8.556	8.035
STD(angle_RL)	mean	15.907	13.974	18.742	18.717	12.053	12.502
STD(angle_RL)	std	11.184	13.479	10.722	9.312	5.349	4.553
MEAN(diameter_AP)	mean	5.673	5.677	5.738	4.477	6.920	7.618
MEAN(diameter_AP)	std	0.835	4.638	1.102	1.752	0.736	1.498
STD(diameter_AP)	mean	1.107	1.863	1.362	1.690	1.127	1.617
STD(diameter_AP)	std	0.572	2.302	0.535	0.652	0.383	0.629
MEAN(diameter_RL)	mean	10.387	9.934	9.955	7.685	12.578	9.410
MEAN(diameter_RL)	std	2.019	6.107	2.701	2.921	1.423	1.537
STD(diameter_RL)	mean	2.346	2.828	2.353	2.834	2.189	1.243
STD(diameter_RL)	std	0.948	2.133	0.798	0.972	0.713	0.495
MEAN(eccentricity)	mean	0.815	0.829	0.792	0.784	0.810	0.683
MEAN(eccentricity)	std	0.057	0.086	0.055	0.054	0.046	0.084
STD(eccentricity)	mean	0.090	0.092	0.116	0.141	0.096	0.121
STD(eccentricity)	std	0.042	0.058	0.054	0.054	0.038	0.037
MEAN(orientation)	mean	9.424	17.098	12.619	15.474	7.805	27.025
MEAN(orientation)	std	8.231	16.024	9.849	9.238	4.850	18.971
STD(orientation)	mean	12.068	15.077	15.893	20.170	10.081	20.863
STD(orientation)	std	8.249	11.239	11.318	8.440	7.103	9.367
MEAN(solidity)	mean	0.938	0.883	0.934	0.908	0.920	0.933
MEAN(solidity)	std	0.017	0.070	0.016	0.031	0.031	0.041
STD(solidity)	mean	0.030	0.063	0.040	0.076	0.046	0.032
STD(solidity)	std	0.012	0.032	0.020	0.027	0.024	0.021
SUM(length)	mean	126.828	63.919	188.960	167.814	167.805	171.913
SUM(length)	std	80.717	57.264	92.204	112.005	55.064	72.697

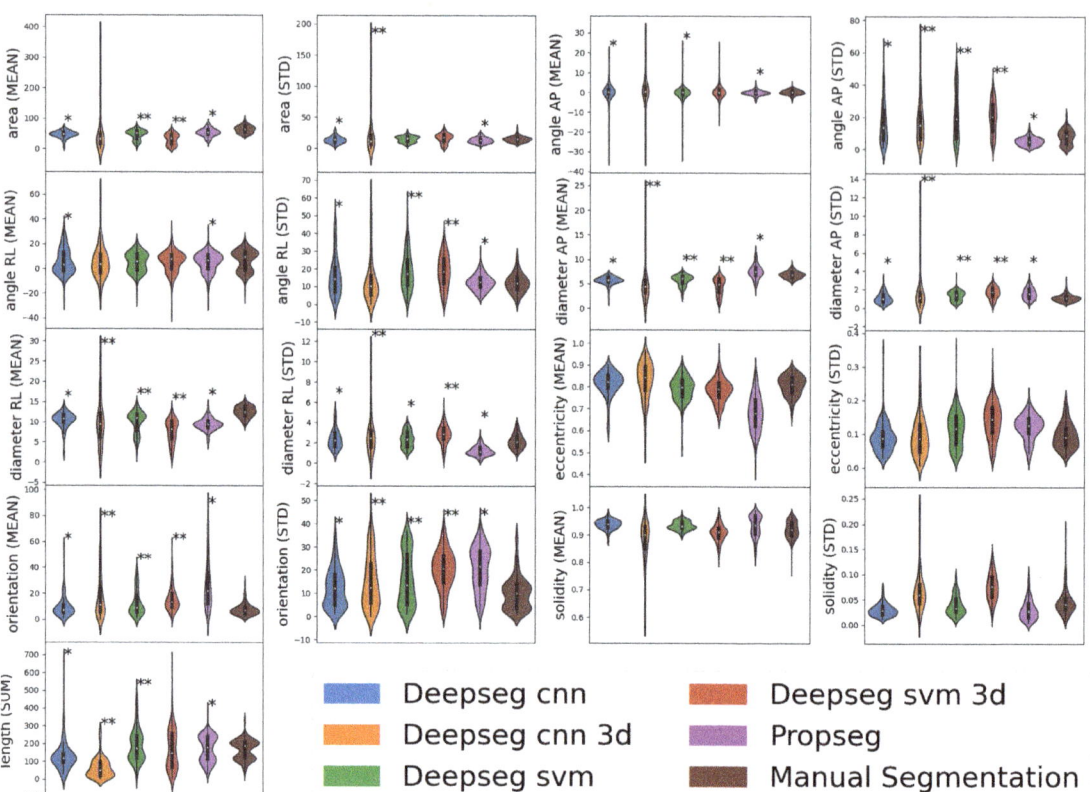

Figure 4. Visualized distributions of various metrics estimated by various segmentation methods for a subset of 50 patient records. Manual segmentation results are shown as the far-right distribution for each metric. Automated segmentation methods (not "Manual Segmentation") are denoted with asterisks denoting how significantly different their distribution is from that of the "Manual Segmentation" distribution; ** for $p < 0.01$, * for $p < 0.05$, as evaluated by one-way ANOVA using SciPy's `f_oneway` function (selected for its ease of implementation). Metrics taken from automated SCT analysis [13] of segmentations from 195 spinal cord MRI images.

3.3. mJOA Score Regression by Assessment Methodology

To assess whether the observed patterns of difference represented diagnostically relevant variation, each metric within each assessment methodology (segmentation algorithm, image contrast, and image orientation) was evaluated for significant regression with patient mJOA score (the distribution of which is shown in Figure 5). Of the metrics extracted from the segmentations, almost every metric was found to be significantly predictive ($p \leq 0.05$) of a patient's mJOA score for at least one assessment methodology (evaluated via SciKit-Learn's `f_regression` function). However, only the T2w contrast, sagittal orientation, and the svm deepseg segmentation algorithm methodology produce a model which had more than 3 parameters significantly related to mJOA score, with 5 total; mean of spinal cross-sectional area ($p = 0.007$), mean of anterior/posterior cross-sectional diameter ($p = 0.001$), mean right/left spinal angle ($p = 0.024$), mean eccentricity ($p = 0.031$), and mean solidity ($p = 0.013$). For all other groups, a combination of these metrics, with the occasional standard deviation of solidity, angle, or diameter was observed to have significant predictive power with the mJOA score. Notably, however, the T2w contrast, sagittal orientation, propseg segmentation algorithm methodology was the only one to find total summed length of the spinal cord as significantly related, despite our assumption that it would not be found as such. A more detailed overview of the distributions of these *p*-values has been visualized by metric (Figure 6) and methodology element (Figure 7).

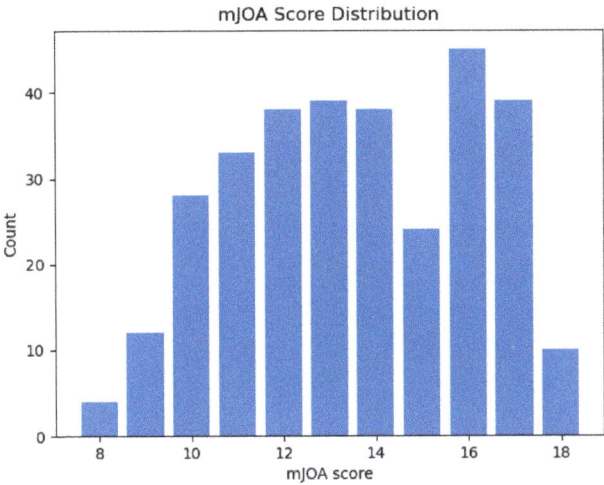

Figure 5. A box plot showing the number of individuals in our study with any given mJOA score. Although not quite ideal, this distribution is relatively balanced across the mid-range of mJOA scores. Note as well that extreme values (mJOA = 18 and mJOA = 8, 9) are rather rare, as would be expected given the acquisition method we used (data taken from those diagnosed with DCM who were undergoing initial assessment).

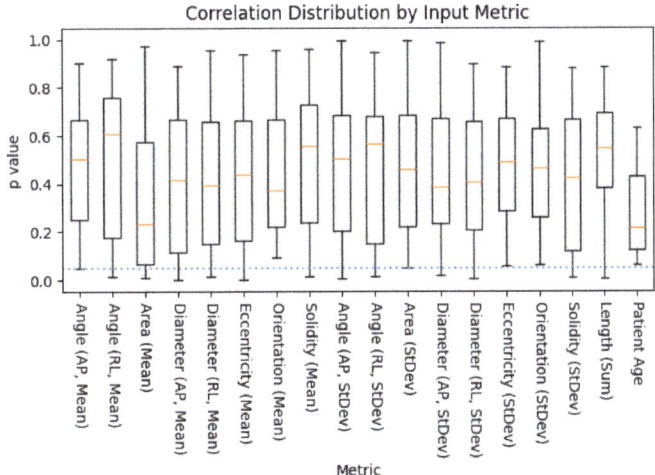

Figure 6. A box plot of the distribution *p*-values of metric to mJOA score correlations, across all combinations of acquisition contrast, orientation, and segmentation algorithm, as evaluated via SciKit-Learn's 'f_regression' algorithm (lower is better). Age was included as a control, as it has been previously shown to be correlated with mJOA score [32]. The dotted blue line represents the threshold of significance for this study ($p < 0.05$), with whiskers representing the maximum/minimum value of the set, or 1.5 times the inter-quartile range, whichever is shorter.

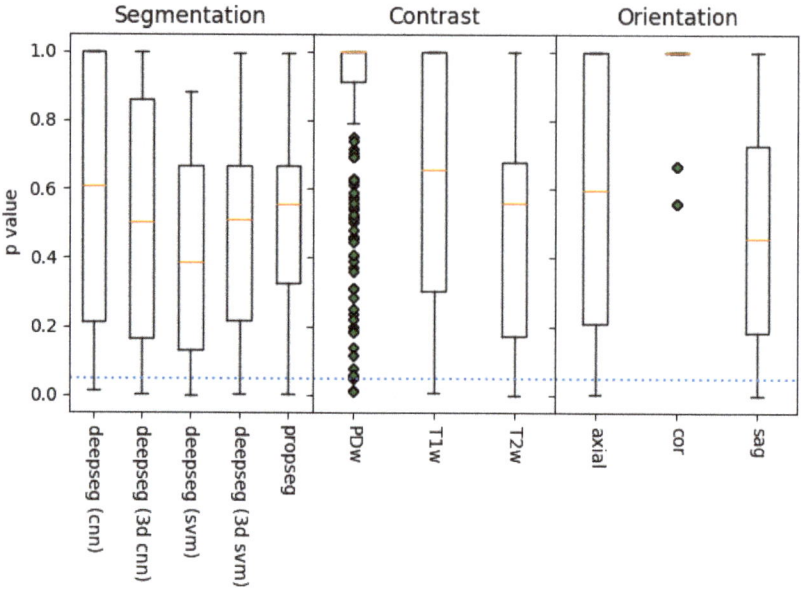

Figure 7. A box plot of the distribution p-values of metric to mJOA score correlations, grouped by acquisition contrast, orientation, and segmentation algorithm, as evaluated via SciKit-Learn's 'f_regression' algorithm (lower is better). The dotted blue line represents the threshold of significance for this study ($p \leq 0.05$), with whiskers representing the maximum/minimum value of the set, or 1.5 times the inter-quartile range, whichever is shorter. Data points outside this range are denoted with green diamonds. Of the methods, it appears that segmentation using deepseg with a svm kernel provided the best results, as did those processed with a T2w contrast along the sagittal plane. However, all but coronal alignment appears capable of statistically significant metric extraction in at least some manner, though the PDw contrast is quite likely a fluke as well (due to its low sample size).

3.4. Linear mJOA Prediction Models

Despite the results prior, none of the assessment methodology models tested produced a multi-parameter linear model that even came close to being remotely accurate, with all performing worse than a 'dummy' random chance-based model ($r^2 = 0$). The r^2 scores for each were evaluated by SciKit-Learn's 'r2_score' function, which can produce negative r^2 scores which imply that the associated model is worse-than-random. For non-batch compensated data, the r^2 scores hovered around -30, while batch compensated metric derived models resulted in r^2 scores ranging from -25 to -10. False Discovery Rate Feature Selection also tended to choose more features for the harmonized data set (with harmonized models having an average of 2 features selected, versus the 1.33 feature average form models trained on standardized metrics alone). This implies that the harmonization processed removed noise which otherwise masked useful trends, though clearly this was still not enough to lead to a valuable model. Tables summarizing these attributes, for both standardized (Table 4) and harmonized (Table 5), are available for further inspection.

Table 4. The attributes of our linear models fit on metric data, which was standardized to a common scale, but did not become harmonized by scanner used via CovBat. Orientation, contrast, and segmentation represent the acquisition methodology associated with the model. Features contains the list of features used to train the model, as selected by SciKit-Learn's `SelectFdr` function.

Orientation	Contrast	Segmentation	Samples No.	Features	r^2
acq-axial	T2w	deepseg_cnn_3d	395	STD(angle_RL), MEAN(angle_AP)	−30.492
acq-sag	T2w	deepseg_svm	329	STD(angle_AP)	−29.873
acq-sag	T2w	propseg	308	MEAN(diameter_AP)	−30.576

Table 5. The attributes of our linear models fit on metric data which was standardized to a common scale and harmonized by scanner used via CovBat. Orientation, contrast, and segmentation represent the acquisition methodology associated with the model. Features contains the list of features used to train the model, as selected by SciKit-Learn's `SelectFdr` function.

Orientation	Contrast	Segmentation	Samples No.	Features	r^2
acq-sag	T2w	deepseg_svm	329	STD(angle_AP), MEAN(angle_AP), STD(angle_RL)	−10.329
acq-sag	T2w	deepseg_svm_3d	329	MEAN(angle_AP), MEAN(diameter_RL)	−15.927
acq-sag	T2w	propseg	308	MEAN(orientation)	−25.549

3.5. Logistic DCM Categorical Models

Overall, the categorization models proved far more effective, with one reaching an ROC AUC of 0.92 (sagittal PDw 3d SVM deepseg methodology, not harmonized), with an average ROC AUC of 0.654 for non-harmonized data trained models and 0.612 for CovBat-harmonized data trained models. The mild mJOA model proved best overall, followed by the severe mJOA model and, finally, the moderate mJOA model. Models with fewer samples also tended to have higher ROC AUC scores, suggesting some level of over-fitting was occurring, as the higher sample count provided more natural noise which the models could erroneously detect as significant. The full results are summarized in Table 6 (non-harmonized) and Table 7 (CovBat-harmonized).

Table 6. The attributes of logistic models fit on metric data, which was standardized to a common scale, but not and harmonized by scanner used via CovBat. Severity indicates the class attempting to be distinguished from all others (binary classification), while orientation, contrast, and segmentation represent the acquisition methodology associated with the model. Features contains the list of features used to train the model, as selected by SciKit-Learn's `SelectFdr` function.

Severity	Orientation	Contrast	Segmentation	Sample No.	Features	AUC
severe	acq-axial	T2w	propseg	413	MEAN(eccentricity), STD (area)	0.713
severe	acq-sag	T2w	deepseg_cnn	269	STD(area)	0.519
moderate	acq-axial	T2w	deepseg_cnn	420	MEAN(area)	0.568
moderate	acq-axial	T2w	deepseg_svm_3d	420	STD(solidity)	0.549
mild	acq-sag	PDw	deepseg_svm_3d	27	MEAN(angle_RL)	0.920

Table 7. The attributes of logistic models fit on metric data which was standardized to a common scale and harmonized by scanner used via CovBat. Severity indicates the class attempting to be distinguished from all others (binary classification), while orientation, contrast, and segmentation represent the acquisition methodology associated with the model. Features contains the list of features used to train the model, as selected by SciKit-Learn's `SelectFdr` function.

Severity	Orientation	Contrast	Segmentation	Samples No.	Features	AUC
severe	acq-sag	T2w	deepseg_svm_3d	329	MEAN(diameter_RL)	0.630
moderate	acq-axial	T2w	deepseg_svm_3d	420	STD(solidity)	0.538
mild	acq-sag	PDw	deepseg_svm_3d	27	STD(diameter_RL)	0.75
mild	acq-sag	T2w	deepseg_svm	329	STD(angle_RL)	0.558
mild	acq-sag	T2w	deepseg_svm_3d	329	STD(orientation), MEAN(eccentricity)	0.592

4. Discussion and Conclusions

In this work, we explored predictive outcome modeling using computationally aided MRI analysis. We attempted to extract metrics used by trained surgeons from MRI images of the human cervical spine to predict disease severity. Most of these derived metrics simply lack sufficient differentiation across mJOA score severity. Variation appears to be mostly patient-specific rather than related to DCM severity. This is likely a result of the metrics being sampled across the entirety of the spinal cord, whereas morphological differences related to DCM often only effect a portion of the spinal cord, with the remainder appearing 'healthy'. Although there were some interesting trends within the data, these useful trends appear to be masked by natural inter-individual variance between each of the patients enrolled in this study. As a result, our machine learning systems had difficulty pulling out said meaningful trends, resulting in over-fitting to patient variation and lower overall accuracy.

Non-imaging metrics, such as age, smoking status, and symptom duration have been shown to be important metrics in the development of models to predict patient outcomes after surgical treatment for DCM [32]. MR imaging of the cervical spine plays a vital role in the diagnosis and surgical treatment planning of this patient population. Although this data is vital to a surgeon's decision-making process, most surgeons would not consider treating a patient without and MRI confirmed diagnosis. Efforts to distill a surgeon's acumen into an 'imaging metric' have fallen short in terms of predictive capabilities. Our work, while novel in computational approach, only adds to this body of literature, bringing us closer to integrating advanced imaging metrics with a patient's clinical presentation. Such a reality could greatly improve a surgeon's ability to treat their patients.

The models we presented in this work highlight some key features which we can use to inform future processes. Given the low accuracy of most assessment methodologies, the vast majority of metrics extracted from these segmentations did not correlate strongly with mJOA scores. However, a handful did, showing that assessment methodologies could identify statistically significant correlations. Spinal cord segmentation metrics chosen via feature selection also showed an interesting trend, with the angle and diameter of the spine being selected most commonly, followed by metrics associated with cross-sectional area and spinal cord solidity/eccentricity. This is unsurprising given that pathology of DCM results in compression of the spinal cord (i.e. reduction in diameter, often resulting in a misshapen cross-section), but it nonetheless highlights the potential for a model which focused solely on identifying key variations in these values derived directly from the image itself. It is plausible that finding a way to normalize these metrics relative to the patient's unique spinal cord variations could be incredibly valuable for creating a diagnostic model. These techniques show potential, but appear to be hampered by the natural variance of DCM patients' spinal cords.

There are several limitations to this study. First, all data comes from central-southern Alberta (Figure 1), potentially leading to some implicit demographic attributes of the region influencing the analyses. Second, only relatively simple models (Linear and Logistic regression) were used, whereas more complex models may have proven more useful. Simple models simply cannot capture any significant interaction effects. Given the complexity of DCM, it is extremely likely at least one such severity influencing 'complex' effect exists. We limited our analyses to these simpler models to focus the study on evaluating major trends in the data to inform future model design. Third, only simple measures of accuracy were used (r^2 simply assesses a model's total explained variance, whereas ROC AUC measures its relative ability to predict true positives over false positives), which are likely to mask important details on how each model functions. More nuanced assessment metrics should be considered for future models aimed at diagnostic application; measurements such as false positive rate vs. false negative rate are likely to be far more significant metrics in these contexts (a false positive will be likely caught and dismissed by a clinician upon review, whereas a false negative could lead to significant health consequences for the patient). Fourth, the cross-validation procedure (5-fold) was chosen for its simple implementation in both linear and logistic regression models. A leave-one-out (linear regression) or leave-one-per-category-out (logistic regression) model would be more appropriate here, as it would replicate how a real-world implementation of similar predictive models would be required to function; with a single new patient record being submitted in varying intervals and predictions made for them. Such cross-validation may result in models more prone to over-fitting noise; however, finding noise-resistant metrics would be a must before this limitation could be resolved. Fifth, we only accounted for metrics directly extracted from MRI images. Prior studies have shown that non-imaging metrics can also influence spinal cord morphometrics within a patient [33], and as a result it is likely some confounding or contributing effect from such non-imaging metrics may have not been accounted for. Finding a way to fold in these metrics could improve future models substantially.

Given these limitations, future studies which aim to model DCM outcomes should aim to identify metrics which are normalized to healthy patient variation. This would reduce the amount new models will overfit to natural patient variation over DCM relevant attributes. Likewise, due in part to the limited number of samples available in our dataset and the fact all were diagnosed with DCM, asymptomatic persons who display traits analogous to those of DCM were not accounted for. Prior work has shown MRI images from asymptomatic persons can appear similar to those taken from DCM patients [34]. Increasing the number of MRIs taken from healthy individuals could reduce the likelihood of future models becoming too liberal with their DCM diagnoses. Finding metrics resilient to these forms of over-fitting is imperative if any resulting model is to be implemented in a fully autonomous manner, as to avoid incorrect diagnostic conclusions which may lead to patient harm.

Several possible solutions exist to address these limitations. First, normalizing metrics to be relative per-patient could greatly mitigate natural patient variance effects. These could include ratio metrics (i.e., minimum over maximum ratio), internal outlier detection (i.e., detecting drastic changes in spinal cord shape relative to the rest of the spine), or even dynamically generated metrics such as those produce by Principle Component Analysis. Such metrics would both provide internal normalization for patients, and (in the case of Principle Component Analysis) would be specifically selected based on their relevance to the DCM severity. Second, experimenting with more complex models stands to capture more nuanced details of DCM, such as those of interaction effects between multiple parameters. This would require said metrics to be refined beforehand, however, as such interaction effects would be particularly prone to natural noise masking true relations. Finally, folding in non-imaging derived metrics could address the issue of 'asymptomatic' false positives mentioned prior. Given these effects would likely need to be considered alongside spinal cord morphology metrics, this should be done after the selection of said morphological metrics and after a suitable model is chosen which can reflect these interactions. The outcome of such research could be particularly enlightening, helping to explain what distinguishes asymptomatic persons from those suffering from DCM, potentially providing improved treatment options for the latter.

Overall, it appears that modern computational methods have unmet potential in diagnostic prediction of DCM severity. With improvement of these models via the integration of external non-imaging derived metrics, deploying additional complex statistical and machine learning models, and improved morphological metric identification, it may be possible to create a system capable of working at least as effectively as the average clinician. The numerous limitations of this study will also need to be addressed should such a system come to fruition, namely the problem of models over-fitting to natural patient variation and other noise rather than DCM specific morphological characteristics. If these challenges are met, such a system being integrated in a fully automated capacity could potentially revolutionize the treatment of DCM. Such a system could allow clinicians to focus on each patient's needs more closely, helping them come to more informed treatment decisions and mitigating risks associated with their chosen treatment. This model could also greatly improve our understanding of DCM, potentially identifying targets for new modes of treatment or discovering novel diagnostic metrics.

Author Contributions: Conceptualization, K.O., D.W.C., W.B.J., N.E. and J.C.-A. methodology, K.O., D.W.C., W.B.J., N.E. and J.C.-A. software, K.O. and J.C.-A. validation, K.O., D.A., D.W.C., J.C.-A. formal analysis, K.O.; investigation, K.O., D.W.C., W.B.J. and N.E.; resources, D.W.C., W.B.J. and N.E.; data curation, K.O. and D.W.C.; writing—original draft preparation, K.O.; writing—review and editing, All Authors; visualization, K.O.; supervision, D.W.C. and D.A.; project administration, D.W.C.; funding acquisition, D.W.C. All authors have read and agreed to the published version of the manuscript.

Funding: This research was funded in part by the Alberta Spine Foundation, Department of Clinical Neurosciences, Cumming School of Medicine and the Hotchkiss Brain Institute.

Institutional Review Board Statement: The study was conducted according to the guidelines of the Declaration of Helsinki. Ethics approval for the following research has been renewed by the Conjoint Health Research Ethics Board (CHREB) at the University of Calgary. The CHREB is constituted and operated in compliance with the Tri-Council Policy Statement: Ethical Conduct for Research Involving Humans (TCPS 2); Health Canada Food and Drug Regulations Division 5; Pact C; ICH Guidance E6: Good Clinical Practice and the provisions and regulations of the Health Information Act, RSA 2000 c H-5. Ethics ID: REB18-1614-REN2 Principal Investigator: David Cadotte. The study was originally approved on December 18, 2018 and renewed on an annual basis thereafter.

Informed Consent Statement: Informed consent was obtained from each patient at the initial point of clinical contact.

Data Availability Statement: The data are not publicly available due to its sensitive nature, to preserve the privacy of those enrolled in our study. However, anonymized data may be made available in the context of a data-sharing agreement in coordination with the corresponding author and appropriate research ethics approval.

Acknowledgments: We would like to acknowledge our funding sources—Alberta Spine Foundation, Department of Clinical Neurosciences, Cumming School of Medicine and the Hotchkiss Brain Institute. There are no conflicts of interest. We would also like to acknowledge the clinicians, imaging technicians, and patients who have improved to our research through their contributions to the Canadian Spine Outcomes and Research project.

Conflicts of Interest: The authors declare no conflict of interest.

Abbreviations

The following abbreviations are used in this manuscript:

DCM	Degenerative Cervical Myelopathy
MRI	Magnetic Resonance Imaging
SCT	Spinal Cord Toolbox
FMRIB	Functional Magnetic Resonance Imaging of the Brain
CSORN	Canadian Spine Outcomes and Research

DICOM	Digital Imaging and Communications in Medicine
CNN	Convolutional Neural Network
SVM	Support Vector Machine
ROC AUC	Receiver Operating Characteristic Area Under Curve

References

1. Nouri, A.; Tetreault, L.; Singh, A.; Karadimas, S.K.; Fehlings, M.G. Degenerative cervical myelopathy: Epidemiology, genetics, and pathogenesis. *Spine* **2015**, *40*, E675–E693. [CrossRef] [PubMed]
2. Davies, B.M.; Mowforth, O.D.; Smith, E.K.; Kotter, M.R. Degenerative cervical myelopathy. *BMJ* **2018**, *360*. [CrossRef]
3. Tracy, J.A.; Bartleson, J. Cervical spondylotic myelopathy. *Neurologist* **2010**, *16*, 176–187. [CrossRef] [PubMed]
4. Kovalova, I.; Kerkovsky, M.; Kadanka, Z.; Kadanka, Z., Jr.; Nemec, M.; Jurova, B.; Dusek, L.; Jarkovsky, J.; Bednarik, J. Prevalence and imaging characteristics of nonmyelopathic and myelopathic spondylotic cervical cord compression. *Spine* **2016**, *41*, 1908–1916. [CrossRef]
5. Bednarik, J.; Kadanka, Z.; Dusek, L.; Kerkovsky, M.; Vohanka, S.; Novotny, O.; Urbanek, I.; Kratochvilova, D. Presymptomatic spondylotic cervical myelopathy: An updated predictive model. *Eur. Spine J.* **2008**, *17*, 421–431. [CrossRef] [PubMed]
6. Kopjar, B.; Bohm, P.E.; Arnold, J.H.; Fehlings, M.G.; Tetreault, L.A.; Arnold, P.M. Outcomes of surgical decompression in patients with very severe degenerative cervical myelopathy. *Spine* **2018**, *43*, 1102. [CrossRef]
7. Boogaarts, H.D.; Bartels, R.H. Prevalence of cervical spondylotic myelopathy. *Eur. Spine J.* **2015**, *24*, 139–141. [CrossRef]
8. Evaniew, N.; Cadotte, D.W.; Dea, N.; Bailey, C.S.; Christie, S.D.; Fisher, C.G.; Paquet, J.; Soroceanu, A.; Thomas, K.C.; Rampersaud, Y.R.; et al. Clinical predictors of achieving the minimal clinically important difference after surgery for cervical spondylotic myelopathy: An external validation study from the Canadian Spine Outcomes and Research Network. *J. Neurosurg. Spine* **2020**, *33*, 129–137. [CrossRef]
9. Jenkinson, M.; Beckmann, C.F.; Behrens, T.E.; Woolrich, M.W.; Smith, S.M. Fsl. *Neuroimage* **2012**, *62*, 782–790. [CrossRef]
10. Penny, W.D.; Friston, K.J.; Ashburner, J.T.; Kiebel, S.J.; Nichols, T.E. *Statistical Parametric Mapping: The Analysis of Functional Brain Images*; Elsevier: Amsterdam, The Netherlands, 2011.
11. Vincent, R.D.; Neelin, P.; Khalili-Mahani, N.; Janke, A.L.; Fonov, V.S.; Robbins, S.M.; Baghdadi, L.; Lerch, J.; Sled, J.G.; Adalat, R.; et al. MINC 2.0: A flexible format for multi-modal images. *Front. Neuroinform.* **2016**, *10*, 35. [CrossRef]
12. Tetreault, L.A.; Kopjar, B.; Vaccaro, A.; Yoon, S.T.; Arnold, P.M.; Massicotte, E.M.; Fehlings, M.G. A clinical prediction model to determine outcomes in patients with cervical spondylotic myelopathy undergoing surgical treatment: Data from the prospective, multi-center AOSpine North America study. *JBJS* **2013**, *95*, 1659–1666. [CrossRef]
13. De Leener, B.; Lévy, S.; Dupont, S.M.; Fonov, V.S.; Stikov, N.; Collins, D.L.; Callot, V.; Cohen-Adad, J. SCT: Spinal Cord Toolbox, an open-source software for processing spinal cord MRI data. *Neuroimage* **2017**, *145*, 24–43. [CrossRef]
14. Martin, A.R.; De Leener, B.; Cohen-Adad, J.; Kalsi-Ryan, S.; Cadotte, D.W.; Wilson, J.R.; Tetreault, L.; Nouri, A.; Crawley, A.; Mikulis, D.J.; et al. Monitoring for myelopathic progression with multiparametric quantitative MRI. *PLoS ONE* **2018**, *13*, e0195733.
15. Perone, C.S.; Cohen-Adad, J. Promises and limitations of deep learning for medical image segmentation. *J. Med. Artif. Intell.* **2019**, *2*. [CrossRef]
16. Thakar, S.; Arun, A.; Aryan, S.; Mohan, D.; Hegde, A. Deep flexor sarcopenia as a predictor of poor functional outcome after anterior cervical discectomy in patients with myelopathy. *Eur. J. Neurosurg.* **2019**, *161*, 2201–2209. [CrossRef]
17. Martin, A.; De Leener, B.; Cohen-Adad, J.; Cadotte, D.W.; Nouri, A.; Wilson, J.; Tetreault, L.; Crawley, A.; Mikulis, D.; Ginsberg, H.; et al. Can microstructural MRI detect subclinical tissue injury in subjects with asymptomatic cervical spinal cord compression? A prospective cohort study. *BMJ Open* **2018**, *8*, e019809. [CrossRef]
18. Kikinis, R.; Pieper, S.D.; Vosburgh, K.G. 3D Slicer: A platform for subject-specific image analysis, visualization, and clinical support. In *Intraoperative Imaging and Image-Guided Therapy*; Springer: Cham, Switzerland, 2014; pp. 277–289.
19. Pedregosa, F.; Varoquaux, G.; Gramfort, A.; Michel, V.; Thirion, B.; Grisel, O.; Blondel, M.; Prettenhofer, P.; Weiss, R.; Dubourg, V.; et al. Scikit-learn: Machine Learning in Python. *J. Mach. Learn. Res.* **2011**, *12*, 2825–2830.
20. Virtanen, P.; Gommers, R.; Oliphant, T.E.; Haberland, M.; Reddy, T.; Cournapeau, D.; Burovski, E.; Peterson, P.; Weckesser, W.; Bright, J.; et al. SciPy 1.0: Fundamental Algorithms for Scientific Computing in Python. *Nat. Methods* **2020**, *17*, 261–272. [CrossRef]
21. Hunter, J.D. Matplotlib: A 2D graphics environment. *Comput. Sci. Eng.* **2007**, *9*, 90–95. [CrossRef]
22. Waskom, M.; Gelbart, M.; Botvinnik, O.; Ostblom, J.; Hobson, P.; Lukauskas, S.; Gemperline, D.C.; Augspurger, T.; Halchenko, Y.; Warmenhoven, J.; et al. Mwaskom/Seaborn. 2020. Available online: seaborn.pydata.org (accessed on 23 February 2021).
23. Harris, C.R.; Millman, K.J.; van der Walt, S.J.; Gommers, R.; Virtanen, P.; Cournapeau, D.; Wieser, E.; Taylor, J.; Berg, S.; Smith, N.J.; et al. Array programming with NumPy. *Nature* **2020**, *585*, 357–362. [CrossRef] [PubMed]
24. Wes McKinney. Data Structures for Statistical Computing in Python. In Proceedings of the 9th Python in Science Conference, Austin, TX, USA, 29 June 2010.
25. Chen, A.; Beer, J.; Tustison, N.; Cook, P.; Shinohara, R.; Shou, H. Removal of Scanner Effects in Covariance Improves Multivariate Pattern Analysis in Neuroimaging Data. *bioRxiv* **2019**, 858415. [CrossRef]
26. Gorgolewski, K.J.; Auer, T.; Calhoun, V.D.; Craddock, R.C.; Das, S.; Duff, E.P.; Flandin, G.; Ghosh, S.S.; Glatard, T.; Halchenko, Y.O.; et al. The brain imaging data structure, a format for organizing and describing outputs of neuroimaging experiments. *Sci. Data* **2016**, *3*, 160044. [CrossRef] [PubMed]

27. De Leener, B.; Kadoury, S.; Cohen-Adad, J. Robust, accurate and fast automatic segmentation of the spinal cord. *Neuroimage* **2014**, *98*, 528–536. [CrossRef] [PubMed]
28. Gros, C.; De Leener, B.; Badji, A.; Maranzano, J.; Eden, D.; Dupont, S.M.; Talbott, J.; Zhuoquiong, R.; Liu, Y.; Granberg, T.; et al. Automatic segmentation of the spinal cord and intramedullary multiple sclerosis lesions with convolutional neural networks. *Neuroimage* **2019**, *184*, 901–915. [CrossRef]
29. Fehlings, M.G.; Tetreault, L.A.; Riew, K.D.; Middleton, J.W.; Aarabi, B.; Arnold, P.M.; Brodke, D.S.; Burns, A.S.; Carette, S.; Chen, R.; et al. A clinical practice guideline for the management of patients with degenerative cervical myelopathy: Recommendations for patients with mild, moderate, and severe disease and nonmyelopathic patients with evidence of cord compression. *Glob. Spine J.* **2017**, *7*, 70S–83S. [CrossRef]
30. Tetreault, L.; Kopjar, B.; Nouri, A.; Arnold, P.; Barbagallo, G.; Bartels, R.; Qiang, Z.; Singh, A.; Zileli, M.; Vaccaro, A.; et al. The modified Japanese Orthopaedic Association scale: Establishing criteria for mild, moderate and severe impairment in patients with degenerative cervical myelopathy. *Eur. Spine J.* **2017**, *26*, 78–84. [CrossRef]
31. Tetreault, L.A.; Côté, P.; Kopjar, B.; Arnold, P.; Fehlings, M.G.; America, A.N.; Network, I.C.T.R. A clinical prediction model to assess surgical outcome in patients with cervical spondylotic myelopathy: Internal and external validations using the prospective multicenter AOSpine North American and international datasets of 743 patients. *Spine J.* **2015**, *15*, 388–397. [CrossRef]
32. Gibson, J.; Nouri, A.; Krueger, B.; Lakomkin, N.; Nasser, R.; Gimbel, D.; Cheng, J. Focus: Sensory Biology and Pain: Degenerative Cervical Myelopathy: A Clinical Review. *Yale J. Biol. Med.* **2018**, *91*, 43.
33. Kameyama, T.; Hashizume, Y.; Ando, T.; Takahashi, A. Morphometry of the normal cadaveric cervical spinal cord. *Spine* **1994**, *19*, 2077–2081. [CrossRef]
34. Nakashima, H.; Yukawa, Y.; Suda, K.; Yamagata, M.; Ueta, T.; Kato, F. Abnormal Findings on Magnetic Resonance Images of the Cervical Spines in 1211 Asymptomatic Subjects. *Spine* **2015**, *40*, 392–398. [CrossRef]

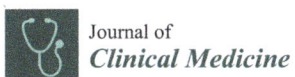

Article

Frailty Is a Better Predictor than Age of Mortality and Perioperative Complications after Surgery for Degenerative Cervical Myelopathy: An Analysis of 41,369 Patients from the NSQIP Database 2010–2018

Jamie R. F. Wilson [1,2,3], Jetan H. Badhiwala [2,3], Ali Moghaddamjou [2,3], Albert Yee [2], Jefferson R. Wilson [2] and Michael G. Fehlings [2,3,*]

1. Nebraska Medical Center, University of Nebraska Medical Center, Omaha, NE 68198, USA; jamie.wilson@unmc.edu
2. Spine Program, Department of Surgery, University of Toronto, Toronto, ON M5T 2S8, Canada; jetan.badhiwala@gmail.com (J.H.B.); Ali.Moghaddamjou@one-mail.on.ca (A.M.); Albert.Yee@sunnybrook.ca (A.Y.); WilsonJeff@smh.ca (J.R.W.)
3. Division of Neurosurgery, Krembil Neuroscience Centre, Toronto Western Hospital, University Health Network, Toronto, ON M5T 2S8, Canada
* Correspondence: Michael.Fehlings@uhn.ca; Tel.: +1-416-603-5627

Received: 22 September 2020; Accepted: 27 October 2020; Published: 29 October 2020

Abstract: Background: The ability of frailty compared to age alone to predict adverse events in the surgical management of Degenerative Cervical Myelopathy (DCM) has not been defined in the literature. Methods: 41,369 patients with a diagnosis of DCM undergoing surgery were collected from the National Surgical Quality Improvement Program (NSQIP) Database 2010–2018. Univariate analysis for each measure of frailty (modified frailty index 11- and 5-point; MFI-11, MFI-5), modified Charlson Co-morbidity index and ASA grade) were calculated for the following outcomes: mortality, major complication, unplanned reoperation, unplanned readmission, length of hospital stay, and discharge to a non-home destination. Multivariable modeling of age and frailty with a base model was performed to define the discriminative ability of each measure. Results: Age and frailty have a significant effect on all outcomes, but the MFI-5 has the largest effect size. Increasing frailty correlated significantly with the risk of perioperative adverse events, longer hospital stay, and risk of a non-home discharge destination. Multivariable modeling incorporating MFI-5 with age and the base model had a robust predictive value (0.85). MFI-5 had a high categorical assessment correlation with a MFI-11 of 0.988 ($p < 0.001$). Conclusions and Relevance: Measures of frailty have a greater effect size and a higher discriminative value to predict adverse events than age alone. MFI-5 categorical assessment is essentially equivalent to the MFI-11 score for DCM patients. A multivariable model using MFI-5 provides an accurate predictive tool that has important clinical applications.

Keywords: degenerative cervical myelopathy; frailty; age; mortality; complications

1. Introduction

Degenerative cervical myelopathy (DCM) is characterized by progressive compression of the spinal cord in the cervical canal, producing debilitating neurological deficits in upper limb function, gait instability, sphincteric disturbance, and ultimately spastic quadriparesis. It is the most common cause of adult spinal cord dysfunction worldwide and its prevalence increases significantly with age [1]. With the projected shift in demographics over the next 30 years, the burden of (potentially treatable) neurological dysfunction in the elderly has become a major public health concern of the 21st century [1–4]. The Institute of Medicine has declared that DCM includes 3 of the top 100 national priorities for comparative effectiveness in research, and efforts to address the rise of disability from DCM have been implemented worldwide, including the establishment of international consensus treatment guidelines [5–7].

DCM is an umbrella term that encompasses a number of degenerative pathologies that include osteoarthritis (spondylosis), ligament disease (ossification of the posterior longitudinal ligament (OPLL), ligament hypertrophy), and degenerative listhesis or instability. These entities have pronounced effects on the functional abilities and quality of life of impaired individuals, which may be comparable to serious health conditions, such as cancer or heart disease [8]. The mainstay of treatment for DCM is decompressive surgery, which arrests the progression of the disease and provides a sustained and meaningful improvement in functional and quality of life measures [2,3,7,9–13]. Clinical factors such as duration of symptoms prior to surgery and severity of baseline functional impairment correlate strongly with the chances of a substantial clinical benefit after intervention [9,11,12,14,15].

Decisions regarding the best application of surgical intervention for DCM have become an important focus of clinical study [3,6]. In the elderly population, this issue becomes complex as the potential impact of preventing neurological disability in the elderly needs to be balanced against the healthcare costs and complication profile [4,6,7,13]. Although increasing age is associated with poorer surgical outcomes, in DCM patients many studies have shown sustained long-term functional and quality of life improvements after surgery [4,10,11,15–17]. Moreover, when elderly patients are matched for co-morbidities and baseline functional impairment, their complication profile is equivalent [3]. This has led to the evolving opinion that age alone has become less relevant for the purpose of estimating perioperative risk profile and prognosis after surgery [18–22].

Efforts to move past age alone as a predictor of outcomes has led to the development of measures of physiological reserve (or 'frailty indices'). The most commonly cited index in spine surgery is the Modified Frailty Index (11-point or 5-point, Table 1) [23–26] which is derived from the original 70-point Canadian Study of Health and Aging Frailty Index (CSHA-FI) [27]. Other measures include the American Society of Anesthesiologists Grading scale (ASA) and the modified Charlson Co-morbidity Index (mCCI). ASA is a well-established subjective estimate of overall illness severity that has an uncertain role in the prediction of perioperative outcomes after spine surgery [18]. The mCCI, like the MFI, is also matched to NSQIP variables but produces different weightings according to increasing age and certain co-morbidities. Although used widely in general surgery, the mCCI has received limited application in spine surgery [19,20,28]. In 2017, Shin et al. published a study of 6965 patients who underwent either anterior cervical discectomy or posterior cervical fusion, and showed frailty (as measured by the 11-point MFI) was associated with an increased risk of adverse events [23]. However, this study did not distinguish between radiculopathy or myelopathy patients, and it has been previously demonstrated that myelopathy patients have a higher risk of perioperative complications compared to patients with purely radicular symptoms [24]. To date, no study exists that models the impact of frailty specifically on surgical DCM patients, or that compares the discriminatory ability of different measures of frailty.

Table 1. NSQIP clinical variables matched from the CSHA-FI used to construct the 11- and 5- item modified frailty index (MFI-11, MFI-5), compared with the modified Charlson Co-morbidity Index (mCCI).

NSQIP Variables		CSHA-FI	mCCI (Weighting)
MFI-11	MFI-5		
Functional health status prior to admission	Functional health status prior to admission	Changes in daily activities	Ascites/Esophageal Varices (3)
Diabetes Mellitus	Diabetes Mellitus	Diabetes Mellitus	Diabetes Mellitus (1)
History of Severe COPD	History of Severe COPD	Respiratory problems	History of Severe COPD (1)
Hypertension requiring medication	Hypertension requiring medication	Arterial hypertension	Renal Failure (2)
Congestive Heart failure within 30 days of admission	Congestive Heart failure within 30 days of admission	Congestive heart failure	Congestive heart failure (1)
Myocardial Infarction within past 6 months prior to surgery		Myocardial Infarction	Prior Myocardial Infarction (1)
Previous Cardiac Surgery OR Angina <1 month prior to surgery		Cardiac problems	Disseminated Cancer (6)
Impaired sensorium		Clouding or delirium	
History of TIA or Cerebrovascular Accident with no deficits		Cerebrovascular problems	Prior TIA or Cerebrovascular Accident (1)
Cerebrovascular Accident with deficits		History of stroke	Hemiplegia (2)
Previous intervention for peripheral vascular disease OR Rest pain/Gangrene secondary to peripheral vascular disease		Decreased peripheral pulses	Peripheral Vascular Disease (1)
			40 years old or less (0)
			41–50 years old (1)
			51–60 years old (2)
			61–70 years old (3)
			71 years old+ (4)

NSQIP, National Surgical Quality Improvement Program; CSHA-FI, Canadian Study of Health and Aging Frailty Index; mCCI, modified Charlson Co-morbidity Index; COPD, chronic obstructive pulmonary disease; MFI, modified frailty index; OR, Odds Ratio; TIA, transient ischemic attack.

The objectives of the current study were to (1) define the effect of age on the perioperative outcomes of mortality, unplanned readmission/reoperation, major complication, length of stay and discharge to non-home destination for patients undergoing surgery for DCM, (2) directly compare measures of frailty in the same cohort to determine which factor exhibits a greater influence on the observed outcomes, and (3) define the potential correlation between MFI-5 and MFI-11 in DCM patients. We hypothesize that after adjustment for common surgical factors, frailty is a better predictor of perioperative complications compared to age alone. Frailty as a predictor of perioperative complications would have important implications for the clinical management of elderly patients with DCM.

2. Experimental Section

2.1. Data Source

The data source for this study was the American College of Surgeons (ACS) National Surgical Quality Improvement Program (NSQIP) database, for years 2010 through 2018 inclusive. The NSQIP datasets encode surgical procedures by Current Procedural Terminology (CPT) codes and diagnoses by International Classification of Diseases, Ninth/Tenth Revision, Clinical Modification (ICD-9/10-CM) codes. NSQIP collects pre-operative through 30-day post-operative data on randomly assigned patients at participating hospitals. Quality and reliability of the data are ensured through rigorous training of data abstractors and inter-rater reliability audits of participating sites [25].

2.2. Patient Population

Eligible patients who had a primary diagnosis of DCM (ICD-9-CM 721.1 or 722.71; ICD-10-CM M47.12 or M50.00, M50.01, M50.02, M50.03) and underwent a cervical decompression and fusion operation, including anterior (CPT 22551, 22554, 63081) and/or posterior (CPT 22600, 63051, 63020) approach. ICD-9/10-CM and CPT codes used for this study are summarized in Table 2.

Table 2. List of ICD-9, ICD-10, and Current Procedural Terminology (CPT) codes used to determine diagnosis, operative approach and number of operated levels.

Coding System	Code	Description
ICD-9-CM	721.1	Cervical spondylosis with myelopathy
	722.71	Intervertebral disc disorder with myelopathy, cervical region
ICD-10-CM	M47.12	Other spondylosis with myelopathy, cervical region
	M50.00, M50.01, M50.02, M50.03	Cervical disc disorder with myelopathy
CPT	22551	Arthrodesis, anterior interbody, including disc space preparation, discectomy, osteophytectomy and decompression of spinal cord and/or nerve roots; cervical below C2+ Each additional interspace 22552
	22600	Arthrodesis, posterior or posterolateral technique, single level; cervical below C2 segment+ Each additional vertebral segment 22614
	22856	Cervical arthroplasty (anterior)
	63081	Cervical corpectomy (anterior)
	63001	Posterior cervical laminoplasty
	63045, 63015	Posterior cervical laminectomy

ICD, International Classification of Diseases; CM, Clinical Modification; CPT, Current Procedural Terminology.

2.3. Baseline Characteristics

Data relating to baseline demographic characteristics and comorbidities were extracted. The number of operated levels was determined by searching the "other procedure" fields for CPT add-on codes specifying each additional level fused (CPT 22552, 22614). Surgical approaches were separated into anterior, posterior, or combined as a categorical variable.

2.4. Calculation of Frailty Indices

The MFI-11 was calculated according to established mapping of existing variables included in the NSQIP database (see Table 1). A total score between zero and one was calculated by dividing the number of variables present (for functional status, partial or complete dependency = 1) by 11. Afterwards, 0.09 was categorized as "Pre-Frail", 0.18 as "Frail", and 0.27 and above as "Severely Frail", in line with previously established standards [26,29]. A modified frailty index (mFI-5) was derived according to the standard methodology described by Searle et al. [30], calculated using NSQIP variables [31]. Specifically, five factors within the NSQIP (functional dependence, diabetes, history of chronic obstructive pulmonary disease (COPD), history of congestive heart failure, and hypertension) map to the original Canadian Study of Health and Aging (CSHA) Frailty Index [27]. For every patient, each of these five factors (deficits) were coded as absent (0) or present (1). The mean score across all deficits was calculated, resulting in an index ranging from 0 (least frail) to 5 (most frail), with a score of

1 as "Pre-Frail", 2 as "Frail", and 3 or more as "Severely Frail" as categorical variables. ASA score was taken directly from the NSQIP database for each patient. The mCCI score was calculated according to previous methods mapped directly from the corresponding NSQIP variables [18], creating a score from 0 to 23 depending on the age and presence of defined co-morbidities.

2.5. Outcomes

Outcomes evaluated were 30-day mortality, unplanned readmission, unplanned reoperation, and major complication, as well as total hospital length of stay (LOS) and routine discharge (home). Major complication was a composite outcome of pneumonia, deep vein thrombosis (DVT), pulmonary embolism, myocardial infarction, cardiac arrest, wound infection or dehiscence, stroke, and sepsis.

2.6. Statistical Analysis

All statistical analyses were performed using Stata 16 (Stata Corp, College Station, TX, USA) with an a priori specified significance level of $p = 0.05$ (two-tailed). Descriptive statistics were by mean and standard deviation (SD) for continuous variables as well as count and percentage for categorical variables.

The effect of age, MFI-5, MFI-11, CCI, and ASA were each analyzed by univariate analysis using simple logistic regression for dichotomous outcomes or linear regression for continuous outcomes. Effect sizes were summarized by odds ratio (OR) (dichotomous outcomes) or beta coefficients (continuous outcomes) and associated 95% confidence intervals (95% CI). The independent effect of age and frailty on outcomes was further evaluated by multivariable regression. Again, for each outcome, a logistic or linear regression model was constructed that included both variables and additionally adjusted for sex, type of fusion, and number of levels as covariates. To weigh the relative importance of age versus frailty in predicting each outcome, standardized regression coefficients were calculated and their magnitudes directly compared. The margins of interaction of the final model of age (by decade) and frailty (continuous variable) were calculated for all adverse events to assess how the burden of frailty was affected by increasing age.

To compare the discriminative ability of age and the various indices of frailty, receiver operating characteristics (ROC) curve analysis was performed for each dichotomous outcome reported. This was done first using a base model that included the type of approach, number of operated levels and gender, and then with the addition of age and each index of Frailty, before comparing to the final multivariable model incorporating age, MFI-5, and the base model. The Kappa correlation coefficient was calculated to assess the discriminative ability of the MFI-5 to predict the categorical assessment of frailty compared to the MFI-11 assessment.

2.7. Ethics Approval

Institutional Review Board approval was not required for this study, which relied on de-identified data derived from a national administrative healthcare dataset.

3. Results

A total of 41,369 patients with the ICD-9/ICD-10 diagnostic code for DCM were identified from the NSQIP database. The mean age was 56.6 (56.5–56.7) years with a range of 18–90, and 46% of patients were female. The majority of patients were Caucasian, although ethnicity metrics were not captured in 9.84% of patients. Data on the surgical approach, based on validated CPT codes, was available for 34,287 patients. Anterior, posterior and combined anterior-posterior surgical approaches were all included; however, 79.86% of the patients underwent anterior surgery. Furthermore, the study included single and multi-level disease, but the majority of cases were single or two-level pathology (39.24% and 31.64% respectively). The ASA grade and mCCI scores were calculated in all patients, and the median was 3 and 2, respectively. MFI-11 was calculated for 11,758 patients with 39.55% and 37.47% in the "Not Frail" or "Pre-Frail" categories. MFI-5 scores were calculated for 41,140 patients, with 44.68% "Not Frail" and 36.03% "Pre-Frail". Complete descriptive statistics for all indices are listed in Table 3.

Table 3. Patient demographics and descriptive statistics.

Age Mean (95% CI)	56.6 (56.5–56.7)
Distribution (n):	
18–30	627
30–40	3728
40–50	8858
50–60	12,427
60–70	9966
70–80	4745
80–90	931
90+	87
Gender	
Male	22,191 (54%)
Female	19,167 (46%)
Ethnicity	
White	30,778 (74%)
Black/African American	5260 (13%)
Asian	897 (2.1%)
American Indian	222 (0.5%)
Native Hawaiian/Pacific Islands	141 (0.4%)
Unknown	4071 (10%)
Approach (where defined)	
Anterior	27,380 (80%)
Posterior	5945 (17%)
Combined	962 (3%)
Distribution of Frailty	
MFI5	
Not frail	18,482 (45%)
Pre-frail	14,904 (36%)
Frail	6816 (16%)
Severely Frail	1167 (3%)
MFI11	
Not frail	4650 (40%)
Pre-frail	4406 (37%)
Frail	2239 (19%)
Severely Frail	463 (4%)
mCCI score	
0	4125 (10%)
1–2	17,613 (43%)
3–4	14,670 (35%)
5–6	4645 (11%)
>6	316 (1%)
ASA	
1	1359 (3%)
2	19,289 (47%)
3	19,354 (47%)
4	1325 (3%)

MFI-5, MFI-11, Modified Frailty Index 5-point or 11-point; mCCI, Modified Charlson Co-morbidity Index; ASA, American Society of Anesthesiology Grade; 95% CI, 95% Confidence Interval.

3.1. Univariate Analysis of Age and Frailty Indices on Outcomes

Univariate analysis demonstrated that age, frailty (MFI-5 or MFI-11), ASA, and mCCI were significantly predictive of perioperative mortality, major complication, unplanned readmission, unplanned reoperation, length of hospital stay, and discharge to non-home destination (Table 4). The OR effect size of age increases by decade for mortality, major complication, length of stay, and discharge to non-home destination (see Table 5). Based on categorical analysis of frailty tiers, increasing frailty was significantly associated with increased risk of all adverse events, increased length of stay and non-home discharge. The effect size of the MFI-5 index on all outcomes was greater than the MFI-11. Categorical correlation between frailty tiers calculated by the MFI-11 and MFI-5 was strongly significant with a kappa coefficient of 0.96 (97.58% agreement) and a spearman rank correlation of 0.988 ($p < 0.001$).

3.2. Multivariable Analysis Adjusting for Approach, Number of Levels Operated and Gender

The results from the multivariable regression analysis (adjusting for sex, surgical approach, and number of operated levels) demonstrate that age and/or frailty (as measured by the mFI) both have significant effects on the outcomes of patient mortality, unplanned readmission, unplanned reoperation, major complication, length of stay, and discharge home (see Table 6). Both increasing age and higher frailty index score were significantly associated with an increased risk of mortality ($p < 0.001$), but the effect size (as demonstrated by the beta coefficient) was greater for frailty (0.53) as compared to age (0.30). The effect size of frailty on the risk of a major complication event and length of stay was also greater than age, but increased frailty and increased age demonstrated equivalent effect sizes on the chance of a routine home discharge (−0.30 vs. −0.28). Increased age appeared to have a greater influence on the risk of unplanned readmission (0.17 compared to 0.14), however, age was not found to have any significant influence on the risk of unplanned reoperation (0.03; $p = 0.676$) and the effect size for frailty was of a magnitude 5.6 times greater (0.17; $p = 0.016$). Similar to the univariate analysis, increasing frailty was associated with a significantly increased risk of all outcomes, with 'Severely Frail' patients demonstrating an effect size 4–5 times larger for some outcomes (mortality, major complication, unplanned reoperation).

ROC area under the curve (AUC) analysis demonstrated the discriminative ability of the base model could be improved across all outcomes with the addition of age or an index of frailty (See Table 7). MFI-5 and CCI appeared to provide the best discriminative ability when added to the base model compared to the other measures of frailty. However, the final multivariable model demonstrated superior discriminative ability for all outcomes above all of the individual frailty measures + base models tested with an AUC range from 0.76–0.84.

Table 4. Univariate analysis for age, MFI-5, MFI-11, mCCI and ASA grade on the outcome of Mortality, Major Complication, Unplanned Readmission, Unplanned Reoperation, Length of Hospital Stay, and Discharge to non-home destination.

	Mortality	Major Complication (Pneumonia, DVT/PE, MI, Cardiac Arrest, Wound Infection/Dehiscence, Sepsis, CVA)	Unplanned Readmission	Reoperation	Length of Hospital Stay (Regression Coefficient)	Discharge to Non-Home Destination
Age	1.09 (1.08–1.11) *	1.06 (1.05–1.06) *	1.05 (1.03–1.07) *	1.07 (0.99–1.04)		1.072 (1.070–1.075) *
MFI5						
Pre-frail	4.89 (2.72–8.79) *	2.40 (2.06–2.80) *	1.30 (0.71–2.40)	0.57 (0.22–1.51)	0.82 (0.70–.94) *	2.22 (2.07–2.38) *
Frail	8.37 (4.58–15.32) *	3.80 (3.22–4.48) *	3.40 (1.89–6.12) *	2.71 (1.26–5.86) *	1.67 (1.52–1.82) *	3.85 (3.56–4.12) *
Severely Frail	27.70 (14.29–53.69) *	11.63 (9.44–14.33) *	6.37 (2.80–14.50) *	8.57 (3.41–21.52) *	3.74 (3.42–4.06) *	8.67 (7.62–9.86) *
MFI11						
Pre-frail	4.45 (1.68–11.81) *	1.87 (1.45–2.41) *	1.11 (0.59–2.09)	0.49 (0.18–1.28)	0.80 (0.47–1.13) *	1.71 (1.53–1.91) *
Frail	7.11 (2.62–19.29) *	2.84 (2.17–3.72) *	2.75 (1.51–5.01) *	1.92 (0.88–4.22)	1.83 (1.42–2.24) *	2.89 (2.56–3.26) *
Severely Frail	20.51 (6.98–60.26) *	7.39 (5.30–10.31) *	3.74 (1.56–8.95) *	4.68 (1.77–12.38) *	4.39 (3.61–5.16) *	7.81 (6.38–9.56) *
mCCI	1.76 (1.62–1.90) *	1.51 (1.47–1.56) *	1.40 (1.25–1.58) *	1.32 (1.11–1.57) *	0.53 (0.50–0.56) *	1.59 (1.56–1.62) *
ASA	4.14 (3.12–5.50) *	3.60 (3.26–3.98) *	1.40 (1.25–1.85) *	1.32 (1.12–1.57) *	1.58 (1.50–1.67) *	3.35 (3.19–3.53) *

MFI-5, MFI-11, Modified Frailty Index 5-point or 11-point; mCCI, Modified Charlson Co-morbidity Index; ASA, American Society of Anesthesiology Grade; DVT, deep vein thrombosis; PE, Pulmonary Embolus; MI, Myocardial Infarction; CVA, Cerebrovascular Accident. * indicates the result is statistically significant (p value < 0.05).

Table 5. Univariate analysis by decade demonstrates increasing effect size (odds ratios) with increasing age for the outcomes of Mortality, Major Complication, Length of Hospital Stay, and Discharge Destination.

Age by Decade	Mortality	Major Complication (Pneumonia, DVT/PE, MI, Cardiac Arrest, Wound Infection/Dehiscence, Sepsis, CVA)	Unplanned Readmission	Reoperation	Length of Hospital Stay (Regression Coefficient)	Discharge to Non-Home Destination
30–40	0.0044 (0.0005–0.038) *	1.04 (0.41–2.70)	0.046 (0.0041–0.51) *	0.32 (0.067–1.50)	−0.13 (−0.59–0.32)	0.84 (0.56–1.25)
40–50	0.015 (0.047–0.046) *	1.55 (0.63–3.81)	0.097 (0.012–0.77) *	0.40 (0.14–1.16) *	0.11 (−0.33–0.55)	1.30 (0.90–1.90)
50–60	0.023 (0.0086–0.066) *	2.87 (1.17–6.97) *	0.12 (0.016–0.90) *	0.76 (0.33–1.78)	0.73 (0.29–1.15) *	2.23 (1.54–3.23) *
60–70	0.073 (0.028–0.19) *	4.93 (2.03–11.96)	0.19 (0.025–1.43)	0.42 (0.15–1.15)	1.23 (0.79–1.67) *	4.29 (2.96–6.21) *
70–80	0.17 (0.065–0.43) *	9.03 (3.72–21.92) *	0.35 (0.046–2.61)	†	2.21 (1.75–2.66) *	9.36 (6.45–13.58) *
80–90	0.21 (0.074–0.63) *	11.69 (4.71–29.04) *	0.27 (0.029–2.70)	†	3.23 (2.68–3.78) *	20.73 (14.05–30.57) *
90+	†	19.90 (6.82–58.05) *	†	†	3.87 (2.65–5.09) *	52.24 (28.78–94.82) *

Correlation between frailty tiers calculated by the MFI-11 and MFI-5 was strongly significant with a kappa coefficient of 0.96 (97.58% agreement) and a spearman rank correlation of 0.988 (p < 0.001). † indicates that this decade was removed from analysis due to collinearity; * indicates the result is statistically significant (p value < 0.05).

Table 6. Multivariable analysis adjusting for age, gender, number of levels and surgical approach including one of either MFI-5, mFI-11, mCCI or ASA as the inter-changeable dependent variable.

	Mortality	Major Complication (Pneumonia, DVT/PE, MI, Cardiac Arrest, Wound Infection/Dehiscence, Sepsis, CVA)	Unplanned Readmission	Reoperation	Length of Hospital Stay (Regression Coefficient)	Discharge to Non-Home Destination
Age	1.08 (1.05–1.10) *	1.04 (1.03–1.05) *	1.02 (0.99–1.04)	0.98 (0.95–1.02)	0.021 (0.015–0.026) *	1.05 (1.05–1.06) *
MFI5 score						
Pre-frail	2.03 (1.65–2.51) *	1.67 (1.54–1.80) *	1.58 (1.14–2.18) *	2.25 (1.51–3.36) *	0.61 (0.53–0.69) *	1.60 (1.53–1.67) *
Frail	2.07 (1.09–3.92) *	1.48 (1.24–1.77) *	0.80 (0.35–1.80)	0.54 (0.15–1.87)	0.31 (0.17–0.45) *	1.28 (1.17–1.40) *
Severely Frail	3.19 (1.64–6.17) *	2.27 (1.87–2.75) *	2.67 (1.27–5.63) *	2.87 (1.06–7.83) *	0.92 (0.74–1.09) *	2.15 (1.94–2.38) *
	10.84 (5.28–22.30) *	5.83 (4.54–7.48) *	3.47 (1.18–10.21) *	10.71 (3.57–32.17) *	2.84 (2.47–3.21) *	4.94 (4.19–5.83) *
MFI11						
Pre-frail	1.70 (0.55–5.32)	1.16 (0.86–1.57)	0.95 (0.42–2.13)	0.56 (0.16–1.91)	0.55 (0.11–0.99) *	1.25 (1.07–1.46) *
Frail	2.81 (0.89–8.88)	1.68 (1.21–2.32) *	2.51 (1.15–5.49) *	2.55 (0.92–7.12)	1.14 (0.86–1.95) *	2.24 (1.90–2.65) *
Severely Frail	7.68 (2.21–26.61) *	4.12 (2.80–6.23) *	3.16 (1.06–9.43) *	7.99 (2.51–25.40) *	4.01 (3.00–5.06) *	5.60 (4.29–7.32) *
mCCI	1.53 (0.35–1.74) *	1.35 (1.28–1.43) *	1.36 (1.10–1.68) *	1.60 (1.25–2.05) *	0.40 (0.34–0.46) *	1.30 (1.26–1.35) *
ASA	2.48 (1.06–1.10) *	2.54 (2.25–2.86) *	1.87 (1.13–3.09) *	1.88 (0.98–3.59)	1.02 (0.92–1.12)	2.49 (2.32–2.66) *

MFI-5, MFI-11, Modified Frailty Index 5-point or 11-point. mCCI, Modified Charlson Co-morbidity Index. ASA, American Society of Anesthesiology Grade; * indicates the result is statistically significant (*p* value < 0.05).

Table 7. Area under Receiver Operating Characteristics curve analysis by model, for each outcome studied.

	Mortality	Major Complication (Pneumonia, DVT/PE, MI, Cardiac Arrest, Wound Infection/Dehiscence, Sepsis, CVA)	Unplanned Readmission	Unplanned Reoperation	Hospital Stay 30 Days or Greater after Index Case	Discharge to Non-Home Destination
Base model (approach, number of levels, gender)	0.68	0.68	0.74	0.77	0.69	0.72
Base model + Age	0.80	0.74	0.77	0.76	0.76	0.80
Base model + MFI5	0.77	0.74	0.78	0.82	0.73	0.78
Base model + MFI11	0.75	0.70	0.73	0.78	0.69	0.76
Base model + mCCI	0.81	0.75	0.79	0.80	0.78	0.80
Base model + ASA	0.76	0.75	0.76	0.78	0.79	0.79
Final multivariable model (age, MFI-5, approach, number of levels, gender)	0.83	0.76	0.79	0.84	0.78	0.81

MFI-5, MFI-11, Modified Frailty Index 5-point or 11-point; mCCI, Modified Charlson Co-morbidity Index; ASA, American Society of Anesthesiology Grade.

4. Discussion

As the burden of age-related degenerative spine conditions becomes an ever-greater public health priority, DCM has the potential to be a major cause of preventable neurological disability and poor quality of life across the world [4,8,16]. Decompressive surgery remains the only treatment proven to arrest or reverse the dysfunction caused by myelopathy and has a proven benefit in the elderly population [3,7,10,32]. The diagnosis of DCM and identification of suitable surgical candidates is therefore of paramount importance, and for this reason, identifying tools to aid risk stratification and predict potential outcomes after surgery is a major focus of clinical research [6,9,13,14].

The evidence for decompressive surgery to improve functional and quality of life impairment in DCM is strong [7,10,32]. Reports on the effect of age on the outcomes after DCM surgery have been variable, with many supporting the notion that increasing age is associated with negative clinical outcomes, whether increased complication rates or functional outcomes [12,13,15,33]. A recent ambispective study has demonstrated a clear and sustained benefit for surgery in DCM for both functional and quality of life outcomes in patients over the age of 70, albeit with an order of magnitude less than their younger surgery- and co-morbidity-matched cohort [3]. The suggested mechanism for this discrepancy has traditionally been the burden of age-related co-morbidities influencing clinical outcomes and reduction of physiological reserve, which has been manifested as measures of frailty or frailty indices in recent years. This hypothesis has been further substantiated with the correlation of worsening frailty to increased complication rate after spine surgery, and poorer recovery after spinal cord injury [28,34,35]. However, despite DCM being the most common indication for cervical spine surgery in North America, the effect of frailty on the outcomes after DCM surgery has not been investigated [16].

This study is one of the most comprehensive investigations of perioperative adverse events after surgery for DCM, and is the first to present a direct comparison of age and frailty indices. Concepts of frailty, although distinct from risk stratification, are increasingly incorporated in the pre-operative assessment as a superior and comprehensive alternative to age alone. Although it is no surprise that increasing age leads to an increased risk of adverse events, it appears the burden of frailty can have an effect up to 28 times the magnitude compared to age alone. On univariate analysis, increasing frailty (MFI-5/MFI-11) had the largest effect size for mortality, major complication and discharge to non-home destination. This effect remained in the multivariable model, but the effect size was largest for mortality and unplanned reoperation. These findings suggest that physiological reserve is much more of a driver of perioperative complications when compared to age alone. This is consistent with previous studies on spine surgical patients, but also other surgical domains [36,37]. The degree to which frailty appears to have an influence on unplanned reoperation rates has a sound pathophysiological basis. Given the usual indications for early reoperation are compressive hematoma, infection, and hardware failure, patients who have a higher mFI score are more likely to develop post-operative infections and a higher risk of osteopenia/osteoporosis.

Frailty significantly affected the risk of perioperative adverse events for patients of all ages, but the burden of frailty becomes greater with increased age. This effect is not linear, as demonstrated by the margins of interaction between age (by decade) and categorical level of frailty (see Figure 1). This effect (for readmission, reoperation, length of stay, and discharge to non-home destination) begins after the age of 60, which is in line with previously reported studies [32,34,35].

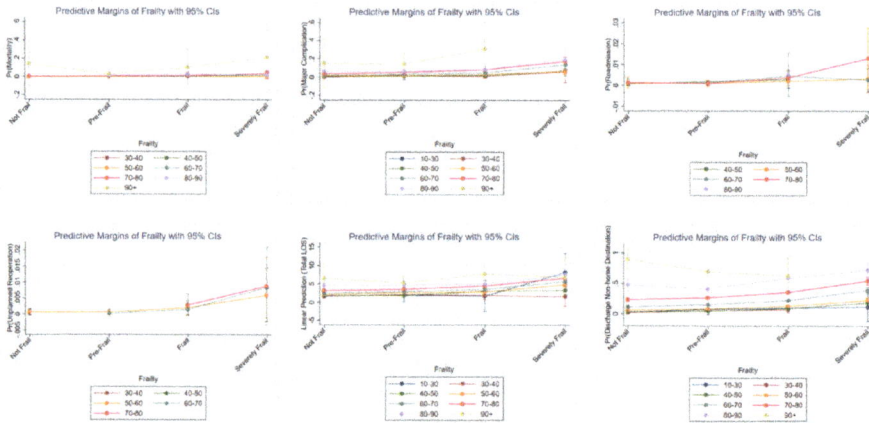

Figure 1. Predictive margins of the final multivariable model for each frailty level stratified per decade of age, for each outcome studied. Decades of age were removed if co-linearity was present. 95% CI, 95% Confidence Interval.

The mCCI proved a significant predictor of all adverse events on univariate and multivariable analysis, and the effect size remained similar for both. This may suggest that it could be a useful tool in the assessment of DCM patients. However, the role of the mCCI in multivariable modeling is unclear due to the inclusion of age-related modifiers. The mCCI incorporates increasing age as a contributor to the overall score, and therefore does not provide an age-independent measure of frailty. It cannot therefore be a definitive frailty assessment when incorporated into a multivariable model that includes age as a continuous variable. The ASA score also proved to be significantly predictive of adverse events on both univariable and multivariable analysis. However, the ASA score is notoriously subjective and its practical use for pre-operative adverse event prediction modeling has not been substantiated.

There was strong correlation between the MFI-11 and MFI-5 assessment of frailty tiers, which has been echoed in previous articles in other spine pathologies [28]. The effect size of the odds ratio or regression coefficients were larger when the MFI-5 was used compared to the MFI-11 for all dichotomous outcomes and length of hospital stay. This would suggest that to achieve an assessment of "Frail" or "Severely Frail" with the MFI-5 this would indicate a greater degree of frailty compared to the MFI-11 equivalent. This is strong evidence that the use of the MFI-5 is an effective determinant of frailty and further substantiates the MFI-5 as the standard of choice for frailty assessment for DCM patients. This has important implications for the use of MFI-5 in clinical practice and for future studies into the effect of frailty in adult spine surgery.

There are limitations to the current study. The NSQIP database carries metrics regarding peri-operative events, but no long term follow up or outcome measures are included. This restricts the analysis to short term follow up only, and therefore long-term outcomes cannot be extrapolated. However, the validity of short-term complication rates and their use for pre-operative decision-making in spine surgery is well published. In a similar vein, there is no measure of baseline functional impairment and therefore there is no way to eliminate the effect of myelopathy severity on the surgical approach, or other covariates applied to the regression model. Pre-operative neurological function is a key predictor of the functional outcomes of DCM surgery, however its relationship to perioperative adverse events and mortality is less clear. It is known that myelopathy patients have increased perioperative complications compared to radiculopathy [26], but there is a paucity of evidence of the effect of functional impairment on perioperative outcomes in DCM.

There was an observed difference in the number of patients that were able to have the MFI-11 calculated ($n = 11{,}758$) compared to the MFI-5 ($n = 41{,}140$). This difference arose arbitrarily due to a reduction in the demographic information collected by NSQIP from 2015 onwards. This difference in numbers has the potential to skew the effects and effect size of the results presented. The authors argue that given the categorical correlation of frailty was excellent between MFI-5 and MFI-11 (97.58% agreement), the large size of the cohorts, the strength of the a priori statistical frameworks and the levels of significance observed, the risk of statistical inaccuracy is low.

The study is a retrospective analysis of prospectively collected nationwide hospital inpatient registry data. As such, it lacks the protection from confounders and bias from a true prospectively-collected data set. However, uniformity across the data collection and homogeneity amongst the selected cohort does reduce the impact of any latent confounding. The cohort selection relied on ICD-9 & 10 diagnostic codes, and therefore the potential risk of not capturing patients if they were inappropriately coded is present. Patients were removed from the final analysis if no reliable CPT code data could identify the surgical approach or number of levels, which led to a reduction in the overall number of patients in the multivariable model. It is unlikely that these occurrences have affected the findings of the study given the levels of significance seen on univariable and multivariable analysis.

The authors note that DCM carries a significant heterogeneity in presenting symptoms ranging from mild sensory disturbance in the fingers through to gait instability and eventual quadriparesis. Traditional measures of frailty, in particular those based on 5- or 11-point scales as used in this study, may not be as accurate when compared to other pathologies not affecting gait or upper limb function. Therefore, developing more appropriate indices of frailty specific to DCM should be a future research priority. Also, the authors wish to state that the purpose of this study is not to prove patients who have an increased frailty score should not be offered surgical management. In contrast, this study should be used to provide further clarification of the factors that go into informed decision-making, which should be a shared process between the patient and clinician. The concept that frailty could potentially be viewed as a modifiable risk factor is also emerging, however evidence that improving frailty index scores prior to planned spine surgery to reduce perioperative complications is not conclusive at this stage [38].

5. Conclusions

Increasing frailty appears to have a greater influence on the risk of perioperative mortality, risk of major complication, unplanned readmission, unplanned reoperation, and longer duration of hospital stay when directly compared to age alone for patients undergoing surgery for DCM. The MFI-5 is a robust predictor of adverse outcomes after DCM surgery and is equivalent to the traditional MFI-11 when categorizing patients as 'Pre-Frail', 'Frail', or 'Severely Frail.' Multivariable models incorporating MFI-5 with age, approach, number of levels, and gender provide an accurate and reliable method of predicting outcomes from DCM surgery. Future work should focus on how to delineate the association of frailty with long term functional and quality of life outcomes after DCM surgery.

Author Contributions: Conceptualization, J.R.F.W., J.H.B., J.R.W., A.Y. and M.G.F.; methodology, J.R.F.W., J.H.B. and A.M.; formal analysis, J.R.F.W., J.H.B., A.M. and M.G.F.; investigation, J.R.F.W., J.H.B. and A.M.; writing—Original draft, J.R.F.W. and J.H.B.; writing—Review and editing, J.R.W., A.Y. and M.G.F.; supervision and administration, J.R.W., A.Y. and M.G.F. All authors have read and agreed to the published version of the manuscript.

Funding: This research received no external funding.

Acknowledgments: J.R.F.W. is the recipient of an award from the Neurosurgery Research and Education Fund (NREF) of the American Association of Neurological Surgeons (AANS). M.G.F. acknowledges support from the Gerry and Tootsie Halbert Chair in Neural Repair and Regeneration and the DeZwirek Family Foundation. This work has been produced with patient information from the National Safety Quality Improvement Program (NSQIP) organization and contributing members.

Conflicts of Interest: The authors declare no conflict of interest.

References

1. Karadimas, S.K.; Erwin, W.M.; Ely, C.G.; Dettori, J.R.; Fehlings, M.G. Pathophysiology and Natural History of Cervical Spondylotic Myelopathy. *Spine* **2013**, *38*, S21–S36. [CrossRef] [PubMed]
2. Nouri, A.; Tetreault, L.; Singh, A.; Karadimas, S.K.; Fehlings, M.G. Degenerative Cervical Myelopathy. *Spine* **2015**, *40*, E675–E693. [CrossRef] [PubMed]
3. Wilson, J.R.F.; Badhiwala, J.; Jiang, F.; Wilson, J.R.; Kopjar, B.; Vaccaro, A.R.; Fehlings, M.G. The Impact of Older Age on Functional Recovery and Quality of Life Outcomes after Surgical Decompression for Degenerative Cervical Myelopathy: Results from an Ambispective, Propensity-Matched Analysis from the CSM-NA and CSM-I International, Multi-Center Studies. *J. Clin. Med.* **2019**, *8*, 1708. [CrossRef]
4. Wilson, J.R.; Badhiwala, J.H.; Moghaddamjou, A.; Martin, A.R.; Fehlings, M.G. Degenerative Cervical Myelopathy; A Review of the Latest Advances and Future Directions in Management. *Neurospine* **2019**, *16*, 494–505. [CrossRef] [PubMed]
5. Institute of Medicine Initial National Priorities for Comparative Effectiveness Research. *Initial National Priorities for Comparative Effectiveness Research*; The National Academies Press: Washington, DC, USA, 2009.
6. Davies, B.M.; Khan, D.Z.; Mowforth, O.D.; McNair, A.G.K.; Gronlund, T.; Kolias, A.G.; Tetreault, L.; Starkey, M.L.; Sadler, I.; Sarewitz, E.; et al. RE-CODE DCM (REsearch Objectives and Common Data Elements for Degenerative Cervical Myelopathy): A Consensus Process to Improve Research Efficiency in DCM, Through Establishment of a Standardized Dataset for Clinical Research and the Definition of the Research Priorities. *Glob. Spine J.* **2019**, *9*, 65S–76S. [CrossRef]
7. Fehlings, M.G.; Tetreault, L.A.; Riew, K.D.; Middleton, J.W.; Aarabi, B.; Arnold, P.M.; Brodke, D.S.; Burns, A.S.; Carette, S.; Chen, R.; et al. A Clinical Practice Guideline for the Management of Patients with Degenerative Cervical Myelopathy: Recommendations for Patients with Mild, Moderate, and Severe Disease and Nonmyelopathic Patients with Evidence of Cord Compression. *Glob. Spine J.* **2017**, *7*, 70S–83S. [CrossRef] [PubMed]
8. Oh, T.; Lafage, R.; Lafage, V.; Protopsaltis, T.; Challier, V.; Shaffrey, C.; Kim, H.J.; Arnold, P.; Chapman, J.R.; Schwab, F.; et al. Comparing Quality of Life in Cervical Spondylotic Myelopathy with Other Chronic Debilitating Diseases Using the Short Form Survey 36-Health Survey. *World Neurosurg.* **2017**, *106*, 699–706. [CrossRef] [PubMed]
9. Badhiwala, J.H.; Witiw, C.D.; Nassiri, F.; A Akbar, M.; Mansouri, A.; Wilson, J.R.; Fehlings, M.G. Efficacy and Safety of Surgery for Mild Degenerative Cervical Myelopathy: Results of the AOSpine North America and International Prospective Multicenter Studies. *Neurosurgery* **2019**, *84*, 890–897. [CrossRef]
10. Fehlings, M.G.; Ibrahim, A.; Tetreault, L.; Albanese, V.; Alvarado, M.; Arnold, P.; Barbagallo, G.M.V.; Bartels, R.H.M.A.; Bolger, C.; Defino, H.L.A.; et al. A Global Perspective on the Outcomes of Surgical Decompression in Patients with Cervical Spondylotic Myelopathy. *Spine* **2015**, *40*, 1322–1328. [CrossRef]
11. Fehlings, M.G.; Wilson, J.R.; Kopjar, B.; Yoon, S.T.; Arnold, P.M.; Massicotte, E.M.; Vaccaro, A.R.; Brodke, D.S.; Shaffrey, C.I.; Smith, J.S.; et al. Efficacy and Safety of Surgical Decompression in Patients with Cervical Spondylotic Myelopathy. *J. Bone Jt. Surg. Am.* **2013**, *95*, 1651–1658. [CrossRef]
12. Tetreault, L.; Palubiski, L.M.; Kryshtalskyj, M.; Idler, R.K.; Martin, A.R.; Ganau, M.; Wilson, J.R.; Kotter, M.; Fehlings, M.G. Significant Predictors of Outcome Following Surgery for the Treatment of Degenerative Cervical Myelopathy. *Neurosurg. Clin. North Am.* **2018**, *29*, 115–127.e35. [CrossRef] [PubMed]
13. Fehlings, M.; Wilson, J.R.F.; Jiang, F. Clinical predictors of complications and outcomes in degenerative cervical myeloradiculopathy. *Indian Spine J.* **2019**, *2*, 59. [CrossRef]
14. Badhiwala, J.; Witiw, C.D.; Nassiri, F.; Jaja, B.N.; Akbar, M.A.; Mansouri, A.; Merali, Z.; Ibrahim, G.M.; Wilson, J.R.; Fehlings, M.G. Patient phenotypes associated with outcome following surgery for mild degenerative cervical myelopathy: A principal component regression analysis. *Spine J.* **2018**, *18*, 2220–2231. [CrossRef]
15. Tetreault, L.; Tan, G.; Kopjar, B.; Côté, P.; Arnold, P.; Nugaeva, N.; Barbagallo, G.M.V.; Fehlings, M.G. Clinical and Surgical Predictors of Complications Following Surgery for the Treatment of Cervical Spondylotic Myelopathy. *Neurosurgery* **2015**, *79*, 33–44. [CrossRef]
16. Fehlings, M.G.; Tetreault, L.; Nater, A.; Choma, T.; Harrop, J.; Mroz, T.; Santaguida, C.; Smith, J.S. The Aging of the Global Population. *Neurosurgery* **2015**, *77*, S1–S5. [CrossRef] [PubMed]

17. Tetreault, L.; Ibrahim, A.K.; Côté, P.; Singh, A.; Fehlings, M.G. A systematic review of clinical and surgical predictors of complications following surgery for degenerative cervical myelopathy. *J. Neurosurg. Spine* **2016**, *24*, 77–99. [CrossRef]
18. Lakomkin, N.; Zuckerman, S.L.; Stannard, B.; Montejo, J.; Sussman, E.S.; Virojanapa, J.; Kuzmik, G.; Goz, V.; Hadjipanayis, C.G.; Cheng, J.S. Preoperative Risk Stratification in Spine Tumor Surgery. *Spine* **2019**, *44*, E782–E787. [CrossRef]
19. Meng, X.; Press, B.; Renson, A.; Wysock, J.S.; Taneja, S.S.; Huang, W.C.; Bjurlin, M.A. Discriminative Ability of Commonly Used Indexes to Predict Adverse Outcomes After Radical Cystectomy: Comparison of Demographic Data, American Society of Anesthesiologists, Modified Charlson Comorbidity Index, and Modified Frailty Index. *Clin. Genitourin. Cancer* **2018**, *16*, e843–e850. [CrossRef]
20. Ondeck, N.T.; Bovonratwet, P.; Ibe, I.K.; Bohl, D.D.; McLynn, R.P.; Cui, J.J.; Baumgaertner, M.R.; Grauer, J.N. Discriminative Ability for Adverse Outcomes After Surgical Management of Hip Fractures. *J. Orthop. Trauma* **2018**, *32*, 231–237. [CrossRef]
21. Shah, R.; Ms, J.D.B.; Ms, J.C.H.; Varley, P.R.; Wisniewski, M.K.; Shinall, M.C.; Arya, S.; Johnson, J.; Nelson, J.B.; Youk, A.; et al. Validation of the Risk Analysis Index for Evaluating Frailty in Ambulatory Patients. *J. Am. Geriatr. Soc.* **2020**, *68*, 1818–1824. [CrossRef]
22. Varley, P.R.; Borrebach, J.D.; Arya, S.; Massarweh, N.N.; Bilderback, A.L.; Wisniewski, M.K.; Nelson, J.B.; Johnson, J.T.; Johanning, J.M.; Hall, D.E. Clinical Utility of the Risk Analysis Index as a Prospective Frailty Screening Tool within a Multi-practice, Multi-hospital Integrated Healthcare System. *Ann. Surg.* **2020**. [CrossRef] [PubMed]
23. Shin, J.I.; Kothari, P.; Phan, K.; Kim, J.S.; Leven, D.; Lee, N.J.; Cho, S.K.-W. Frailty Index as a Predictor of Adverse Postoperative Outcomes in Patients Undergoing Cervical Spinal Fusion. *Spine* **2017**, *42*, 304–310. [CrossRef]
24. Lukasiewicz, A.M.; Basques, B.A.; Bohl, D.D.; Webb, M.L.; Samuel, A.M.; Grauer, J.N. Myelopathy Is Associated with Increased All-Cause Morbidity and Mortality Following Anterior Cervical Discectomy and Fusion. *Spine* **2015**, *40*, 443–449. [CrossRef] [PubMed]
25. Shiloach, M.; Frencher, S.K.; Steeger, J.E.; Rowell, K.S.; Bartzokis, K.; Tomeh, M.G.; Richards, K.E.; Ko, C.Y.; Hall, B.L. Toward Robust Information: Data Quality and Inter-Rater Reliability in the American College of Surgeons National Surgical Quality Improvement Program. *J. Am. Coll. Surg.* **2010**, *210*, 6–16. [CrossRef] [PubMed]
26. Yagi, M.; Michikawa, T.; Hosogane, N.; Fujita, N.; Okada, E.; Suzuki, S.; Tsuji, O.; Nagoshi, N.; Asazuma, T.; Tsuji, T.; et al. The 5-Item Modified Frailty Index Is Predictive of Severe Adverse Events in Patients Undergoing Surgery for Adult Spinal Deformity. *Spine* **2019**, *44*, E1083–E1091. [CrossRef]
27. Rockwood, K.; Song, X.; Macknight, C.; Bergman, H.; Hogan, D.B.; McDowell, I.; Mitnitski, A. A global clinical measure of fitness and frailty in elderly people. *Can. Med. Assoc. J.* **2005**, *173*, 489–495. [CrossRef]
28. Ondeck, N.T.; Bohl, D.D.; Bovonratwet, P.; Anandasivam, N.S.; Cui, J.J.; McLynn, R.P.; Grauer, J.N. Predicting Adverse Outcomes After Total Hip Arthroplasty. *J. Am. Acad. Orthop. Surg.* **2018**, *26*, 735–743. [CrossRef]
29. Miller, E.; Lenke, L.G.; Espinoza-Rebmann, K.; Neuman, B.J.; Sciubba, D.M.; Smith, J.S.; Qiu, Y.; Dahl, B.; Matsuyama, Y.; Fehlings, M.G.; et al. Use of the Adult Spinal Deformity (ASD) Frailty Index (ASD-FI) to Predict Major Complications in the Scoli-Risk 1 Multicenter, International Patient Database. *Spine J.* **2016**, *16*, S131–S132. [CrossRef]
30. Searle, S.D.; Mitnitski, A.; Gahbauer, E.A.; Gill, T.M.; Rockwood, K. A standard procedure for creating a frailty index. *BMC Geriatrics* **2008**, *8*, 24. [CrossRef]
31. Subramaniam, S.; Aalberg, J.J.; Soriano, R.P.; Divino, C.M. New 5-Factor Modified Frailty Index Using American College of Surgeons NSQIP Data. *J. Am. Coll. Surg.* **2018**, *226*, 173–181.e8. [CrossRef]
32. Fehlings, M.G.; Barry, S.; Kopjar, B.; Yoon, S.T.; Arnold, P.; Massicotte, E.M.; Vaccaro, A.; Brodke, D.S.; Shaffrey, C.; Smith, J.S.; et al. Anterior Versus Posterior Surgical Approaches to Treat Cervical Spondylotic Myelopathy. *Spine* **2013**, *38*, 2247–2252. [CrossRef] [PubMed]
33. Evaniew, N.; Belley-Côté, E.P.; Fallah, N.; Noonan, V.K.; Rivers, C.S.; Dvorak, M.F. Methylprednisolone for the Treatment of Patients with Acute Spinal Cord Injuries: A Systematic Review and Meta-Analysis. *J. Neurotrauma* **2016**, *33*, 468–481. [CrossRef]

34. Banaszek, D.; Inglis, T.; Marion, T.; Charest-Morin, R.; Moskven, E.; Rivers, C.S.; Kurban, D.; Flexman, A.M.; Ailon, T.; Dea, N.; et al. Effect of Frailty on Outcome after Traumatic Spinal Cord Injury. *J. Neurotrauma* **2020**, *37*, 839–845. [CrossRef] [PubMed]
35. Charest-Morin, R.; Street, J.T.; Zhang, H.; Roughead, T.; Ailon, T.; Boyd, M.; Dvorak, M.F.; Kwon, B.K.; Paquette, S.; Dea, N.; et al. Frailty and sarcopenia do not predict adverse events in an elderly population undergoing non-complex primary elective surgery for degenerative conditions of the lumbar spine. *Spine J.* **2017**, *18*, 245–254. [CrossRef] [PubMed]
36. Al Shakarchi, J.; Fairhead, J.; Rajagopalan, S.; Pherwani, A.; Jaipersad, A. Impact of Frailty on Outcomes in Patients Undergoing Open Abdominal Aortic Aneurysm Repair. *Ann. Vasc. Surg.* **2020**, *67*, 100–104. [CrossRef] [PubMed]
37. Pandit, V.; Lee, A.; Zeeshan, M.; Goshima, K.; Tan, T.-W.; Jhajj, S.; Trinidad, B.; Weinkauf, C.; Zhou, W. Effect of frailty syndrome on the outcomes of patients with carotid stenosis. *J. Vasc. Surg.* **2020**, *71*, 1595–1600. [CrossRef]
38. Yagi, M.; Michikawa, T.; Hosogane, N.; Fujita, N.; Okada, E.; Suzuki, S.; Tsuji, O.; Nagoshi, N.; Asazuma, T.; Tsuji, T.; et al. Treatment for Frailty Does Not Improve Complication Rates in Corrective Surgery for Adult Spinal Deformity. *Spine* **2019**, *44*, 723–731. [CrossRef]

Publisher's Note: MDPI stays neutral with regard to jurisdictional claims in published maps and institutional affiliations.

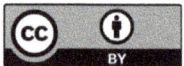

© 2020 by the authors. Licensee MDPI, Basel, Switzerland. This article is an open access article distributed under the terms and conditions of the Creative Commons Attribution (CC BY) license (http://creativecommons.org/licenses/by/4.0/).

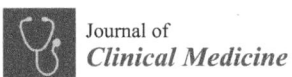

Review

The Role of Magnetic Resonance Imaging to Inform Clinical Decision-Making in Acute Spinal Cord Injury: A Systematic Review and Meta-Analysis

Arash Ghaffari-Rafi [1,2], Catherine Peterson [1], Jose E. Leon-Rojas [3,4], Nobuaki Tadokoro [5], Stefan F. Lange [6], Mayank Kaushal [7], Lindsay Tetreault [8], Michael G. Fehlings [8] and Allan R. Martin [1,8,*]

1. Department of Neurological Surgery, University of California, Davis, CA 95817, USA; aghaffarirafi@ucdavis.edu (A.G.-R.); catpeterson@ucdavis.edu (C.P.)
2. John A. Burns School of Medicine, University of Hawai'i at Mānoa, Honolulu, HI 96813, USA
3. NeurALL Research Group, Escuela de Medicina, Universidad Internacional del Ecuador, Quito 170411, Ecuador; joleonro@uide.edu.ec
4. Queen Square Institute of Neurology, University College London, London WC1N 3BG, UK
5. Department of Orthopaedic Surgery, Kochi University, Nankoku 783-0000, Japan; nobuaki.tadokoro@gmail.com
6. Department of Neurosurgery, University Medical Centre Groningen, 9713 GZ Groningen, The Netherlands; stefanlange@hotmail.nl
7. Department of Neurosurgery, Medical College of Wisconsin, Milwaukee, WI 53226, USA; mayankkaushal@yahoo.com
8. Department of Neurosurgery, Toronto Western Hospital, University of Toronto, Toronto, ON M5T 2S8, Canada; lindsay.tetreault89@gmail.com (L.T.); michael.fehlings@uhn.ca (M.G.F.)
* Correspondence: armartin@ucdavis.edu

Abstract: The clinical indications and added value of obtaining MRI in the acute phase of spinal cord injury (SCI) remain controversial. This review aims to critically evaluate evidence regarding the role of MRI to influence decision-making and outcomes in acute SCI. A systematic review and meta-analysis were performed according to PRISMA methodology to identify studies that address six key questions (KQs) regarding diagnostic accuracy, frequency of abnormal findings, frequency of altered decision-making, optimal timing, and differences in outcomes related to obtaining an MRI in acute SCI. A total of 32 studies were identified that addressed one or more KQs. MRI showed no adverse events in 156 patients (five studies) and frequently identified cord compression (70%, 12 studies), disc herniation (43%, 16 studies), ligamentous injury (39%, 13 studies), and epidural hematoma (10%, two studies), with good diagnostic accuracy (seven comparative studies) except for fracture detection. MRI findings often altered management, including timing of surgery (78%, three studies), decision to operate (36%, 15 studies), and surgical approach (29%, nine studies). MRI may also be useful to determine the need for instrumentation (100%, one study), which levels to decompress (100%, one study), and if reoperation is needed (34%, two studies). The available literature consistently concluded that MRI was useful prior to surgical treatment (13 studies) and after surgery to assess decompression (two studies), but utility before/after closed reduction of cervical dislocations was unclear (three studies). One study showed improved outcomes with an MRI-based protocol but had a high risk of bias. Heterogeneity was high for most findings ($I^2 > 0.75$). MRI is safe and frequently identifies findings alter clinical management in acute SCI, although direct evidence of its impact on outcomes is lacking. MRI should be performed before and after surgery, when feasible, to facilitate improved clinical decision-making. However, further research is needed to determine its optimal timing, effect on outcomes, cost-effectiveness, and utility before and after closed reduction.

Keywords: spinal cord injury; SCI; spine trauma; magnetic resonance imaging; MRI

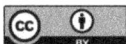

1. Introduction

Traumatic injury to the spine is common and can have devastating consequences when resulting in spinal cord injury (SCI). Acute SCI has an estimated incidence of 750 cases per million annually, often affecting younger individuals and resulting in a substantial impact upon families and society [1]. Evidence-based management of SCI is primarily focused on the acute period, including careful immobilization and transport, avoidance of hypotension and hypoxia, and early surgical decompression [2–5].

Imaging plays a critical role in the initial evaluation of spinal trauma, and computed tomography (CT) has largely supplanted radiography in modern clinical algorithms [6]. CT is widely available and can quickly screen trauma patients for numerous injuries (head, spine, thorax, and abdomen), but the visualization of the spinal soft tissues is poor, including the spinal cord, intervertebral discs, and ligaments. In contrast, magnetic resonance imaging (MRI) provides detailed views of these structures, allowing detection of spinal cord compression, acute disc herniation, ligamentous injury, and epidural hemorrhage. However, MRI has not been widely incorporated into trauma protocols due to concerns over safety, availability, inconvenience, cost, time required, and the argument that MRI findings rarely change clinical decision-making. Surprisingly, in spite of numerous manuscripts investigating MRI in spinal trauma and SCI, high-quality studies that compare clinical decision-making with and without MRI are lacking [6–8]. The American Association of Neurological Surgeons (AANS) and Congress of Neurological Surgeons (CNS) published guidelines for acute cervical spine trauma and SCI in 2002 and updated these in 2013, but offered limited recommendations regarding the use of MRI beyond its utility for cervical collar clearance—no recommendations on the use of MRI in adult patients with SCI were offered [6]. A systematic review performed by Bozzo et al. (2011) [8] took a broader approach in evaluating the clinical utility of MRI, by considering various indirect lines of evidence; based on low-quality evidence, the authors offered a weak recommendation that MRI be performed in all patients with SCI when feasible, to direct management [8]. More recently, a multi-disciplinary group sponsored by AOSpine, AANS/CNS, and Ontario Neurotrauma Foundation developed clinical practice guidelines (CPGs) on five controversial topics in SCI that included a similarly weak recommendation based on very weak evidence that MRI should be used when feasible, to guide clinical decision-making in SCI [9]. However, this CPG was primarily based on expert opinion, as the systematic review that formed its evidentiary basis found only one study that examined MRI for clinical decision-making, and it had a high risk of bias due to methodological issues [7,10]. Overall, the efforts to synthesize the evidence have not provided sufficient guidance on the routine use of MRI in acute SCI; as a result, clinical practice among spinal surgeons and other clinicians remains highly variable.

The overarching aim of this review was to determine if performing an MRI in the acute phase of SCI yields useful clinical information, leading to improvements in patient care and outcomes. However, in view of previous reviews that revealed the paucity of literature directly addressing this question, we aimed to perform a more inclusive review seeking indirect evidence that answers the key questions (KQs) listed in Table 1. Hence, our review aims to synthesize the available direct and indirect evidence regarding the utility of MRI, to guide decision-making in the acute phase of SCI.

Table 1. Key Questions of Systematic Review.

Key Questions (KQ)
KQ1: What is the diagnostic accuracy of MRI to detect the following features that are likely to alter clinical management in patients with acute SCI?
1.1 Ongoing spinal cord compression 1.2 Disc herniation 1.3 Ligamentous injury 1.4 Epidural hematoma 1.5 Fracture 1.6 SCIWORA
KQ2: What is the frequency of abnormal MRI findings (from KQ1) in patients with acute SCI?
KQ3: How often does obtaining an MRI alter clinical decision-making in acute SCI??
3.1 If surgery is required 3.2 When to operate 3.3 Surgical approach (e.g., anterior vs. posterior) 3.4 Need for instrumentation 3.5 Which levels to decompress 3.6 Need for reoperation after surgery
KQ4: When should MRI be performed in acute SCI?
4.1 Before closed reduction 4.2 Before surgery 4.3 After closed reduction/surgery to assess decompression 4.4 Within a specific time period (e.g., 24 h)
KQ5: What is the frequency of adverse events when performing MRI in acute SCI patients?
KQ6: How does obtaining an MRI (compared with not obtaining MRI) affect neurological, functional, and health-related quality of life outcomes?

2. Materials and Methods

The systematic review was designed in accordance with the Preferred Reporting Items for Systematic Reviews and Meta-Analyses (PRISMA) and the Cochrane Handbook of Systematic Reviews of Interventions [11–13].

Only studies with human subjects published in the English language were included, with the search confined to randomized controlled trials (RCTs), cohort studies, case series, and case-control studies. Reviews, opinion articles, case reports, and case series with less than ten patients were excluded. A summary of the study's design in PICO format (population, intervention, comparison, outcome), including inclusion and exclusion criteria, is found in Table 2. Studies of interest were those that included adults (16 years or older) with SCI in the acute phase (within 7 days of injury). Relevant studies that also included a small proportion of pediatric patients (<20%) were allowed after consideration by the authors, but were marked with an asterisk (*) in all tables. Relevant studies were required to utilize MRI in the acute phase (within 7 days) for the purpose of clinical decision-making (Table 1). Investigations that only examined the role of MRI for prognostication were excluded. The outcomes of interest were selected a priori based on previous studies, and are specified as KQs 1–6 listed in Table 1.

For KQ1, studies were only included if they calculated the diagnostic accuracy of MRI in reference to a gold standard measure (e.g., intraoperative findings) for the detection of specific pathological entities (spinal cord compression, disc herniation, ligamentous injury, epidural hematoma, fracture, or a spinal cord lesion/edema/contusion in the context of SCI without radiologic abnormality [SCIWORA]). For KQ2, studies were included that simply reported the frequency of abnormal MRI findings among the entities included in KQ1. For KQ3, studies were included if they examined how often obtaining an MRI alters clinical decision-making in SCI, including if surgery is required, when to operate, surgical approach, the need for instrumentation, which levels to decompress, or the need for reoperation after surgery. Comparative studies were also included that evaluated differences in decision-making between groups that did and did not undergo MRI. For KQ4, studies were included that reported data on the optimal timing of MRI in acute SCI, including before or after closed reduction, before or after surgery, within a certain time period, or studies that compared differences in timing of MRI between groups. Regarding KQ5, studies that reported the frequency of adverse events when performing MRI in SCI were included. Finally, for KQ6, comparative studies were included that evaluated differences in outcomes (neurological, functional, health-related quality of life) between patients that received an MRI versus those that did not.

Table 2. PICO Summary of Inclusion and Exclusion Criteria.

	Inclusion	Exclusion
Patient		
	Adult human population (≥16 years old) Studies that include patients in the acute phase of SCI (within 7 days of injury)	Pediatric population (age < 16)
Intervention		
	MRI scan within 7 days of injury to inform one or more clinical decisions	MRI purely for prognosis
Outcome		
	Addresses one or more key questions in Table 1	
Comparison		
	MRI vs. no MRI MRI vs. CT No comparison (MRI alone)	
Study Design		
	Studies designed to assess the detection of a specific imaging feature and/or its relationship to alter decision-making or outcomes	Review articles Opinions Case reports or series < 10 patients Animal or biomechanical studies

Medical subheadings (MeSH) and text words related to acute spinal cord injury and magnetic resonance imaging were utilized for the search strategy. Medline, Embase, and Cochrane Central Register for Controlled Trials (CENTRAL, Wiley interface) were searched. A first search was performed between 1 January 1980 to 30 April 2016. The project was subsequently postponed, and a second search from 1 January 2016 to 26 August 2020 was completed with some overlap in dates to ensure no relevant studies were missed. The starting year of 1980 for the search was based on the timing of the first clinical MRI manuscripts being published in the 1980s [14]. In relevant literature and reviews, references were manually searched for additional studies, while use of Embase ensured gray literature was also screened. Other than dates, no database search limitations were utilized. The Appendix A provides the search protocols, including keywords. Specific search strategies were developed under guidance of library/information scientists with expertise in systemic review searches. Search results were imported to EndNote (Clarivate Analytics, Philadelphia, PA, USA) for the first search and Covidence (Covidence A/S, Melbourne, Australia) for the second search, to reduce data entry errors and bias (i.e., deduplicating references). All investigation reports were assessed for inconsistencies (e.g., design description, outcome presentation, total patients analyzed).

Two authors independently screened all titles and abstracts based on the eligibility criteria. Two authors reviewed each manuscript in full-text for inclusion, to assess eligibility for final inclusion and data extraction. Any discordances between reviewers during the abstract screening, full-text screening, or data-extraction phases were resolved with discussion and review by a third author. In compliance with recommendations from the Cochrane Handbook for Systematic Reviews of Interventions, the following data were compiled into a Microsoft Excel spreadsheet: author, publication year, journal citation, setting, inclusion and exclusion criteria, study design, study population, KQs addressed, and outcomes.

Data were placed into tables stratified by the KQ, enabling qualitative assessment. For simplicity, studied populations were categorized as SCIWORA when CT or radiographs showed no evidence of traumatic injury; otherwise, they were labeled as SCI (i.e., including cases with fracture or malalignment). For quantitative outcome data that were similarly reported across studies and their populations, a meta-analysis was conducted to calculate pooled results. In these cases, a chi-squared test for heterogeneity was performed and the I^2 statistic was calculated. Analysis was conducted using R v4.0.2 Statistical Software (R Foundation for Statistical Computing, Vienna, Austria) [15].

Two authors independently performed risk of bias assessment according to the National Institutes of Health (NIH) Quality Assessment Tool [16]. Studies appraised as good had minimally low risk of bias, studies appraised as fair had moderately low risk of bias, and those appraised as poor had high risk of bias.

3. Results

The two electronic database searches yielded a total of 21,323 unique citations (Figure 1). After title and abstract review, 268 manuscripts were selected. Following full-text review, 32 studies were identified that met eligibility criteria and were included in the qualitative synthesis in the form of Tables 3–8. Three studies were prospective, while the remainder were retrospective case series, cohort studies, or case-control studies (Table 9). Risk of bias assessment found a high risk of bias in two studies, moderately low in 17, and minimally low in 13 (Table 9).

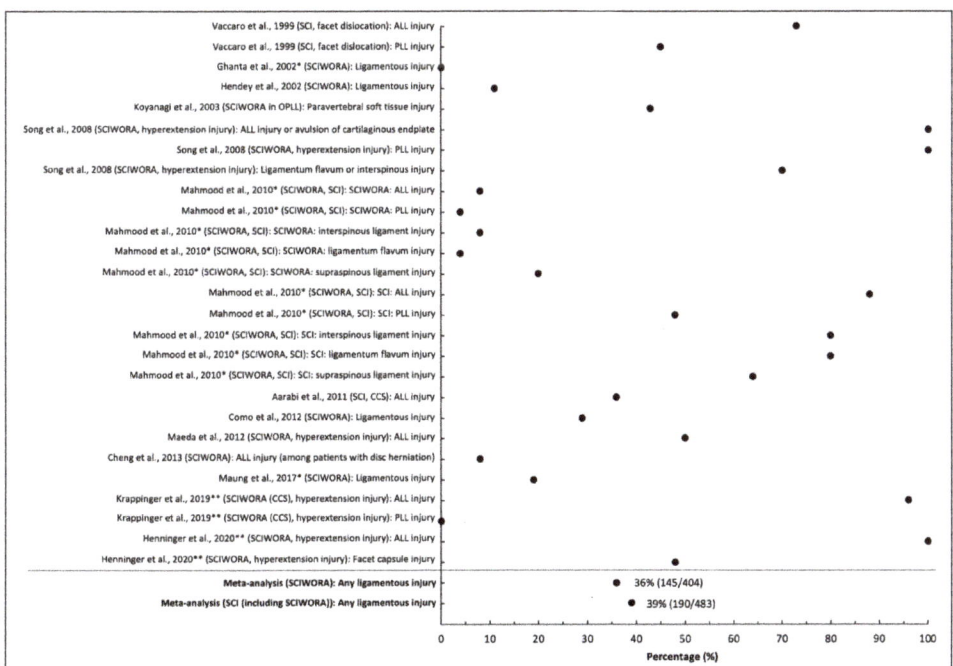

Figure 1. Frequency of ligamentous injury on MRI in patients with acute spinal cord injury. * Studies that include pediatric patients (<16) or unspecified age range. ** Studies with overlapping cohorts.

Table 3. Key Question 1: What is the diagnostic accuracy of MRI to detect specific features of spinal injury that are likely to alter clinical management in patients with acute SCI.

Citation	Disease	Sample Size	Age (Years)	SCI Level	Sequence	Field Strength	Injury	Comparison		Outcome
Ligamentous Injury										
Maeda et al., 2012	SCIWORA, hyperextension injury	n = 88	Mean: 64, range: 33–89	Cervical	NS	NS	ALL injury	Instability on flexion/extension radiographs		Unstable: 23/28 (sensitivity: 0.82) Stable: 39/60 (specificity: 0.65)
Krappinger et al., 2019 **	SCIWORA, CCS, hyperextension injury	n = 23	Mean: 62.7, range: 38–87	Cervical	T1W, T2W, STIR	1.5T	ALL injury PLL injury	Intraoperative findings Intraoperative findings	Radiologist On-Call Specialized MRI Radiologist	Injured: 15/22 patients (sensitivity: 0.68), 15/25 segments (sensitivity: 0.60) Uninjured: 0, denominator NS (specificity: 1.0) Injured: 19/22 patients (sensitivity: 0.86), 22/25 segments (sensitivity: 0.88) Uninjured: 0, denominator NS (specificity: 1.0)
Henninger et al., 2020 **	SCIWORA, hyperextension injury	n = 21	Mean: 62, range: 38–87	Cervical	T1W, STIR	1.5T	ALL injury PLL injury	Intraoperative findings Intraoperative findings	STIR T2 Any sequence Any sequence	100% agreement, no injury in 23/23 patients 88% agreement 61% agreement 88% agreement PLL injured: 1/2 (sensitivity: 0.50)
Fracture										
Mirvis et al., 1988 *	SCI	n = 21	Mean: 42.5, range: 17–66	Cervical	T1W, T2W	1.5T	Fracture	CT myelography		Fracture: 2/5 (sensitivity: 0.40) No fracture: 14/14 (specificity: 1.0)

Table 3. Cont.

Citation	Disease	Sample Size	Age (Years)	SCI Level	Sequence	Field Strength	Injury	Comparison	Outcome
Disc Injury/ Herniation									
Kalfas et al., 1988 *	SCI	n = 62	NS	Cervical (n = 40), Thoracic (n = 17), Lumbar (n = 5)	T1W, T2W	0.5T	Disc herniation with cord compression	Intraoperative findings	2/2 (sensitivity: 1.0)
Maeda et al., 2012	SCIWORA, hyperextension injury	n = 88	Mean: 64, range: 33–89	Cervical	NS	NS	Intervertebral disc injury	Instability on flex-ion/extension radiographs	Unstable: 18/28 (sensitivity: 0.64) Stable: 41/60 (specificity: 0.68)
Bao et al., 2020	SCIWORA	n = 16	Mean: 51.1, range: 30–73	Cervical	T1W, T2W	3.0T	Intervertebral disc injury	Intraoperative findings	5/5 (sensitivity: 1.0)
Henninger et al., 2020 **	SCIWORA, hyperextension injury	n = 21	Mean: 62, range: 38–87	Cervical	T1W, STIR	1.5T	Intervertebral disc injury	Intraoperative findings	STIR 88% agreement T2W 61% agreement Any sequence 79% agreement
Cord Contusion/Edema									
Zhu et al., 2019	SCIWORA	n = 16	Mean: 47.5, range: 22–65	Cervical	T2W	NS	Hemorrhage, contusion, or edema	Intraoperative findings	100% (16/16) MRI

ALL, anterior longitudinal ligament; MRI, magnetic resonance imaging; CT, computed tomography; STIR, short T1 inversion recovery. * Studies that include pediatric patients (<16) or unspecified age range. ** Studies with overlapping cohorts.

Table 4. Key Question 2: What is the frequency of abnormal MRI findings of specific features of spinal injury that are likely to alter clinical management in patients with acute SCI?

Citation	Disease State	Sample Size	Age (Years)	SCI Level	Sequence	Field Strength	Injury	Outcome
Ligamentous Injury								
Vaccaro et al., 1999	SCI, facet dislocation	n = 11	Mean: 46, range: 17–84	Cervical	T1W, T2W	1.5T	ALL injury	73% (8/11)
							PLL injury	45% (5/11)
Ghanta et al., 2002 *	SCIWORA	n = 13 (subgroup)	Mean: 28.5, range: 0.4–78	Cervical	NS	NS	Ligamentous injury	0% (0/13)
Hendey et al., 2002	SCIWORA	n = 27	Median: 42, range: 21–89	Cervical	NS	NS	Ligamentous injury	11% (3/27)
Koyanagi et al., 2003	SCIWORA in OPLL	n = 28	Mean: 63.0, range: 45–78	Cervical	T2W	NS	Paravertebral soft tissue injury	43% (12/28)
Song et al., 2008	SCIWORA, hyperextension injury	n = 27	Mean: 54.1, range: 21–72	Cervical	T1W, T2W	1.5T	ALL injury or avulsion of cartilaginous endplate	100% (27/27)
							PLL injury	100% (27/27)
							Ligamentum flavum or interspinous injury	70% (19/27)
							SCIWORA: ALL injury	8% (2/25)
							SCIWORA: PLL injury	4% (1/25)
							SCIWORA: interspinous ligament injury	8% (2/25)
							SCIWORA: ligamentum flavum injury	4% (1/25)
Mahmood et al., 2010 *	SCIWORA, SCI	SCIWORA: n = 25, SCI: n = 25	Mean: 45, range: 12–64	Cervical	T1W, T2W	0.5T	SCIWORA: supraspinous ligament injury	20% (5/25)
							SCI: ALL injury	88% (22/25)
							SCI: PLL injury	48% (12/25)
							SCI: interspinous ligament injury	80% (20/25)
							SCI: ligamentum flavum injury	80% (20/25)
							SCI: supraspinous ligament injury	64% (16/25)
Aarabi et al., 2011	SCI, CCS	n = 42	Mean: 58.3, range: 32–87	Cervical	T2W, STIR	NS	ALL injury	36% (15/42)
Como et al., 2012	SCIWORA	n = 24	Mean: 60.5, range: 34–83	Cervical	T1W, T2W	1.5T	Ligamentous injury	29% (7/24)

Table 4. Cont.

Citation	Disease State	Sample Size	Age (Years)	SCI Level	Sequence	Field Strength	Injury	Outcome
Maeda et al., 2012	SCIWORA, hyperextension injury	n = 88	Mean: 64, range: 33–89	Cervical	NS	NS	ALL injury	50% (44/88)
Cheng et al., 2013	SCIWORA	n = 70	Mean: 57.7, range: 36–79	Cervical	T1W, T2W	NS	ALL injury (among patients with disc herniation)	8% (2/26)
Maung et al., 2017 *	SCIWORA	n = 123	NS	Cervical	NS	NS	Ligamentous injury	19% (23/123)
Krappinger et al., 2019 **	SCIWORA (CCS), hyperextension injury	n = 23	Mean: 62.7, range: 38–87	Cervical	T1W, T2W, STIR	1.5T	ALL injury PLL injury	96% (22/23) 0% (0/23)
Henninger et al., 2020 **	SCIWORA, hyperextension injury	n = 21	Mean: 62, range: 38–87	Cervical	T1W, STIR	1.5T	ALL injury Facet capsule injury	100% (21/21) 48% (10/21)
Meta-analysis ***	SCIWORA SCI (including SCIWORA)	n = 404 n = 482	Range: 0.4–89 Range: 0.4–89	Cervical Cervical			Any ligamentous injury Any ligamentous injury	36% (145/404), $I^2 = 0.94, p < 0.001$ 39% (190/483), $I^2 = 0.93, p < 0.001$
Disc Injury or Herniation								
Kalfas et al., 1988 *	SCI	n = 62	NS	Cervical (n = 40), Thoracic (n = 17), Lumbar (n = 5)	T1W, T2W	0.5T	Disc herniation with cord compression	3% (2/62)
Mirvis et al., 1988	SCI	n = 21	Mean: 42.5, range: 17–66	Cervical	T1W, T2W	1.5T	Disc herniation	57% (12/21) 37% (7/19) on CT Myelography
Doran et al., 1993	SCI, facet dislocation	n = 12	Mean: 34.1, range: 18–59	Cervical	NS	NS	Disc herniation with cord compression Disc bulge or herniation	83% (10/12) 100% (12/12)
Gupta et al., 1999	SCIWORA	n = 15	Range: 20–60	Cervical	NS	NS	Disc herniation	40% (6/15)
Selden et al., 1999	SCI	n = 55	Mean: 29.2, range: 2–92	Cervical	T1W, T2W	1.5T	Disc herniation	42% (23/55)

Table 4. Cont.

Citation	Disease State	Sample Size	Age (Years)	SCI Level	Sequence	Field Strength	Injury	Outcome
Vaccaro et al., 1999	SCI, facet dislocation	n = 11	Mean: 46, range: 17-84	Cervical	T1W, T2W	1.5T	Disc herniation	Pre-Reduction:18% (2/11) Post-Reduction: 45% (5/11)
Ghanta et al., 2002 *	SCIWORA	n = 13 (subgroup)	Mean: 28.5, range: 0.4-78	Cervical	NS	NS	Disc herniation	15% (2/13)
Hendey et al., 2002	SCIWORA	n = 27	Median: 42, range: 21-89	Cervical	NS	NS	Disc herniation	48% (13/27)
Tewari et al., 2004	SCIWORA	n = 40	Mean: 42.1, range: 16-70	Cervical	T1W, T2W	NS	Disc herniation	38% (15/40)
Darsaut et al., 2006	SCI, fracture-dislocation	n = 17	Mean: 40.2, range: 19-78	Cervical	T1W, T2W	1.5T	Disc injury Disc herniation Disc herniation	Pre-Traction: 88% (15/17) Pre-Traction: 24% (4/17) Post-Traction: 0% (0/17)
Song et al., 2008	SCIWORA, hyperextension injury	n = 27 (subgroup)	Mean: 54.1, range: 21-72	Cervical (Lower)	T1W, T2W	1.5T	Disc herniation	100% (27/27)
Sharma et al., 2009	SCIWORA	n = 12	Mean: 38.66, range: 22-58	Cervical	T1W, T2W	NS	Disc herniation	17% (2/12)
Mahmood et al., 2010 *	SCIWORA, SCI	SCIWORA: n = 25, SCI: n = 25	Mean: 45, range: 12-64	Cervical	T1W, T2W	0.5T	SCIWORA: disc injury SCIWORA: disc herniation SCI: disc injury SCI: disc herniation	16% (4/25) 44% (11/25) 40% (10/25) 16% (4/25)
Maeda et al., 2012	SCIWORA	n = 88	Mean: 64, range: 33-89	Cervical	NS	NS	Disc injury	42% (37/88)
Cheng et al., 2013	SCIWORA	n = 70	Mean: 57.7, range: 36-79	Cervical	T1W, T2W	NS	Disc herniation	37% (26/70)
Maung et al., 2017 *	SCIWORA	n = 123	NS	Cervical	NS	NS	Disc injury	4% (5/123)

Table 4. Cont.

Citation	Disease State	Sample Size	Age (Years)	SCI Level	Sequence	Field Strength	Injury	Outcome
Meta-analysis	SCIWORA SCI (including SCIWORA)	n = 400 n = 577		Mixed			SCIWORA: disc injury SCIWORA: disc herniation SCI: disc injury SCI: disc herniation SCI: Disc herniation with cord compression	20% (46/230), $I^2 = 0.96$, $p < 0.001$ 45% (102/229), $I^2 = 0.84$, $p < 0.001$ 26% (71/278), $I^2 = 0.95$, $p < 0.001$ 43% (159/370), $I^2 = 0.83$, $p < 0.001$ 16% (12/74), $I^2 = 0.98$, $p < 0.001$
Cord Compression								
Kalfas et al., 1988 *	SCI	n = 62	NS	Cervical (n = 40), Thoracic (n = 17), Lumbar (n = 5)	T1W, T2W	0.5T	Cord compression	45% (28/62)
Doran et al., 1993	SCI, facet dislocation	n = 12 (subgroup)	Mean: 34.1, range: 18–59	Cervical	NS	NS	Cord compression	83% (10/12)
Fehlings et al., 1999	SCI	n = 71	Mean: 39.7, range: 17–96	Sub-axial (C3-T1)	T1W, T2W	NS	Cord compression	T1W: 89% (63/71) T2W: 92% (65/71) Either: 96% (68/71)
Selden et al., 1999	SCI	n = 55	Mean: 29.2, range: 2–92	Cervical	T1W, T2W	1.5T	Cord compression	89% (49/55)
Hendey et al., 2002	SCIWORA	n = 27	Median: 42, range: 21–89	Cervical	NS	NS	Cord compression	15% (4/27)
Koyanagi et al., 2003	SCIWORA in OPLL	n = 28	Mean: 63.0, range: 45–78	Cervical	T2W	NS	Cord compression	100% (28/28)
Darsaut et al., 2006	SCI, fracture-dislocation	n = 17	Mean: 40.2, range: 19–78	Sub-axial (C3-T1)	T1W, T2W	1.5T	Cord compression	Pre-Traction: 65% (11/17) Post-Traction 6% (2/17)
Sharma et al., 2009	SCIWORA	n = 12	Mean: 38.66, range: 22–58	Cervical	T1W, T2W	NS	Cord compression	16% (2/12)

Table 4. Cont.

Citation	Disease State	Sample Size	Age (Years)	SCI Level	Sequence	Field Strength	Injury	Outcome
Mahmood et al., 2010 *	SCIWORA, SCI	SCIWORA: n = 25, SCI: n = 25	Mean: 45, range: 12–64	Cervical	T1W, T2W	0.5T	SCIWORA: cord compression SCI: cord compression	0% (0/25) 20% (5/25)
Aarabi et al., 2011	SCI, CCS	n = 211	Mean: 58.3, range: 32–87	Cervical	T2W, STIR	NS	Cord compression	88% (185/211)
Como et al., 2012	SCIWORA	n = 24	Mean: 60.5, range: 34–83	Cervical	T1W, T2W	1.5T	Cord compression	54% (13/24)
D'Souza et al., 2017	SCI	n = 20	Mean: 35.95, range: 17–54	Cervical	T1W, T2W	3T	Cord compression	50% (10/20)
Meta-analysis	SCIWORA SCI (including SCIWORA)	n = 116 n = 589	Range: 17–96	Mixed			Cord compression Cord compression	41% (47/116), $I^2 = 0.94, p < 0.001$ 70% (413/589), $I^2 = 0.95, p < 0.001$
Epidural Hematoma								
Selden et al., 1999	SCI	n = 55	Mean: 29.2, range: 2–92	Cervical	T1W, T2W	1.5T	Extra-axial hemorrhage	27% (15/55)
D'Souza et al., 2017	SCI	n = 20	Mean: 35.95, range: 17–54	Cervical	T1W, T2W, DTI	3T	Epidural hemorrhage	5% (1/20)
Maung et al., 2017 *	SCIWORA	n = 123	NS	Cervical	NS	NS	Epidural hemorrhage	3% (4/123)
Meta-analysis	SCI (including SCIWORA)	n = 143	Range: 17–54	Cervical			Epidural/extra-axial hemorrhage	10% (20/198), $I^2 = 0.92, p < 0.001$
Fracture								
Mirvis et al., 1988	SCI	n = 21	Mean: 42.5, range: 17–66	Cervical	T1W, T2W	1.5T	Fracture	10% (2/21)
D'Souza et al., 2017	SCI	n = 20	Mean: 35.95, range: 17–54	Cervical	T1W, T2W, DTI	3T	Fracture	20% (4/20)
Meta-analysis	SCI	n = 41	Range: 17–66	Cervical			Fracture	15% (6/41), $I^2 = 0$, $p = 0.61$

Table 4. Cont.

Citation	Disease State	Sample Size	Age (Years)	SCI Level	Sequence	Field Strength	Injury	Outcome
Intramedullary Lesion (SCIWORA)								
Fehlings et al., 1999	SCIWORA	n = 14 (subgroup)	Mean: 39.7, range: 17–96	Sub-axial (C3–T1)	T2W	NS	Edema or contusion	100% (14/14)
Gupta et al., 1999	SCIWORA	n = 15	Range: 20–60	Cervical	NS	NS	Edema only	27% (4/15)
							Edema or contusion	53% (8/15)
Ghanta et al., 2002 *	SCIWORA	n = 13 (subgroup)	Mean: 28.5, range: 0.4–78	Cervical	NS	NS	Edema only	8% (1/13)
							Edema or contusion	23% (3/13)
Koyanagi et al., 2003	SCIWORA in OPLL	n = 28	Mean: 63.0, range: 45–78	Cervical	T2W	NS	Edema or contusion	75% (21/28)
Tewari et al., 2004	SCIWORA	n = 40	Mean: 42.1, range: 16–70	Cervical	T1W, T2W	NS	Edema or contusion	90% (36/40)
Sharma et al., 2009	SCIWORA	n = 12	Mean: 38.66, range: 22–58	Cervical	T1W, T2W	NS	Edema only	42% (5/12)
							Edema, contusion, or hemorrhage	100% (12/12)
Mahmood et al., 2010 *	SCIWORA	n = 25 (subgroup)	Mean: 45, range: 12–64	Cervical	T1W, T2W	0.5T	Edema only	36% (9/25)
							Edema or contusion	100% (25/25)
Machino et al., 2011	SCIWORA	n = 100	Mean: 55, range: 16–87	Cervical	T2W	1.5T	Edema or contusion	92% (92/100)
Como et al., 2012	SCIWORA	n = 24	Mean: 60.5, range: 34–83	Cervical	T1W, T2W	1.5T	Edema	100% (24/24)
Liu et al., 2015	SCIWORA	n = 59	Mean: 41.1, range: 21–68	Cervical (n = 19), Thoracic (n = 40)	NS	3T	Edema only	12% (7/59)
							Edema or contusion	36% (21/59)
Boese et al., 2016	SCIWORA	n = 23	Mean: 53.7, range: 22–80	Cervical	T1W, T2W	1.5T	Edema only	65% (15/23)
							Edema or contusion	65% (15/23)
Asan et al., 2018	SCIWORA	n = 11	Range: 28–81	Cervical (n = 7), Thoracic (n = 4)	NS	NS	Contusion, cavitation, or edema	36% (4/11)
Zhu et al., 2019	SCIWORA	n = 16	Mean: 47.5, range: 22–65	Cervical	T2W	NS	Edema only	56% (9/16)
							Edema or contusion	100% (16/16)
Meta-Analysis *	SCIWORA	n = 380	Range: 12–87	Cervical (n = 336), Thoracic (n = 44)			Edema only	40% (74/187), $I^2 = 0.90$, $p < 0.001$
							Any intramedullary abnormality	77% (291/380), $I^2 = 0.91$, $p < 0.001$

* Studies that include pediatric patients (<16) or unspecified age range. ** Studies with overlapping cohorts. *** Henninger et al., 2020 was excluded from meta-analysis due to overlapping cohort with Krappinger et al., 2019.

Table 5. Key Question 3: How often does obtaining an MRI alter clinical decision-making in acute SCI.

Citation	Disease State	Sample Size	Age (Years)	SCI Level	Sequence	Field Strength	MRI Finding and Change in Decision-Making	Outcome
If Surgery Is Required								
Kalfas et al., 1988	SCI	n = 62	NS	Cervical (n = 40), Thoracic (n = 17), Lumbar (n = 5)	T1W, T2W	0.5T	2 patients had cord compression due to acute disc herniation leading to anterior surgery	3% (2/62)
Mirvis et al., 1988	SCI	n = 21	Mean: 42.5, range: 17–66	Cervical	T1W, T2W	1.5T	3 patients with disc herniation were managed with anterior decompression	14% (3/21)
Doran et al., 1993	SCI	n = 12 (subgroup)	Mean: 34.1, range: 18–59	Cervical	NS	NS	10 patients with frank disc herniation and severe cord compression were managed with anterior cervical discectomy	83% (10/12)
Gupta et al., 1999	SCIWORA	n = 15	Range: 20–60	Cervical	NS	NS	6 patients had intervertebral disc prolapse, all underwent anterior surgery	40% (6/15)
Selden et al., 1999 **	SCI	n = 55	Mean: 29.2, range: 2–92	Cervical	T1W, T2W	1.5T	Among 18 patients with bilateral dislocated facets, acute disc herniation in 10/18 led to anterior surgery. Among 26 patients who underwent successful closed reduction, ongoing cord compression in 13/26 led to surgery	56% (10/55) 50% (13/26)
Ghanta et al., 2002 *	SCIWORA	n = 13 (subgroup)	Mean: 28.5, range: 0.4–78	Cervical	NS	NS	1 patient with disc herniation was managed with anterior decompression	8% (1/13)
Papadopoulos et al., 2002 **	SCI	n = 66	Mean: 32, range: 2–92	Cervical	T1W, T2W	1.5T	34 patients had cord compression leading to emergent surgery	51% (34/66)
Tewari et al., 2004 **	SCIWORA	n = 40	Mean: 42.1, range: 16–70	Cervical	T1W, T2W	NS	3 patients with disc herniation were managed with anterior decompression	8% (3/40)
Sharma et al., 2009	SCIWORA	n = 12	Mean: 38.66, range: 22–58	Cervical	T1W, T2W	NS	2 patients had disc prolapse and underwent surgery due to this finding	17% (2/12)

Table 5. Cont.

Citation	Disease State	Sample Size	Age (Years)	SCI Level	Sequence	Field Strength	MRI Finding and Change in Decision-Making	Outcome
Machino et al., 2011	SCIWORA	n = 100	Mean: 55, range: 16–87	Cervical	T2W	1.5T	100 patients had profound neurological deficits and cord compression requiring surgical decompression	100% (100/100)
Como et al., 2012	SCIWORA	n = 24	Mean: 60.5, range: 34–83	Cervical	T1W, T2W	1.5T	13 patients required operative decompression	54% (13/24)
Boese et al., 2016	SCIWORA	n = 23	Mean: 53.7, range: 22–80	Cervical	T1W, T2W	1.5T	Only patients with both cord compression and intramedullary edema (classified as Type IIc) were considered for surgery. 8/15 of these underwent surgery	35% (8/23)
Maung et al., 2017	SCIWORA	n = 123	NS	Cervical	NS	NS	6 patients had MRI findings that led to surgical treatment (ligamentous injury, epidural hematoma)	5% (6/123)
Bao et al., 2020	SCIWORA	n = 16	Mean: 51.1, range: 30–73	Cervical	T1W, T2W	3.0T	10 patients received surgical treatment based upon neutral MRI results (cord compression, disc injury) and another 2 patients had surgery based on kinetic MRI showing instability	75% (12/16)
Huang et al., 2020 *	SCI, SCIWORA	SCIWORA: n = 42, SCI: n = 12	NS	Cervical	NS	3T, 1.5T	10 patients had MRI findings that led to surgical treatment (cord compression, ligamentous injury, disc herniation)	19% (10/54)
Meta-analysis ***	SCI, SCIWORA	n = 611		Mixed			Any finding leading to surgery	36% (223/611), $I^2 = 0.96$, $p < 0.001$

Table 5. Cont.

Citation	Disease State	Sample Size	Age (Years)	SCI Level	Sequence	Field Strength	MRI Finding and Change in Decision-Making	Outcome
Surgical Approach								
Kalfas et al., 1988	SCI	n = 62	NS	Cervical (n = 40), Thoracic (n = 17), Lumbar (n = 5)	T1W, T2W	0.5T	2 patients had cord compression due to acute disc herniation leading to anterior surgery	3% (2/62)
Mirvis et al., 1988	SCI	n = 21	Mean: 42.5, range: 17–66	Cervical	T1W, T2W	1.5T	3 patients with disc herniation were managed with anterior decompression	14% (3/21)
Doran et al., 1993	SCI	n = 12 (subgroup)	Mean: 34.1, range: 18–59	Cervical	NS	NS	10 patients with frank disc herniation and severe cord compression were managed with anterior cervical discectomy	83% (10/12)
Selden et al., 1999 **	SCI	n = 55	Mean: 29.2, range: 2–92	Cervical	T1W, T2W	1.5T	Among 18 patients with bilateral dislocated facets, acute disc herniation in 10/18 led to anterior surgery	18% (10/55)
Ghanta et al., 2002 *	SCIWORA	n = 13 (subgroup)	Mean: 28.5, range: 0.4–78	Cervical	NS	NS	1 patient with disc herniation was managed with anterior decompression	8% (1/13)
Tewari et al., 2004 **	SCIWORA	n = 40	Mean: 42.1, range: 16–70	Cervical	T1W, T2W	NS	3 patients with disc herniation were managed with anterior decompression	8% (3/40)
Sharma et al., 2009	SCIWORA	n = 12	Mean: 38.66, range: 22–58	Cervical	T1W, T2W	NS	2 patients had disc prolapse and underwent surgery due to this finding	17% (2/12)
Aarabi et al., 2011	SCIWORA, CCS	n = 211	Mean: 58.3, range: 32–87	Cervical	T2W, STIR	NS	Among 42 patients that required surgery, anterior approach was chosen in 28 due to anterior compression limited to 1–3 segments and/or kyphosis, while the posterior was chosen in the remaining 14	20% (42/211)

Table 5. Cont.

Citation	Disease State	Sample Size	Age (Years)	SCI Level	Sequence	Field Strength	MRI Finding and Change in Decision-Making	Outcome
Cheng et al., 2013	SCIWORA	n = 70	Mean: 57.7, range: 36-79	Cervical	T1W, T2W	NS	Among 70 patients treated surgically, MRI findings dictated surgical approach: 45 underwent anterior surgery due to anterior cord compression (disc, osteophytes, or OPLL); the remaining 25 underwent posterior procedures	100% (70/70)
Meta-analysis *	SCI, SCIWORA	n = 500		Mixed			Any finding leading to difference in surgical approach	29% (143/500), I² = 0.97, p < 0.001
When to Operate								
Selden et al., 1999 **	SCI	n = 55	Mean: 29.2, range: 2-92	Cervical	T1W, T2W	1.5T	27 patients had cord compression leading to emergent surgery 34 patients had cord compression leading to emergent surgery	49% (27/55)
Papadopoulos et al., 2002 **	SCI	n = 66	Mean: 32, range: 2-92	Cervical	T1W, T2W	1.5T	No cord compression in 32 patients after traction, allowing delayed surgery in 22 Total	51% (34/66) 33% (22/66) 85% (56/66)
Darsaut et al., 2006	SCI, fracture-dislocation	n = 17	Mean: 40.2; range: 19-78	Sub-axial (C3-T1)	T2W, T1W	1.5T	Among 11 patients with cord compression pre-reduction, MRI showed decompression in 9/11, leading to delayed surgery	53% (9/17)
Meta-analysis ***	SCI, SCIWORA	n = 83		Mixed			Any finding leading to difference in surgical timing	78% (65/83), I² = 0.84, p = 0.01

Table 5. Cont.

Citation	Disease State	Sample Size	Age (Years)	SCI Level	Sequence	Field Strength	MRI Finding and Change in Decision-Making	Outcome
Need for Instrumentation								
Krappinger et al., 2019 **	SCIWORA, CCS, hyperextension injury	n = 23	Mean: 62.7, range: 38–87	Cervical	T1W, T2W, STIR	1.5T	Findings of cord edema in all 23 patients and ligamentous injury (suggesting segmental instability) in 19 patients (including instability at a different level in several patients) led to decompression and instrumented fusion	100% (23/23)
Which Levels or How Many Levels to Decompress								
Krappinger et al., 2019 **	SCIWORA, CCS, hyperextension injury	n = 23	Mean: 62.7, range: 38–87	Cervical	T1W, T2W, STIR	1.5T	Findings of cord edema in all 23 patients and ligamentous injury (suggesting segmental instability) in 19 patients (including instability at a different level in several patients) led to decompression and instrumented fusion	100% (23/23)
Need for Re-operation After Surgery								
Aarabi et al., 2011 **	SCIWORA, CCS	n = 211	Mean: 58.3, range: 32–87	Cervical	T2W, STIR	NS	Among 28 patients that underwent anterior surgery, post-operative MRI found ongoing cord compression in 11, leading to additional posterior surgery	5% (11/211)
Aarabi et. al., 2019 **	SCI	n = 184	Mean: 43.5	Cervical	T1W, STIR	NS	Ongoing cord compression after surgery (inadequate decompression), but rates of re-operation were not reported	34% (63/184)

* Studies that include pediatric patients (<16) or unspecified age range. ** Studies with overlapping cohorts. *** Selden et al., 1999 was excluded from meta-analysis due to overlapping cohort with Papadopoulos et al., 2002.

Table 6. Key Question 4: When should MRI be performed in acute spinal cord injury?

Citation	Disease State	Sample Size	Age (Years)	SCI Level	Sequence	Field Strength	Evidence Regarding Timing of MRI
Performance of MRI on Initial Assessment (Prior to Intervention)?							
Kalfas et al., 1988	SCI	n = 62	NS	Cervical (n = 40), Thoracic (n = 17), Lumbar (n = 5)	T1W, T2W	0.5T	Useful to detect disc herniation, cord compression (if to operate, surgical approach)
Doran et al., 1993	SCI, facet dislocation	n = 12	Mean: 34.1, range: 18–59	Cervical	NS	NS	Useful to detect disc herniation, cord compression (if to operate, surgical approach)
Gupta et al., 1999	SCIWORA	n = 15	Range: 20–60	Cervical	NS	NS	Useful to detect disc herniation, cord compression (if to operate, surgical approach)
Selden et al., 1999 **	SCI	n = 55	Mean: 29.2, range: 2–92	Cervical	T1W, T2W	1.5T	Useful to detect disc herniation, cord compression (if to operate vs. closed reduction, surgical approach, timing of surgery)
Vaccaro et al., 1999	SCI, facet dislocation	n = 11	Mean: 46, range: 17–84	Cervical	T1W, T2W	1.5T	Unclear if pre-reduction MRI has utility: 2 patients had disc herniations prior to closed reduction but did not deteriorate after reduction
Papadopoulos et al., 2002 **	SCI	n = 66	Mean: 32, range: 2–92	Cervical	T1W, T2W	1.5T	Useful to detect cord compression (if to operate, timing of surgery)
Darsaut et al., 2006	SCI, fracture-dislocation	n = 17	Mean: 40.2, range: 19–78	Cervical	T1W, T2W	1.5T	Unclear if pre-reduction MRI has utility: 11 patients had cord compression prior to traction/reduction but did not deteriorate after reduction
Sharma et al., 2009	SCIWORA	n = 12	Mean: 38.66, range: 22–58	Cervical	T1W, T2W	NS	Useful to detect disc herniation, cord compression (if to operate, surgical approach)
Aarabi et al., 2011	SCIWORA, CCS	n = 211	Mean: 58.3, range: 32–87	Cervical	T2W, STIR	NS	Useful to detect anterior cord compression (surgical approach)
Como et al., 2012	SCIWORA	n = 24	Mean: 60.5, range: 34–83	Cervical	T1W, T2W	1.5T	Useful to detect cord compression (if to operate)
Cheng et al., 2013	SCIWORA	n = 70	Mean: 57.7, range: 36–79	Cervical	T1W, T2W	NS	Useful to detect anterior cord compression (surgical approach)

Table 6. Cont.

Citation	Disease State	Sample Size	Age (Years)	SCI Level	Sequence	Field Strength	Evidence Regarding Timing of MRI
Boese et al., 2016	SCIWORA	n = 23	Mean: 53.7, range: 22–80	Cervical	T1W, T2W	1.5T	Useful to detect cord compression and edema (if to operate), but authors state "our results cannot provide guidance on therapeutic management"
Maung et al., 2017	SCIWORA	n = 123	NS	Cervical	NS	NS	Useful to detect ligamentous injury, epidural hematoma (if to operate)
Bao et al., 2020	SCIWORA	n = 16	Mean: 51.1, range: 30–73	Cervical	T1W, T2W	3.0T	Useful to detect cord compression, disc injury, instability (if to operate)
Huang et al., 2020 *	SCI, SCIWORA	SCIWORA: n = 42, SCI: n = 12	NS	Cervical	NS	3T, 1.5T	Useful to detect cord compression, ligamentous injury, disc herniation (if to operate)
Performance of MRI After Closed Reduction to Assess Decompression?							
Selden et al., 1999 **	SCI	n = 55	Mean: 29.2, range: 2–92	Cervical	T1W, T2W	1.5T	Useful to detect post-reduction cord compression (if to operate)
Vaccaro et al., 1999	SCI, facet dislocation	n = 11	Mean: 46, range: 17–84	Cervical	T1W, T2W	1.5T	Unclear if post-reduction MRI has utility: 5 patients had disc herniations after closed reduction but did not deteriorate
Darsaut et al., 2006	SCI, fracture-dislocation	n = 17	Mean: 40.2, range: 19–78	Cervical	T1W, T2W	1.5T	Useful to detect post-reduction cord compression (if to operate)
Performance of MRI After Surgery to Assess Decompression?							
Aarabi et al., 2011 **	SCIWORA, CCS	n = 211	Mean: 58.3, range: 32–87	Cervical	T2W, STIR	NS	Useful to detect post-operative cord compression (if to re-operate)
Aarabi et al., 2019 **	SCI	n = 184	Mean: 43.5	Cervical	T1W, STIR	NS	Useful to detect post-operative cord compression (if to re-operate), but rates of re-operation were not reported
Performance of MRI within a Specific Time Period (e.g., 24 h)							
Aarabi et al., 2019 *	SCI	n = 184	Mean: 43.5	Cervical	T1W, STIR	NS	Time interval to pre-operative MRI did not differ between successfully (8.3 +/− 7.7 h) and unsuccessfully (8.6 +/− 8.7 h) decompressed patients

* Studies that include pediatric patients (<16) or unspecified age range. ** Studies with overlapping cohorts.

Table 7. Key Question 5: What is the frequency of adverse events when performing MRI in acute SCI patients?

Citation	Disease	Sample Size	Age (Years)	SCI Level	Sequence	Field Strength	Activity/Imaging	Adverse Event	Outcome
Kalfas et al., 1988 *	SCI	$n = 62$	NS	Cervical ($n = 40$) Thoracic ($n = 17$) Lumbar ($n = 5$)	T1W, T2W	0.5T	MRI within first 36 h of injury	Any adverse event	0% (0/62)
Selden et al., 1999 **	SCI	$n = 18$	Mean: 29.2, range: 2–92	Cervical	T1W, T2W	1.5T	MRI within first 21 h of injury	Any adverse event	0% (0/55)
Papadopoulos et al., 2002 **	SCI	$n = 66$	Mean: 32, range: 2–92	Cervical	T1W, T2W	1.5T	Emergent MRI (average: 4.1 h)	Neurological deterioration Permanent neurological	0% (0/66)
Darsaut et al., 2006	SCI, fracture-dislocation	$n = 17$	Mean: 40.2, range: 19–78	Cervical	T1W, T2W	1.5T	MRI during closed reduction	deterioration during reduction/MRI Burning sensation at pin sites	0% (0/12) 0% (0/12)
Bao et al., 2020	SCIWORA	$n = 16$	Mean: 51.1, range: 30–73	Cervical	T1W, T2W	3.0T	Neutral, flexion, and extension MRI Neutral and flexion MRI	Neurological deterioration Neurological deterioration	0% (0/14) 0% (0/2)
Meta-analysis ***	SCI	$n = 156$	NS	Mixed	NS	NS		Any adverse event	0% (0/156), $I^2 = 0$, $p = 1$

* Studies that include pediatric patients (<16) or unspecified age range. ** Studies with overlapping cohorts. *** Selden et al., 1999 was excluded from meta-analysis due to overlapping cohort with Papadopoulos et al., 2002.

Table 8. Key Question 6: How does obtaining an MRI (compared with not obtaining MRI) affect neurological, functional, and health-related quality of life outcomes? (Differences in outcome between patients receiving MRI and those not receiving MRI).

Citation	Disease State	Sample Size	Age (Years)	SCI Level	Sequence	Field Strength	Outcome	Imaging/Treatment Group	Result	
Improvement in Frankel Grade from Admission										
Papadopoulos et al., 2002 **	SCI	n = 91	Mean: 32, range: 2–92	Cervical	T1W, T2W	1.5T	Any Frankel Grade improvement	MRI-protocol	50% (30/66)	p < 0.006
								Reference group	24% (6/25)	
							Grade A/B improvement to D/E	MRI-protocol	16% (8/50)	p = 0.09 ***
								Reference group	0% (0/20)	
Length of Stay										
Papadopoulos et al., 2002 **	SCI	n = 91	Mean: 32, range: 2–92	Cervical	T1W, T2W	1.5T	ICU stay	MRI-protocol	9.9 ± 1.7 days	p < 0.001
								Reference group	23.8 ± 3.7 days	
							General care duration	MRI-protocol	8.4 ± 1.7 days	p = 0.31
								Reference group	9.3 ± 3.0 days	
							Rehabilitation duration	MRI-protocol	58.1 ± 5.6 days	p = 0.47
								Reference group	66.0 ± 10.7 days	
							Total length of stay	MRI-protocol	71.4 ± 5.9 days	p = 0.02
								Reference group	99.9 ± 13.1 days	

** This study assigned patients non-randomly to either (1) an MRI-based protocol that included urgent imaging and treatment, or (2) a reference group that did not receive MRI or emergent surgical treatment. This study was deemed to have a high risk of bias, primarily due to selection. *** p value calculated using Fisher exact test, not reported by authors.

Table 9. Risk of bias assessment. Studies arranged alphabetically by the last name of the first author. Risk of bias assessment was performed according to the National Institutes of Health (NIH) Quality Assessment Tool. Studies appraised as good had minimally low risk of bias, studies appraised as fair had moderately low risk of bias, and those appraised as poor had high risk of bias.

	Study	Year	Study Design	Risk of Bias
1	Aarabi et al.	2011	Retrospective case series	Minimally low
2	Aarabi et al.	2019	Retrospective case series	Minimally low
3	Asan et al.	2018	Prospective case series	Moderately low
4	Bao et al.	2020	Retrospective case series	Moderately low
5	Boese et al.	2016	Retrospective case series	Moderately low
6	Cheng et al.	2012	Retrospective case series	Moderately low
7	Como et al.	2012	Retrospective case series	Moderately low
8	Darsaut et al.	2006	Prospective case series	Moderately low
9	Doran et al.	1993	Retrospective case series	High
10	D'Souza et al.	2017	Retrospective case control study	Moderately low
11	Fehlings et al.	1999	Retrospective case series	Moderately low
12	Ghanta et al.	2002	Retrospective case series	Moderately low
13	Gupta et al.	1999	Retrospective case series	Moderately low
14	Hendey et al.	2002	Retrospective case series	Moderately low
15	Henninger et al.	2020	Retrospective case series	Moderately low
16	Huang et al.	2020	Retrospective case series	Minimally low
17	Kalfas et al.	1988	Retrospective case series	Moderately low
18	Koyanagi et al.	2003	Retrospective case series	Moderately low
19	Krappinger et al.	2019	Retrospective case series	Minimally low
20	Liu et al.	2015	Retrospective case series	Minimally low
21	Machino et al.	2019	Retrospective case series	Minimally low
22	Maeda et al.	2012	Retrospective case series	Minimally low
23	Mahmood et al.	2010	Retrospective case control study	Moderately low
24	Maung et al.	2016	Retrospective case series	Moderately low
25	Mirvis et al.	1988	Retrospective case series	Moderately low
26	Papadopoulos et al.	2002	Prospective cohort study	High
27	Selden et al.	1999	Retrospective case series	Minimally low
28	Sharma et al.	2009	Retrospective case series	Minimally low
29	Song et al.	2008	Retrospective case series	Minimally low
30	Tewari et al.	2005	Retrospective case series	Minimally low
31	Vaccaro et al.	1999	Retrospective case series	Minimally low
32	Zhu et al.	2019	Retrospective case series	Minimally low

3.1. KQ1: Diagnostic Accuracy of MRI

Seven studies involving SCI were identified that addressed KQ1 (Table 3) [17–23]. Five studies calculated the diagnostic accuracy of MRI in relation to intraoperative findings [17–19,22,23], one compared against flexion/extension radiographs [20], and one against CT myelography [21]. Two studies with overlapping cohorts focused on hyperextension injuries and central cord syndrome [17,18]; both studies investigated detection of ALL injury, demonstrating superior sensitivity of STIR over T2-weighted (T2w) images (88% vs. 61%) [18] and a specialized MRI radiologist over a general radiologist (86% vs. 68%) [17]. In addition, one study also reported improved sensitivity of STIR over T2w images (82% vs. 61%) to identify intervertebral disc injury/herniation [18]. Two studies found 2 and 5 cases, respectively, of acute disc herniation on MRI that were verified by intraoperative findings [22,23]. Another study investigated the diagnostic accuracy of T2w images to detect intramedullary hemorrhage/contusion/edema in patients with SCIWORA compared with direct visualization of the spinal cord, reporting a sensitivity of 100% [19]. One study compared MRI against flexion/extension radiographs for segmental instability [20]; the MRI finding of ALL injury was present in 23/28 patients with instability (sensitivity: 0.82) and absent in 39/60 patients without instability (specificity: 0.65), while the finding of disc injury was present in 18/28 patients with instability (sensitivity: 0.64) and absent in 41/60 patients without instability (specificity: 0.68). One study found that MRI had only 40% (2/5) sensitivity to detect fracture, but 100% specificity (14/14) compared with CT myelography [21]. Meta-analysis was not possible for KQ1 findings due to the limited data available.

3.2. KQ2: Frequency of Abnormal Findings

Overall, 28 studies relevant to KQ2 were identified, reporting the frequency of certain pathological MRI findings in various types of SCI (Table 4) [17–21,23–45].

3.2.1. Ligamentous Injury

Thirteen studies provided data on the frequency of ligamentous injury, all in patients with cervical SCI [17,18,20,24–29,34,37,41,43]. Among these studies, nine focused on patients with SCIWORA, in which the frequency of ligamentous injury ranged from 0 to 100% [20,24–28,34,37,41]. The pooled frequency of ligamentous injury in SCIWORA was 36% (145/404 across eight studies excluding [18] due to overlapping cohort with [17]), but heterogeneity across studies was high ($I^2 = 0.94$, $p < 0.001$). Similarly, the pooled frequency of ligamentous injury was 39% in all patients with SCI (190/483 across 12 studies), with high heterogeneity ($I^2 = 0.93$, $p < 0.001$; Figure 1).

3.2.2. Disc Injury/Herniation

Sixteen studies provided data on the frequency of disc herniation and/or injury in SCI, including 15 in cervical injuries and one including all spinal levels [20,21,23,25–28,30–33,37,41–44]. The rate of disc injury ranged from 4% to 42% in studies involving cervical SCIWORA, whereas it was 40% to 88% in other SCI studies [20,21,23,25–28,30–33,37,41–44]. Disc herniation was present in 37% to 100% of patients with SCIWORA, whereas it was present in 24% to 100% in SCI [20,21,23,25–28,30–33,37,41–44]. Disc herniation causing cord compression varied from 3% to 83% in two studies involving SCI [23,30]. In SCIWORA, the aggregate rate of disc injury was 20% (46/230), while disc herniation was more frequent at 45% (102/229); both results showed high heterogeneity across studies ($I^2 = 0.96, 0.84$, respectively, both $p < 0.001$). The pooled frequency of disc injury, disc herniation, and disc herniation causing cord compression across all studies (SCIWORA and SCI) was 26% (71/278), 43% (159/370), and 16% (12/74), respectively, while heterogeneity was high for all analyses ($I^2 = 0.95, 0.83$, and 0.98, respectively, all $p < 0.001$; Figure 2).

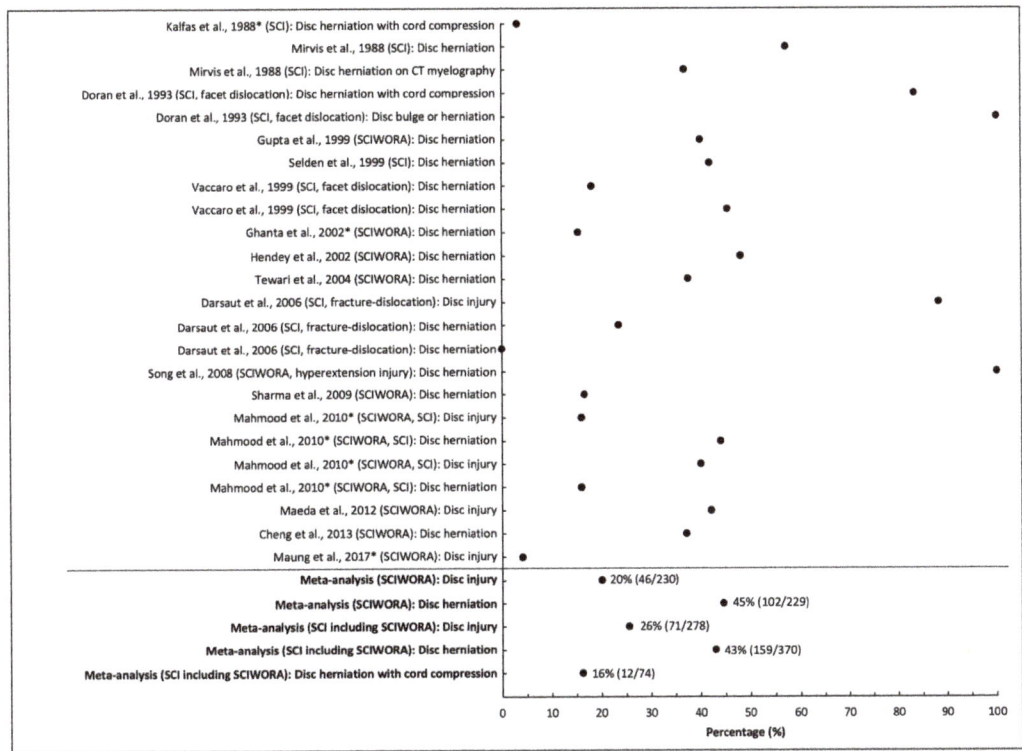

Figure 2. Frequency of disc injury or herniation on MRI in patients with acute spinal cord injury. * Studies that include pediatric patients (<16) or unspecified age range.

3.2.3. Cord Compression

Twelve studies reported the frequency of ongoing spinal cord compression in SCI, including nine that included only cervical injuries, two that had sub-axial injuries (C3-T1), and one that included all levels [23–25,29–31,33,34,38,39,41,44]. A cohort examining sub-axial SCI found cord compression frequency at 89% (63/71) with a T1w sagittal sequence, but 92% (65/71) with T2w sagittal and 96% (68/71) when either result was positive [38]. In SCIWORA, cord compression was identified in 0% to 100% of patients in five studies [24,25,33,34,41]. In two studies involving cervical dislocations, cord compression was noted in 65% to 83% [30,31]. For fracture-dislocation patients, cord compression frequency was 65% (11/17) pre-traction, but 12% (2/17) post-traction according to one study [31]. The pooled frequency of cord compression across studies in patients with SCIWORA was 41% (47/116), whereas it was 70% (413/589) among all cases of SCI; heterogeneity across studies was high in both groups (I^2 = 0.94, 0.95, respectively, both $p < 0.001$; Figure 3).

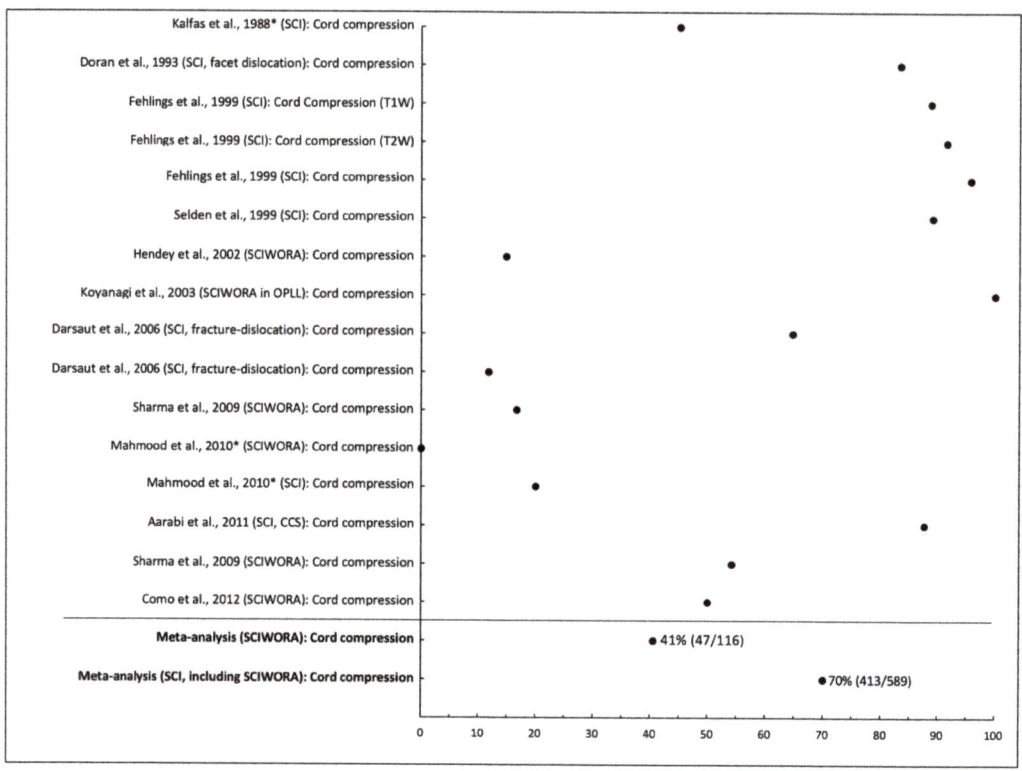

Figure 3. Frequency of cord compression on MRI in patients with acute spinal cord injury. * Studies that include pediatric patients (<16) or unspecified age range.

3.2.4. Epidural Hematoma

Three investigations in cervical SCI reported epidural hematoma in 3% to 27% of patients, resulting in a pooled frequency of 10% (20/198) [26,39,44]; the results showed high heterogeneity ($I^2 = 0.92$, $p < 0.001$; Figure 4).

3.2.5. Fracture

Two small studies provided data on the frequency of identifying fractures in patients with SCI, with a range of 10% to 20% and a pooled frequency of 15% (6/41) [21,39]; the results were homogeneous across these two studies, with $I^2 = 0$, $p = 0.61$ (Figure 4).

3.2.6. Intramedullary Lesions in SCIWORA

Thirteen studies provided data on the frequency of intramedullary signal change in patients with SCIWORA, including 336 cervical injuries and 44 thoracic injuries [19,24,32–38,40–42,45]. The pooled frequency of simple edema was 40% (74/187), while the rate of any intramedullary lesion (including edema, contusion, hemorrhage, or cavitation) was 77% (291/380) [19,24,32–38,40–42,45]; heterogeneity between studies was high ($I^2 = 0.90, 0.91$ respectively, both $p < 0.001$; Figure 4).

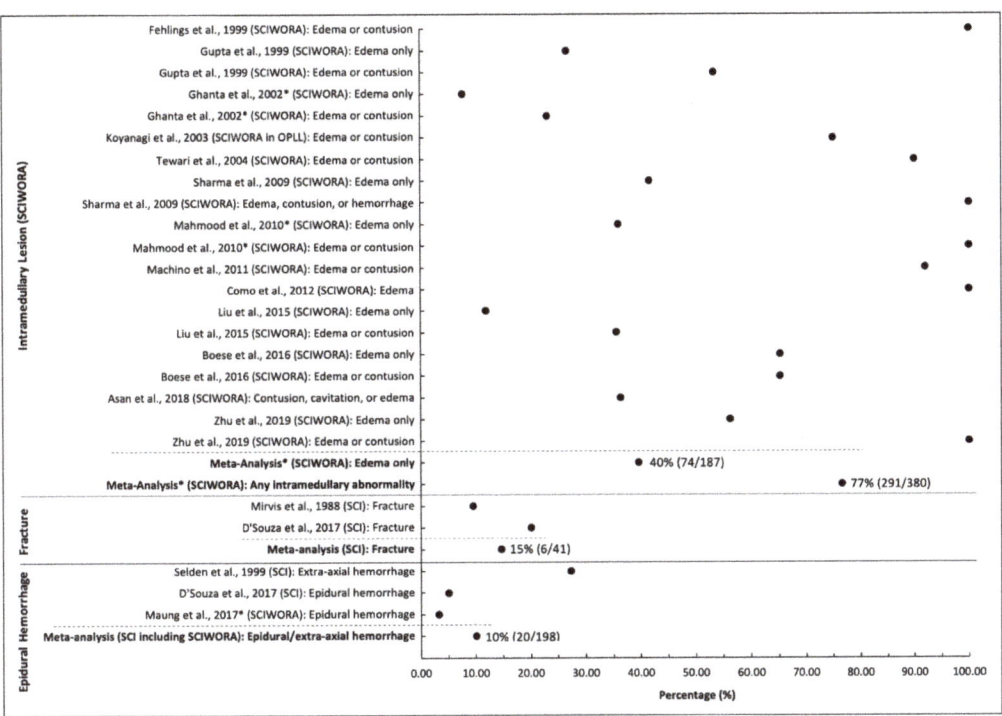

Figure 4. Frequency of Epidural Hemorrhage, Fracture, and Intramedullary Lesions (SCIWORA) on MRI in patients with acute spinal cord injury. * Studies that include pediatric patients (<16) or unspecified age range.

3.3. KQ3: Influence of MRI on Clinical Decision-Making

Twenty studies provided data relevant to KQ3, regarding if surgery is required, surgical approach, when to operate, determining the need for instrumentation, which levels to decompress, and the need for reoperation after surgery, based upon MRI findings in acute SCI (Table 5) [10,17,21–24,26,28–33,37,40,42,44–47].

3.3.1. If Surgery Is Required

Fifteen studies reported that MRI results directly influenced the decision of whether surgery was required in acute SCI [10,21–24,26,30,32,33,37,40,42,44–46]. Specific MRI findings that reportedly led to the decision for surgical treatment included cord compression, disc herniation, ligamentous injury, instability, and intramedullary edema (in conjunction with cord compression in SCIWORA). The frequency of MRI results reportedly leading to a decision to operate ranged from 3% to 100% across studies, with a pooled average of 36% (223/611) and high heterogeneity across studies ($I^2 = 0.96$, $p < 0.001$).

3.3.2. Surgical Approach

Nine studies reported on the influence of MRI findings on surgical approach [21,23,28–30,33,37,42,44]. Seven studies cited acute disc herniations with cord compression as the rationale for performing anterior surgery, at a rate of 3% to 83% of cases across studies [21,23,30,33,37,42,44]. Two additional studies of SCIWORA noted that MRI dictated surgical approach in all patients requiring surgery (42/211 and 70/70 patients, respectively), listing anterior compression, anterior compression limited to 1–3 segments, and kyphosis as reasons for selecting anterior surgery [28,29]. Overall, MRI was reported to affect the surgical approach in 29% (143/500) of patients in the included studies, with high heterogeneity ($I^2 = 0.97$, $p < 0.001$).

3.3.3. When to Operate

Three investigations examined the role of MRI in determining when to operate [10,31,44]. In two studies with overlapping datasets, 49% to 52% of patients required emergent surgery due to MRI-documented cord compression [10,44]. Two studies found that after traction/closed reduction, 33% to 82% of patients had good decompression and could undergo delayed surgery to perform definitive fixation [10,31]. Meta-analysis found that MRI affected surgical timing in 78% (65/83) of patients, with high heterogeneity ($I^2 = 0.84$, $p = 0.01$).

3.3.4. Need for Instrumentation

One study reported on the need for instrumented fusion due to the finding of segmental instability [17]. This study reported that the level of injury in SCIWORA (showing edema on MRI) and any levels showing ligamentous injury on MRI (19/23 patients) or segmental instability intraoperatively (22/23 patients) would be decompressed and fused.

3.3.5. Which Levels to Decompress

A single study reported that MRI findings of edema and ligamentous injury, and intraoperative findings of instability, dictated which level(s) would be decompressed and fused [17].

3.3.6. Need for Re-Operation after Surgery

Two studies reported the use of post-operative MRI to determine if adequate cord compression had been achieved after SCI [29,47]. One study found that 11/28 patients undergoing anterior surgery had residual cord compression, and this finding led to additional posterior surgical decompression [29]. Another study found that 63/184 patients had inadequate decompression following surgery for acute SCI, highlighting the role of cord swelling and the possible need for multi-level laminectomy and expansile duraplasty [47].

3.4. KQ4: When to Perform MRI

Sixteen studies provided data addressing KQ4 (Table 6) [10,22–24,26,28–33,43–47]. Fourteen studies concluded that MRI was useful during the initial assessment for the purpose of decision-making (related to one or more aspects of KQ3) [10,22–24,26,28–30,32,33,44–47]. However, two studies found that MRI prior to closed reduction of cervical facet dislocation was of unclear utility, with one study finding that two patients with pre-reduction disc herniation did not deteriorate after closed reduction [43], while another study similarly reported that 11 patients with pre-reduction cord compression did not deteriorate during closed reduction [31]. In contrast, Selden et al. found acute disc herniation in 10/18 patients with cervical dislocations, prompting a decision for immediate anterior surgery as the authors felt that closed reduction was unsafe [44]. Furthermore, Doran et al. reported neurological complications in three patients undergoing closed reduction of cervical dislocations that did not have pre-reduction MRI, and subsequent MRI showed disc herniations in all cases [30]. Three studies yielded data on MRI after closed-reduction, with two finding that it was helpful to identify ongoing spinal cord compression [31,44], whereas the third study found no neurological deterioration in spite of disc herniations in five of nine patients [43]. Two studies with overlapping cohorts reported that post-operative MRI was useful to identify inadequate decompression of the cord for consideration of re-operation [29,47]. No studies specifically recommended MRI within a set time period, but one study found no difference in the time interval from injury to pre-operative MRI between patients that were completely and incompletely decompressed [47].

3.5. KQ5: Frequency of Adverse Events When Performing MRI

Five investigations reported on frequency of adverse events when performing an MRI in patients with acute SCI (Table 7) [10,22,23,31,44]. Bao et al. examined patients receiving neutral, flexion, and extension MRIs for cervical SCI without fracture and dislocation, and amongst the cohort of 16 patients found no deterioration of neurological functions [22]. Similarly, when closed reduction for cervical dislocation was performed during MRI, no patients (*n* = 12) experienced permanent neurological deterioration or burning sensations at pin sites [31]. Pooled results found a 0% rate of adverse events (0/156 patients, 95% CI: 0% to 2.4%), with homogeneity across studies ($I^2 = 0$, $p = 1$).

3.6. KQ6: Effect of MRI on Outcomes

One investigation addressed KQ6, evaluating differences in outcome between 66 patients assigned to an MRI-based treatment protocol (including urgent surgery) and 25 who were not assigned (due to a "contraindication to MRI, the need for an emergent surgical procedure, or the bias of specific admitting attending neurosurgeons regarding the 'futility' of emergent surgical treatment") [10]. In patients assigned to the protocol group, Frankel grade improved from admission in 50%, relative to 24% in the non-protocol group ($p < 0.006$). Furthermore, eight of 50 patients from the protocol group presenting with complete motor quadriplegia (grade A or B) improved to independent ambulation (grade D or E), compared with none of the 20 reference patients ($p = 0.09$, Fisher exact test, not reported in original manuscript). MRI protocol patients also had shorter ICU stay (9.9 ± 1.7 days vs. 23.8 ± 3.7 days, $p < 0.001$) and total length of stay (71.4 ± 5.9 days vs. 99.9 ± 13.1 days, $p = 0.02$) [10]. Unfortunately, this study was deemed to have a high risk of bias due to non-random assignment to treatment groups and the confounding effect of more urgent spinal cord decompression in the protocol group compared with the reference group.

4. Discussion

This systematic review and meta-analysis addressed the role of MRI to inform clinical decision-making for patients with acute SCI, offering several lines of evidence supporting its use in routine practice. First, obtaining an MRI in the acute phase of SCI appears to be safe, with no adverse events reported in greater than 150 patients across five studies. This finding confirms the safety of obtaining an MRI in acute SCI, in spite of limited monitoring, additional transfers, and positioning the patient flat and supine for 30 to 45 min. MRI also demonstrates good diagnostic accuracy for ligamentous injury, instability, disc injury, disc herniation, and intramedullary tissue changes, albeit in a small number of comparative studies. Despite substantial heterogeneity between manuscripts, it is clear based on the large number of subjects and studies included in this meta-analysis that MRI frequently identified important pathological findings in patients with SCI, including spinal cord compression in 70%, disc herniation in 43%, ligamentous injury in 39%, and epidural hematoma in 10%. In patients with SCIWORA, MRI demonstrated intramedullary signal change in 77%, disc herniation in 45%, cord compression in 41%, and ligamentous injury in 36%. In contrast, evidence for the utility of MRI in detecting fractures in acute SCI was limited, with a low frequency of positive findings (15%) and poor diagnostic accuracy.

In terms of clinical decision-making, a large number of studies were identified that consistently reported evidence of clinical utility, influencing the decision to operate in 36% of patients, surgical approach in 29%, and the timing of surgery in 78%. Limited evidence also suggested that MRI is useful to determine the need for instrumentation, which levels to decompress, and if re-operation is needed for inadequate decompression. In terms of timing of MRI, most studies concluded that MRI should be performed on initial evaluation, prior to surgery. However, in cases of cervical dislocations, the utility of MRI prior to and after closed reduction remained unclear, due to conflicting results between studies regarding both the frequency and clinical significance of disc herniations; some reports suggest that MRI may be useful to avoid secondary injury due to a large disc herniation, but this area requires further study to draw conclusions. Finally, the results of this review confirm that evidence is lacking to directly show if obtaining an MRI improves outcomes; the only study addressing this topic had a high risk of bias due to non-randomized selection and a confounding effect of earlier spinal cord decompression in patients in the MRI-protocol group. Overall, the body of literature offers moderate evidence that (1) MRI is safe in the acute phase of SCI, (2) MRI has good diagnostic accuracy to detect certain features that are potentially useful for decision-making, (3) these features occur frequently, (4) these features often affect clinical decision-making, and (5) MRI should be performed prior to surgical treatment, whenever possible. However, further studies that investigate management decisions and clinical outcomes with and without MRI, the role of MRI in cervical dislocations, the time delay incurred by obtaining an MRI, and the cost-effectiveness of MRI are required to fully define its utility in acute SCI.

The novelty of the current study is that the review was broadly inclusive, looking for both direct and indirect evidence, while focusing narrowly on the topic of the role of MRI to facilitate clinical decision-making in patients with acute SCI. This review involved a comprehensive search of the literature that considered a large number of citations and full-text articles, and was designed to directly answer a common question that faces surgeons when a patient presents with acute SCI: should I get an MRI first, or just proceed directly to the operating room? The 2002 and 2013 AANS/CNS guidelines for the management of SCI also attempted to address the utility of MRI, but circumvented the main topic with only peripheral recommendations that MRI should be used in pediatric patients to assess SCI, or in adults for collar clearance, for the diagnosis of vertebral artery injury, or to assess patients with ankylosing spondylitis or SCIWORA [6]. Subsequently, AOSpine sponsored an effort to develop five guidelines for controversial topics in SCI, including one on the role of MRI in acute SCI, which provided a weak recommendation that MRI should be used in acute SCI to facilitate improved decision-making and prognostication [9]. These recommendations were based on a systematic review by Kurpad et al. (2017), which was unfortunately hampered by restrictive inclusion criteria yielding only one relevant study (which was deemed to have a high risk of bias) regarding the utility of MRI to guide acute SCI management, thus resulting in a vacuum of relevant evidence [7]. Conversely, Bozzo et al. (2011) utilized liberal inclusion criteria, involving the broader population of all spinal trauma, but was less focused and potentially lacked external validity. Furthermore, the review did not explore how individual studies reported changes in management based on MRI results, nor did it explore the importance of MRI in detection of spinal cord compression, which was the most common entity cited in the current review to affect management. In addition, the vast majority of studies included in both Bozzo et al. (2011) and Kurpad et al. (2017) investigated the use of MRI for prognostication, which we feel is of secondary importance, compared to the imperative task of deciding upon and planning surgical treatment. As a result, a knowledge gap currently exists regarding the optimal use of MRI, with highly variable practice patterns between surgeons. In summary, this systematic review provides a focused synthesis of the literature that clarifies the utility of MRI, while highlighting several areas that require further investigation.

SCI is an inherently difficult condition to study, due to profound heterogeneity in demographics, patterns of injury, timing after injury, neurological presentation, biomechanical stability, comorbidities, concomitant injuries, treatments performed, outcome measures, and MRI methods. The current study performed meta-analyses that clearly reflected this heterogeneity, providing aggregate results that may be helpful to provide general insights, but must be interpreted with caution as the frequency of findings varied with several factors. Complicating matters, the literature uses inconsistent definitions of terms such as SCIWORA, which was originally described in the pediatric population based on radiographs, but has increasingly been used to describe adult SCI without CT evidence of trauma (sometimes dubbed SCIWOCTET). Adult SCIWORA is widely felt to be considerably different than pediatric SCIWORA, with the former frequently involving degenerative spondylosis, ossification of posterior longitudinal ligament, and disc herniations, whereas the latter typically involves ligamentous laxity; therefore, it was not surprising that the SCIWORA results presented in this study also showed high heterogeneity. Furthermore, patients presenting with acute SCI frequently have concomitant injuries, hemodynamic instability, altered mental status, and/or undefined neurological deficits, making it difficult to develop recommendations that are universally applicable. However, the findings of this study are sufficiently compelling to suggest that MRI should be obtained during initial assessment of most patients with acute SCI, in the absence of a contraindication.

Looking ahead, further investigations should focus on several areas to elucidate the role of MRI in acute SCI. First, studies are needed that directly compare outcomes with and without MRI, while implementing similar management otherwise. However, it is doubtful that a randomized study can be ethically performed, as there was a perceived lack of equipoise expressed by expert clinicians in a recent guidelines effort [9]. Furthermore, emerging evidence suggests that earlier decompression has an hour-by-hour benefit on outcomes for the first 36 h after injury [48], suggesting that delays incurred in obtaining an MRI may counteract the benefits. Thus, future studies should include an analysis of the timing of surgery and the related impact of obtaining an MRI. On this topic, institutional protocols such as a "Code SCI" that streamline the care of SCI patients to minimize delays in imaging and definitive treatment should be developed [10,49], akin to "Code Stroke" protocols that have transformed stroke care. Future research is required that prospectively investigates the utility of MRI to make specific decisions on the need for surgery, surgical approach, the number of levels of decompression, and the need for instrumentation. Aarabi et al. (2019) demonstrated that decompressing more levels (up to five) with laminectomy showed higher rates of complete spinal cord decompression, likely due to greater alleviation of spinal cord swelling and secondary injury [47]; identifying pre-operative MRI features that predict spinal cord swelling could inform the need for additional levels of decompression and/or expansile duraplasty. In addition, the vast majority of previous studies have focused on cervical SCI, while the utility of MRI in thoracolumbar injuries is poorly defined, such as burst fractures with SCI. Evaluation of the cost-effectiveness of MRI is also needed to justify its widespread use, particularly in health systems and regions with scarce resources. Finally, emerging microstructural MRI techniques that measure specific physical properties such as axonal injury, demyelination, and perfusion should be studied for their potential value in prognostication [50].

This study is subject to several limitations. The systematic review involved two separate literature searches that were conducted using different interfaces and software tools, which occurred because the authors paused the initial project; this could have resulted in missed citations, although the literature search was comprehensive and overlapping dates were used to mitigate this risk. The large number of citations and full-text articles that were reviewed could also lead to errors, but we had multiple authors reviewing at each step to avoid errors. After careful consideration, we also modified the original inclusion criteria to allow studies with a small number of pediatric patients, as we felt that exclusion of certain key studies would result in a failure to identify important evidence; however, this decision potentially degrades the internal validity, as the small number of pediatric patients could mildly influence the overall results. There also exists the possibility of publication bias, which may have influenced our results. Our approach also excluded studies of spinal trauma without SCI or those that did not perform subgroup analyses with and without SCI; this approach omitted a large number of studies that offered substantial data on the diagnostic accuracy of MRI to detect ligamentous injury and fractures; however, we felt that it was essential to focus the current study on the specific clinical population of acute SCI.

5. Conclusions

MRI is safe and frequently identifies important findings with good diagnostic accuracy that alter clinical management in patients with acute SCI of all presentations, and thus, should be utilized when feasible. Therefore, pessimism that some surgeons feel toward obtaining MRI for the purpose of informing decision-making in acute SCI appears to be unjustified. Although the evidence is imperfect and indirect, it confirms the prior CPG recommendation "that MRI be performed in adult patients with acute SCI prior to surgical intervention, when feasible, to facilitate improved clinical decision-making". Future prospective studies are needed to fully define the utility and cost-effectiveness of

MRI in specific types of SCI, to allow for stronger recommendations that improve and standardize clinical practice.

Author Contributions: Conceptualization, A.R.M., N.T. and M.G.F.; Methodology, A.R.M. and L.T.; Formal analysis, A.R.M. and A.G.-R.; Investigation, A.G.-R., J.E.L.-R., C.P., N.T., S.F.L. and M.K.; Data curation, A.G.-R., J.E.L.-R., C.P., N.T., S.F.L., M.K. and A.R.M.; Writing—original draft preparation, A.R.M. and A.G.-R.; Writing—review and editing, A.R.M., A.G.-R. and M.G.F.; Supervision, A.R.M.; Project administration, A.R.M. All authors have read and agreed to the published version of the manuscript.

Funding: Martin received support from Canadian Institutes of Health Research (CIHR) Fellowship (2016–2017) and Neurosurgery Research and Education Foundation (NREF) Clinical Fellowship (2019–2020). Fehlings was supported by the Halbert Chair in Neural Repair and Regeneration (MGF).

Institutional Review Board Statement: Not applicable.

Informed Consent Statement: Not applicable.

Data Availability Statement: All data supporting reported results can be found within the manuscript.

Conflicts of Interest: The authors declare no conflict of interest.

Appendix A

Pubmed (MEDLINE) Search Strategy

(((magnetic resonance imaging) OR (MRI)) AND (((((((SCI) OR (spinal cord injury)) OR (spinal trauma)) OR (spine fracture)) OR (spine trauma)) OR (cervical fracture)) OR (cervical trauma))) AND (((((((outcome) OR (recovery)) OR (management)) OR (decision-making)) OR (decision)) OR (surgery)) OR (surgical)) OR (treatment))

Embase Ovid Search Strategy

(magnetic AND resonance AND imaging OR mri) AND (((((((sci OR spinal) AND cord AND injury OR spinal) AND trauma OR spine) AND fracture OR spine) AND trauma OR cervical) AND fracture OR cervical) AND trauma) AND ((outcome OR recovery OR management OR decision) AND making OR decision OR surgery OR surgical OR treatment)

CENTRAL Search Strategy

[Magnetic Resonance Imaging] explode all trees OR MRI AND [Spinal Cord Injuries] explode all trees OR spinal cord injury OR SCI OR spinal trauma OR spine trauma OR spine fracture OR cervical fracture OR cervical trauma AND [Outcome Assessment, Health Care] explode all trees OR outcome OR recovery OR management OR MeSH descriptor: [Clinical Decision-Making] explode all trees OR decision-making OR decision OR MeSH descriptor: [General Surgery] explode all trees OR surgery OR surgical OR treatment OR MeSH descriptor: [Therapeutics] explode all trees.

References

1. Wyndaele, M.; Wyndaele, J.J. Incidence, prevalence and epidemiology of spinal cord injury: What learns a worldwide literature survey? *Spinal Cord* **2006**, *44*, 523–529. [CrossRef]
2. Fehlings, M.G.; Vaccaro, A.; Wilson, J.R.; Singh, A.; Cadotte, D.W.; Harrop, J.S.; Aarabi, B.; Shaffrey, C.; Dvorak, M.; Fisher, C.; et al. Early versus Delayed Decompression for Traumatic Cervical Spinal Cord Injury: Results of the Surgical Timing in Acute Spinal Cord Injury Study (STASCIS). *PLoS ONE* **2012**, *7*, e32037. [CrossRef]
3. Fehlings, M.G.; Tetreault, L.A.; Wilson, J.R.; Kwon, B.K.; Burns, A.S.; Martin, A.R.; Hawryluk, G.; Harrop, J.S. A Clinical Practice Guideline for the Management of Acute Spinal Cord Injury: Introduction, Rationale, and Scope. *Glob. Spine J.* **2017**, *7*, 84s–94s. [CrossRef] [PubMed]
4. Hadley, M.N.; Walters, B.C.; Grabb, P.A.; Oyesiku, N.M.; Przybylski, G.J.; Resnick, D.K.; Ryken, T.C. Guidelines for management of acute cervical spinal injuries. Introduction. *Neurosurgery* **2002**, *50*, S1.
5. Walters, B.C.; Hadley, M.N.; Hurlbert, R.J.; Aarabi, B.; Dhall, S.S.; Gelb, D.E.; Harrigan, M.R.; Rozelle, C.J.; Ryken, T.C.; Theodore, N. Guidelines for the management of acute cervical spine and spinal cord injuries: 2013 update. *Neurosurgery* **2013**, *60*, 82–91. [CrossRef]
6. Ryken, T.C.; Hadley, M.N.; Walters, B.C.; Aarabi, B.; Dhall, S.S.; Gelb, D.E.; Hurlbert, R.J.; Rozzelle, C.J.; Theodore, N. Radiographic assessment. *Neurosurgery* **2013**, *72* (Suppl. 2), 54–72. [CrossRef]

7. Kurpad, S.N.; Martin, A.R.; Tetreault, L.A.; Fischer, D.J.; Skelly, A.C.; Mikulis, D.; Flanders, A.E.; Aarabi, B.; Mroz, T.; Tsai, E.C.; et al. Impact of baseline magnetic resonance imaging on neurologic, functional, and safety outcomes in patients with acute traumatic spinal cord injury. *Glob. Spine J.* **2017**, *7*, 151S–174S.
8. Bozzo, A.; Marcoux, J.; Radhakrishna, M.; Pelletier, J.; Goulet, B. The role of magnetic resonance imaging in the management of acute spinal cord injury. *J. Neurotrauma* **2011**, *28*, 1401–1411. [PubMed]
9. Fehlings, M.G.; Martin, A.R.; Tetreault, L.; Aarabi, B.; Anderson, P.; Arnold, P.M.; Broke, D.; Burns, A.; Chiba, K.; Hawryluk, G.; et al. A Clinical Practice Guideline for the Management of Patients with Acute Spinal Cord Injury: Recommendations on the Role of Baseline Magnetic Resonance Imaging in Clinical Decision Making and Outcome Prediction. *Glob. Spine J.* **2017**, *7*, 221S–230S.
10. Papadopoulos, S.M.; Selden, N.R.; Quint, D.J.; Patel, N.; Gillespie, B.; Grube, S. Immediate spinal cord decompression for cervical spinal cord injury: Feasibility and outcome. *J. Trauma* **2002**, *52*, 323–332. [CrossRef] [PubMed]
11. Moher, D.; Shamseer, L.; Clarke, M.; Ghersi, D.; Liberati, A.; Petticrew, M.; Shekelle, P.; Stewart, L.A.; PRISMA-P Group. Preferred reporting items for systematic review and meta-analysis protocols (PRISMA-P) 2015 statement. *Syst. Rev.* **2015**, *4*, 1. [CrossRef] [PubMed]
12. Shamseer, L.; Moher, D.; Clarke, M.; Ghersi, D.; Liberati, A.; Petticrew, M.; Shekelle, P.; Stewart, L.A. Preferred reporting items for systematic review and meta-analysis protocols (PRISMA-P) 2015: Elaboration and explanation. *BMJ* **2015**, *349*, g7647. [CrossRef]
13. Higgins, J.P.T.; Thomas, J.; Chandler, J.; Cumpston, M.; Li, T.; Page, M.J.; Welch, V.A. (Eds.) *Cochrane Handbook for Systematic Reviews of Interventions*; Version 6.2; Cochrane: Oxford, UK, 2021.
14. Edelman, R.R. The History of MR Imaging as Seen through the Pages of Radiology. *Radiology* **2014**, *273*, S181–S200. [CrossRef] [PubMed]
15. R Core Team. *R: A Language and Environment for Statistical Computing*; R Core Team: Vienna, Austria, 2013.
16. National Heart, Lung, and Blood Institute. *National Institute of Health: Quality Assessment Tool for Observational Cohort and Cross-Sectional Studies*; National Heart, Lung, and Blood Institute: Bethesda, MD, USA, 2014.
17. Krappinger, D.; Lindtner, R.A.; Zegg, M.J.; Henninger, B.; Kaser, V.; Spicher, A.; Schmid, R. Spondylotic traumatic central cord syndrome: A hidden discoligamentous injury? *Eur. Spine J.* **2019**, *28*, 434–441. [CrossRef]
18. Henninger, B.; Kaser, V.; Ostermann, S.; Spicher, A.; Zegg, M.; Schmid, R.; Kremser, C.; Krappinger, D. Cervical Disc and Ligamentous Injury in Hyperextension Trauma: MRI and Intraoperative Correlation. *J. Neuroimaging* **2020**, *30*, 104–109. [CrossRef]
19. Zhu, F.; Yao, S.; Ren, Z.; Telemacque, D.; Qu, Y.; Chen, K.; Yang, F.; Zeng, L.; Guo, X. Early durotomy with duroplasty for severe adult spinal cord injury without radiographic abnormality: A novel concept and method of surgical decompression. *Eur. Spine J.* **2019**, *28*, 2275–2282. [CrossRef] [PubMed]
20. Maeda, T.; Ueta, T.; Mori, E.; Yugue, I.; Kawano, O.; Takao, T.; Sakai, H.; Okada, S.; Shiba, K. Soft-tissue damage and segmental instability in adult patients with cervical spinal cord injury without major bone injury. *Spine* **2012**, *37*, E1560–E1566. [CrossRef]
21. Mirvis, S.E.; Geisler, F.H.; Jelinek, J.J.; Joslyn, J.N.; Gellad, F. Acute cervical spine trauma: Evaluation with 1.5-T MR imaging. *Radiology* **1988**, *166*, 807–816.
22. Bao, Y.; Zhong, X.; Zhu, W.; Chen, Y.; Zhou, L.; Dai, X.; Liao, J.; Li, Z.; Hu, K.; Bei, K.; et al. Feasibility and Safety of Cervical Kinematic Magnetic Resonance Imaging in Patients with Cervical Spinal Cord Injury without Fracture and Dislocation. *Orthop. Surg.* **2020**, *12*, 570–581. [CrossRef] [PubMed]
23. Kalfas, I.; Wilberger, J.; Goldberg, A.; Prostko, E.R. Magnetic resonance imaging in acute spinal cord trauma. *Neurosurgery* **1988**, *23*, 295–299. [CrossRef]
24. Como, J.J.; Samia, H.; Nemunaitis, G.A.; Jain, V.; Anderson, J.S.; Malangoni, M.A.; Claridge, J.A. The misapplication of the term spinal cord injury without radiographic abnormality (SCIWORA) in adults. *J. Trauma Acute Care Surg.* **2012**, *73*, 1261–1266. [CrossRef] [PubMed]
25. Hendey, G.W.; Wolfson, A.B.; Mower, W.R.; Hoffman, J.R. Spinal cord injury without radiographic abnormality: Results of the National Emergency X-Radiography Utilization Study in blunt cervical trauma. *J. Trauma* **2002**, *53*, 1–4. [CrossRef]
26. Maung, A.A.; Johnson, D.C.; Barre, K.; Peponis, T.; Mesar, T.; Velmahos, G.C.; McGrail, D.; Kasotakis, G.; Gross, R.I.; Rosenblatt, M.S.; et al. Cervical spine MRI in patients with negative CT: A prospective, multicenter study of the Research Consortium of New England Centers for Trauma (ReCONECT). *J. Trauma Acute Care Surg.* **2017**, *82*, 263–269. [CrossRef] [PubMed]
27. Song, K.J.; Kim, G.H.; Lee, K.B. The efficacy of the modified classification system of soft tissue injury in extension injury of the lower cervical spine. *Spine* **2008**, *33*, E488–E493. [CrossRef]
28. Cheng, X.; Ni, B.; Liu, Q.; Chen, J.; Guan, H.; Guo, Q. Clinical and radiological outcomes of spinal cord injury without radiologic evidence of trauma with cervical disc herniation. *Arch. Orthop. Trauma Surg.* **2013**, *133*, 193–198. [CrossRef] [PubMed]
29. Aarabi, B.; Alexander, M.; Mirvis, S.E.; Shanmuganathan, K.; Chesler, D.; Maulucci, C.; Iguchi, M.; Aresco, C.; Blacklock, T. Predictors of outcome in acute traumatic central cord syndrome due to spinal stenosis. *J. Neurosurg. Spine* **2011**, *14*, 122–130. [CrossRef]
30. Doran, S.E.; Papadopoulos, S.M.; Ducker, T.B.; Lillehei, K.O. Magnetic resonance imaging documentation of coexistent traumatic locked facets of the cervical spine and disc herniation. *J. Neurosurg.* **1993**, *79*, 341–345. [PubMed]
31. Darsaut, T.E.; Ashforth, R.; Bhargava, R.; Broad, R.; Emery, D.; Kortbeek, F.; Lambert, R.; Lavoie, M.; Mahood, J.; MacDowell, I.; et al. A pilot study of magnetic resonance imaging-guided closed reduction of cervical spine fractures. *Spine* **2006**, *31*, 2085–2090. [CrossRef]

32. Gupta, S.K.; Rajeev, K.; Khosla, V.K.; Sharma, B.S.; Paramjit; Mathuriya, S.N.; Pathak, A.; Tewari, M.K.; Kumar, A. Spinal cord injury without radiographic abnormality in adults. *Spinal Cord* **1999**, *37*, 726–729. [PubMed]
33. Sharma, S.; Singh, M.; Wani, I.H.; Sharma, S.; Sharma, N.; Singh, D. Adult Spinal Cord Injury without Radiographic Abnormalities (SCIWORA): Clinical and Radiological Correlations. *J. Clin. Med. Res.* **2009**, *1*, 165–172. [CrossRef]
34. Koyanagi, I.; Iwasaki, Y.; Hida, K.; Imamura, H.; Fujimoto, S.; Akino, M. Acute cervical cord injury associated with ossification of the posterior longitudinal ligament. *Neurosurgery* **2003**, *53*, 887–891. [CrossRef] [PubMed]
35. Asan, Z. Spinal Cord Injury without Radiological Abnormality in Adults: Clinical and Radiological Discordance. *World Neurosurg.* **2018**, *114*, e1147–e1151. [CrossRef] [PubMed]
36. Liu, Q.; Liu, Q.; Zhao, J.; Yu, H.; Ma, X.; Wang, L. Early MRI finding in adult spinal cord injury without radiologic abnormalities does not correlate with the neurological outcome: A retrospective study. *Spinal Cord* **2015**, *53*, 750–753. [CrossRef]
37. Ghanta, M.K.; Smith, L.M.; Polin, R.S.; Marr, A.B.; Spires, W.V. An analysis of Eastern Association for the Surgery of Trauma practice guidelines for cervical spine evaluation in a series of patients with multiple imaging techniques. *Am. Surg.* **2002**, *68*, 563–567. [PubMed]
38. Fehlings, M.G.; Rao, S.C.; Tator, C.H.; Skaf, G.; Arnold, P.; Benzel, E.; Dickman, C.; Cuddy, B.; Green, B.; Hitchon, P.; et al. The optimal radiologic method for assessing spinal canal compromise and cord compression in patients with cervical spinal cord injury. Part II: Results of a multicenter study. *Spine* **1999**, *24*, 605–613. [CrossRef]
39. D'Souza, M.M.; Choudhary, A.; Poonia, M.; Kumar, P.; Khushu, S. Diffusion tensor MR imaging in spinal cord injury. *Injury* **2017**, *48*, 880–884. [CrossRef]
40. Machino, M.; Yukawa, Y.; Ito, K.; Nakashima, H.; Kanbara, S.; Morita, D.; Kato, F. Can magnetic resonance imaging reflect the prognosis in patients of cervical spinal cord injury without radiographic abnormality? *Spine* **2011**, *36*, E1568–E1572. [CrossRef] [PubMed]
41. Mahmood, N.; Rajagopal, K.; Ramesh, A. Cervical spinal cord injury with and without the radiographical evidence of trauma–A retrospective comparative study in adults. *J. Clin. Diagn. Res.* **2010**, *4*, 2183–2189.
42. Tewari, M.K.; Gifti, D.S.; Singh, P.; Khosla, V.K.; Mathuriya, S.N.; Gupta, S.K.; Pathak, A. Diagnosis and prognostication of adult spinal cord injury without radiographic abnormality using magnetic resonance imaging: Analysis of 40 patients. *Surg. Neurol.* **2005**, *63*, 204–209. [CrossRef]
43. Vaccaro, A.R.; Falatyn, S.P.; Flanders, A.E.; Balderston, R.A.; Northrup, B.E.; Cotler, J.M. Magnetic resonance evaluation of the intervertebral disc, spinal ligaments, and spinal cord before and after closed traction reduction of cervical spine dislocations. *Spine* **1999**, *24*, 1210–1217. [CrossRef] [PubMed]
44. Selden, N.R.; Quint, D.J.; Patel, N.; d'Arcy, H.S.; Papadopoulos, S.M. Emergency magnetic resonance imaging of cervical spinal cord injuries: Clinical correlation and prognosis. *Neurosurgery* **1999**, *44*, 785–792. [CrossRef] [PubMed]
45. Boese, C.K.; Müller, D.; Bröer, R.; Eysel, P.; Krischek, B.; Lehmann, H.C.; Lechler, P. Spinal cord injury without radiographic abnormality (SCIWORA) in adults: MRI type predicts early neurologic outcome. *Spinal Cord* **2016**, *54*, 878–883. [CrossRef] [PubMed]
46. Huang, R.; Ryu, R.C.; Kim, T.T.; Alban, R.F.; Margulies, D.R.; Ley, E.J.; Barmparas, G. Is magnetic resonance imaging becoming the new computed tomography for cervical spine clearance? Trends in magnetic resonance imaging utilization at a Level I trauma center. *J. Trauma Acute Care Surg.* **2020**, *89*, 365–370. [CrossRef] [PubMed]
47. Aarabi, B.; Olexa, J.; Chryssikos, T.; Galvagno, S.M.; Hersh, D.S.; Wessell, A.; Sansur, C.; Schwartzbauer, G.; Crandall, K.; Shanmuganathan, K.; et al. Extent of Spinal Cord Decompression in Motor Complete (American Spinal Injury Association Impairment Scale Grades A and B) Traumatic Spinal Cord Injury Patients: Post-Operative Magnetic Resonance Imaging Analysis of Standard Operative Approaches. *J. Neurotrauma* **2019**, *36*, 862–876. [CrossRef]
48. Badhiwala, J.H.; Wilson, J.R.; Witiw, C.D.; Harrop, J.S.; Vaccaro, A.R.; Aarabi, B.; Grossman, R.G.; Geisler, F.H.; Fehlings, M.G. The influence of timing of surgical decompression for acute spinal cord injury: A pooled analysis of individual patient data. *Lancet Neurol.* **2021**, *20*, 117–126. [CrossRef]
49. Masterson, K. A New Spinal Cord Injury Treatment is Getting Patients Back on Their Feet. 2018. Available online: https://www.ucsf.edu/news/2018/09/411471/new-spinal-cord-injury-treatment-getting-patients-back-their-feet (accessed on 10 October 2021).
50. Martin, A.R.; Aleksanderek, I.; Cohen-Adad, J.; Tarmohamed, Z.; Tetreault, L.; Smith, N.; Cadotte, D.W.; Crawley, A.; Ginsberg, H.; Mikulis, D.J.; et al. Translating state-of-the-art spinal cord MRI techniques to clinical use: A systematic review of clinical studies utilizing DTI, MT, MWF, MRS, and fMRI. *NeuroImage* **2016**, *10*, 192–238. [CrossRef]

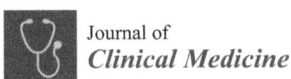 Journal of
Clinical Medicine

Review

The Relative Merits of Posterior Surgical Treatments for Multi-Level Degenerative Cervical Myelopathy Remain Uncertain: Findings from a Systematic Review

Xiaoyu Yang [1,2], Aref-Ali Gharooni [1], Rana S. Dhillon [3], Edward Goacher [4], Edward W. Dyson [5], Oliver Mowforth [1], Alexandru Budu [6], Guy Wynne-Jones [7], Jibin Francis [1], Rikin Trivedi [1], Marcel Ivanov [6], Sashin Ahuja [8], Kia Rezajooi [9], Andreas K. Demetriades [10], David Choi [11], Antony H. Bateman [12], Nasir Quraishi [13], Vishal Kumar [14], Manjul Tripathi [15], Sandeep Mohindra [15], Erlick A. Pereira [16], Giles Critchley [17], Michael G. Fehlings [18], Peter J. A. Hutchinson [1], Benjamin M. Davies [1,*] and Mark R. N. Kotter [1,19]

1. Division of Neurosurgery, Department of Clinical Neurosciences, University of Cambridge, Cambridge CB0 0GG, UK; xy393@outlook.com (X.Y.); aag56@cam.ac.uk (A.-A.G.); om283@cam.ac.uk (O.M.); Jibin.Francis@gmail.com (J.F.); RikinTrivedi@hotmail.com (R.T.); pjah2@cam.ac.uk (P.J.A.H.); mrk25@cam.ac.uk (M.R.N.K.)
2. Department of Neurosurgery, Leiden University Medical Centre, 2333ZA Leiden, The Netherlands
3. Department of Neurosurgery, St Vincent's Hospital Melbourne, Melbourne, VIC 3065, Australia; ranadhillon@email.com
4. Department of Neurosurgery, Royal Hallamshire Hospital, Sheffield S10 2JF, UK; edward.goacher@doctors.org.uk
5. Victor Horsley Department of Neurosurgery, National Hospital for Neurology & Neurosurgery, London WC1N 3BG, UK; edwarddyson@nhs.net
6. Department of Neurosurgery, Sheffield Teaching Hospitals National Health Service Foundation Trust, Sheffield S10 2JF, UK; budu.alexandru@gmail.com (A.B.); marcel.ivanov@nhs.net (M.I.)
7. Department of Orthopaedics, The Newcastle upon Tyne Hospitals NHS Foundation Trust, Newcastle upon Tyne NE7 7DN, UK; GuyWynneJones@gmail.com
8. Welsh Centre for Spinal Surgery & Trauma, University hospital of Wales, Cardiff CF14 4XW, UK; sashinahuja@gmail.com
9. Spinal Surgery Unit, Royal National Orthopaedic Hospital, Stanmore HA7 4LP, UK; kia.rezajooi@rnoh.nhs.uk
10. Edinburgh Spinal Surgery Outcome Studies Group, Department of Neurosurgery, Royal Infirmary of Edinburgh, Edinburgh EH16 4SA, UK; demetriades@gmail.com
11. Department of Neurosurgery, National Hospital for Neurology and Neurosurgery, University College London Hospitals, London WC1N 3BG, UK; david.choi@nhs.net
12. Royal Derby Spinal Centre, Royal Derby Hospital, Derby DE22 3NE, UK; abateman@doctors.org.uk
13. Nottingham Centre for Spinal Studies and Surgery, Queens Medical Centre, Nottingham University Hospitals, Nottingham NG7 2UH, UK; Nasir.Quraishi@nuh.nhs.uk
14. Department of Orthopaedics, Post Graduate Institute of Medical Education and Research (PGIMER), Chandigarh 160012, India; drkumarvishal@gmail.com
15. Department of Neurosurgery, Post Graduate Institute of Medical Education and Research (PGIMER), Chandigarh 160012, India; drmanjultripathi@gmail.com (M.T.); sandeepneuro@gmail.com (S.M.)
16. Neurosciences Research Centre, Institute of Molecular and Clinical Sciences, St George's, University of London, London WC1E 7HU, UK; erlick.pereira2@nhs.net
17. Brighton and Sussex Medical School, South East Neurosurgery and South East Spinal Surgery, University Hospitals Sussex NHS Foundation Trust, Brighton BN1 9PX, UK; giles.critchley@nhs.net
18. Division of Neurosurgery, Toronto Western Hospital, University Health Network, Toronto, ON M5T 2S8, Canada; Michael.Fehlings@uhn.ca
19. Anne McLaren Laboratory for Regenerative Medicine, Welcome Trust MRC Cambridge Stem Cell Institute, University of Cambridge, Cambridge CB2 0PY, UK
* Correspondence: bd375@cam.ac.uk

Citation: Yang, X.; Gharooni, A.-A.; Dhillon, R.S.; Goacher, E.; Dyson, E.W.; Mowforth, O.; Budu, A.; Wynne-Jones, G.; Francis, J.; Trivedi, R.; et al. The Relative Merits of Posterior Surgical Treatments for Multi-Level Degenerative Cervical Myelopathy Remain Uncertain: Findings from a Systematic Review. *J. Clin. Med.* **2021**, *10*, 3653. https://doi.org/10.3390/jcm10163653

Academic Editors: Allan R. Martin and Aria Nouri

Received: 4 July 2021
Accepted: 17 August 2021
Published: 18 August 2021

Publisher's Note: MDPI stays neutral with regard to jurisdictional claims in published maps and institutional affiliations.

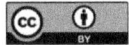

Copyright: © 2021 by the authors. Licensee MDPI, Basel, Switzerland. This article is an open access article distributed under the terms and conditions of the Creative Commons Attribution (CC BY) license (https://creativecommons.org/licenses/by/4.0/).

Abstract: Objectives: To assess the reporting of study design and characteristics in multi-level degenerative cervical myelopathy (DCM) treated by posterior surgical approaches, and perform a comparison of clinical and radiographic outcomes between different approaches. Methods: A literature search was performed in Embase and MEDLINE between 1995–2019 using a sensitive search string combination. Studies were selected by predefined selection criteria: Full text articles in English, with >10 patients (prospective) or >50 patients (retrospective), reporting outcomes of multi-level DCM treated by posterior surgical approach. Results: A total of 75 studies involving 19,510 patients, conducted worldwide, were identified. Laminoplasty was described in 56 studies (75%), followed by laminectomy with (36%) and without fusion (16%). The majority of studies were conducted in Asia (84%), in the period of 2016–2019 (51%), of which laminoplasty was studied predominantly. Twelve (16%) prospective studies and 63 (84%) retrospective studies were identified. The vast majority of studies were conducted in a single centre (95%) with clear inclusion/exclusion criteria and explicit cause of DCM. Eleven studies (15%) included patients with ossification of the posterior longitudinal ligament exclusively with cohorts of 57 to 252. The clinical and radiographic outcomes were reported with heterogeneity when comparing laminoplasty, laminectomy with and without fusion. Conclusions: Heterogeneity in the reporting of study and sample characteristics exists, as well as in clinical and radiographic outcomes, with a paucity of studies with a higher level of evidence. Future studies are needed to elucidate the clinical effectiveness of posterior surgical treatments.

Keywords: cervical spine; multi-level; myelopathy; laminoplasty; laminectomy; fusion; degenerative cervical myelopathy

1. Introduction

Degenerative cervical myelopathy (DCM) is a common and disabling condition, caused by arthritic changes in the cervical spine that compress and injure the cervical spinal cord. This results in functional impairment of the spinal cord that progresses at various rates and patterns, most commonly in a stepwise deterioration with periods of stable symptoms [1]. DCM is estimated to affect up to 2.3% [2] of adults and leads to progressive loss of dexterity, gait disturbance, imbalance, bladder disturbance, and occasionally incontinence and tetraplegia [1]. Surgery is currently the only treatment shown to alter the natural history of the disease: removing the mechanical compression on the spinal cord can stop disease progression and typically offer meaningful, albeit incomplete, recovery. There are a number of different surgical approaches and techniques in use. International guidelines currently recommend surgery for moderate (mJOA 12–14) to severe impairment (mJOA $\leq$ 11) and any progressive disease [3].

These guidelines leave the choice of procedure at the discretion of the operating surgeon, which reflects an uncertainty within scientific evidence over the relative merits and contra/indications for specific procedures [4]. Understanding these nuances is a recognised research priority by AO Spine RECODE DCM (aospine.org/recode) [5]; 'Individualising Surgery', and the need to address specific sub-questions of surgery, for example as is being evaluated in cervical spondylotic myelopathy (CSM) surgery, a randomised controlled trial (RCT) of anterior versus posterior surgery [6].

A further area of uncertainty remains the role of stabilisation or reconstruction after decompression. For DCM treated posteriorly, the typically used techniques are laminectomy, laminoplasty or laminectomy and fusion [7]. These techniques all provide posterior decompression but have differing approaches to stabilisation: laminectomy includes no stabilisation [8], laminoplasty (with several variations) uses a construct to float and retain the dorsal elements posteriorly [9] whilst laminectomy and fusion uses instrumentation to rigidly stabilise the spinal column [10–14]. These techniques therefore represent contrasting views on the contribution of dynamic instability to the pathogenesis of DCM, and the significance and role of retaining range of motion (ROM) versus preventing secondary cervical deformity.

Whether or not this is significant to patients is uncertain [10,15], with conflicting evidence [16–19] and recommendations [8,14,20,21], leading to widespread variation in clinical practice [22,23]. Although widely used, there has been no prospectively powered comparison of these techniques [4]. Furthermore, much of the evidence comes from cohorts including single level disease [24,25]. One assumption is the inherent biomechanical implications for posterior surgery are magnified when treating multiple levels, and this is most likely where any divergence would be most significant. This subgroup of multi-level DCM is therefore underrepresented in DCM literature [24,25] and represents an important knowledge gap in particular given the popularity of a global preference for posterior techniques for multi-level DCM [7].

The objectives of this study were therefore to describe the current evidence for posterior surgical treatment of multi-level DCM in terms of the range of outcome measures and the manner in which they were reported to inform the design of a prospective trial. Furthermore, where possible, to compare the clinical and radiographic outcomes between different posterior approaches.

2. Materials and Methods

The systematic review was conducted in accordance with the Preferred Reporting Items for Systematic Reviews and Meta-Analyses: the PRISMA Statement [26]. Due to heterogenous outcome reporting, a formal meta-analysis was not possible in this study and comparisons were made descriptively [27].

2.1. Literature Search and Selection

Up to 11th November 2019, the electronic databases Embase [Ovid] and MEDLINE [Ovid] were searched using the search strategies as shown in Table S1. Two of the authors (XY and AG) independently evaluated the articles by title, abstract, or full article, where necessary, to select the studies that met the predefined selection criteria. Selection criteria were stated as follows:

- Prospective study with more than 10 patients or retrospective study with more than 50 patients;
- Including multi-level DCM, defined as 2 or more levels;
- Including posterior surgical treatment;
- English, full text;
- Articles published since 1st January 1995.

Animal studies, letters and editorials were excluded from this study. Reference screening and citation tracking were performed on the identified articles and as a final check, the reviews found in the search were studied to make sure no relevant articles were missed. Any discrepancy in selection between the two reviewers was resolved by a third reviewer (BD). Descriptive statistics were used to report frequency and proportion of outcome measures. Statistical comparisons were made using the Chi-Squared test, with significance set at $p = 0.05$.

2.2. Data Extraction

Data extraction was performed by two independent reviewers (XY and AG), using a piloted extraction template covering study characteristics, design, participant characteristics, clinical outcome and radiographic outcome. Extracted data underwent a narrative synthesis and was presented with summary tables.

2.3. Quality Assessment

Two reviewers (XY and AG) independently appraised each publication according to study design. None of the studies found in our review of the literature were randomised trials. Nonrandomised observational studies were evaluated utilising the New Castle Ottawa Scale to evaluate the validity of each. Discrepancies between the two reviewers were addressed by a joint re-evaluation of the original article.

3. Results

3.1. Characteristics of Studies

Of the 1322 articles identified, 1074 original articles were left after removing duplicates. Following abstract and title review, 124 articles were shortlisted. After reviewing the full text, 75 articles were included in this study, assessing 19,510 patients (Figure 1). Of the 75 included articles, 18 studies reported the comparison between anterior and posterior approach, of which the data regarding posterior approach was extracted and included in this review.

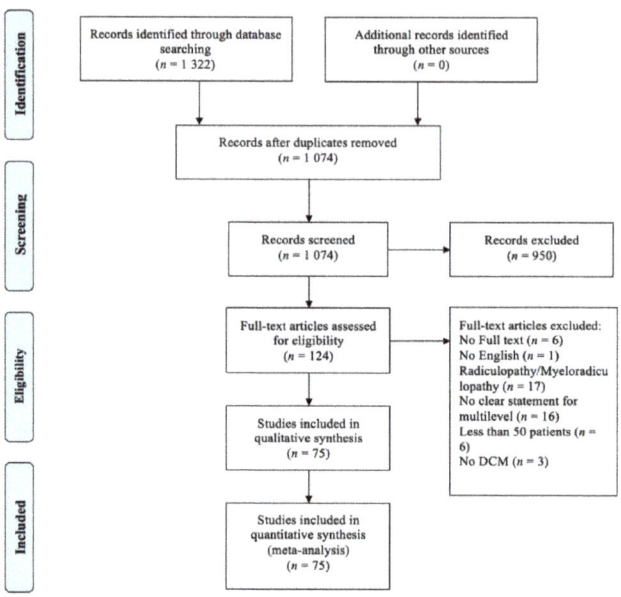

Figure 1. PRISMA flow diagram of search strategy.

Laminoplasty was described in 56 studies (75%), whereas laminectomy with fusion in 27 (36%), and laminectomy without fusion in 12 (16%). The majority of studies were conducted in Asia ($n = 63$, 84%), followed by North America ($n = 8$, 11%) and Europe ($n = 4$, 5%) (Figure 2A). The articles were mainly published in the period of 2016–2019 ($n = 38$, 51%) and 2011–2015 ($n = 26$, 35%), of which laminoplasty was studied predominantly (Figure 2B). The sample size ranged from 51 to 1025.

3.2. Data Quality

The New Castle Ottawa Scale was used to assess the quality of each study due to its high content validity and inter-rater reliability. One study was allotted three stars, three studies four stars, five studies five stars, and two studies were assessed and awarded six stars (Table 1).

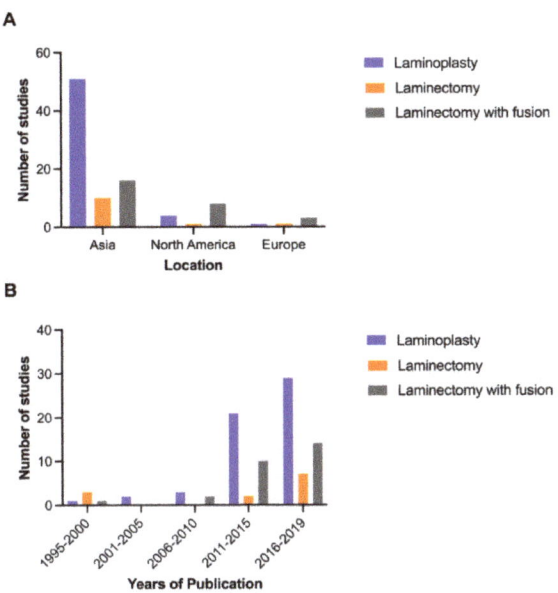

Figure 2. Location (**A**) and trend (**B**) of published research.

Table 1. Study Quality.

Article	Years of Publication	Selection				Comparability	Outcome			Total Score
		Exposed Cohort	Non-Exposed Cohort	Ascertainment of Exposure	Outcome of Interest		Assessment of Outcome	Length of Follow-Up	Adequacy of Follow-Up	
Ajiboye et al.	2017	-	-	*	-	*	-	-	-	3 *
Chang et al.	2017	-	-	*	-	*	-	*	*	5 *
Du et al.	2013	-	-	*	-	*	*	*	*	5 *
Ha et al.	2019	*	*	*	-	*	-	*	*	6 *
Highsmith et al.	2011	-	-	*	-	*	-	*	*	4 *
Lee et al.	2016	-	-	*	-	*	-	*	*	4 *
Lee et al.	2018	-	-	*	-	*	-	*	*	4 *
Li et al.	2019	-	-	*	-	*	-	*	*	5 *
Stephens et al.	2017	*	*	*	-	*	-	*	*	5 *
Yang et al.	2013	-	-	*	-	**	*	*	*	6 *
Yoo et al.	2017	-	-	*	-	**	-	*	*	5 *

3.3. Study Design, Patient Selection and Reporting Differences

Twelve (16%) studies were conducted prospectively, and 63 (84%) retrospective studies were identified. The vast majority of studies were conducted in a single centre ($n = 71$, 95%), three were in multiple centres, and the design of the other study is unknown. Of the 75 studies, 45 (60%) documented that ethical approval was obtained, including one study which held the waiver for ethical approval. Clear inclusion and exclusion criteria were defined in 72 (96%) and 59 (79%) studies, respectively. All of the included studies described the cause of cervical myelopathy, of which 11 (15%) studies included patients suffering ossification of the posterior longitudinal ligament (OPLL) exclusively with sample sizes of 57 to 252, while other studies comprised patients with DCM. The number of levels involved in the diagnosis of multi-DCM was specified in 36 studies describing it as two or more than two levels ($n = 3$, 4%), three or more than three levels ($n = 28$, 37%), four levels ($n = 4$, 5%) and five levels ($n = 1$, 1%).

Reporting differences were noted when comparing prospective with retrospective studies (Tables S2–S4). When compared to retrospective studies, prospective studies were more likely to report the duration of symptom ($p = 0.047$) and the result of dynamic X-rays ($p = 0.023$).

3.4. Comparison between Laminoplasty and Laminectomy with Fusion

Six retrospective studies [28–33] compared laminoplasty to laminectomy with fusion with sample sizes ranging from 56 to 141 patients (Table 2). The surgical treatment was decided based on (1) surgeon's choice: Highsmith et al. [30] chose patients with more facet pathology to undergo laminectomy and fusion, while Yang et al. [33] preferred patients with large anterior osteophytes, facet degeneration, and the continuous type of OPLL to receive laminectomy and fusion; (2) radiographic parameters: Ha et al. [29] preferred laminectomy with fusion for patients with straight or lordotic cervical curvature and segmental instability, and those with severe cord compression caused by OPLL, while Stephens et al. [32] preferred those who demonstrated any amount of C2–7 kyphosis to undergo laminectomy and fusion; or (3) the combination of both (further details were not available) [31]. Of the six studies, two [29,31] included patients with exclusively OPLL, while others comprised patients with DCM.

Table 2. Studies describing laminoplasty versus laminectomy with fusion.

Article	Years of Publication	Sample Size	Study Design	Allocation Basis	Cause of Myelopathy	Function Outcome	Time Point	Radiographic Outcome	Time Point
Ajiboye et al.	2007	70	Retro	NA	CSM	mJOA	Pre- and post-operation	Disc-osteophyte complex size	Baseline and 10 months
Ha et al.	2019	91	Retro	Radiological factors and age	OPLL	NDI JOA	Pre- and 2 years post-operation	Cobb angle C2–7 SVA C0–2 Cobb angle C2–7 Cobb angle T1 slope Total ROM	Pre-operation Pre-operation and 6,12,24 months
								Occupying ratio of the spinal canal The thickness of the OPLL	Pre-operation
								Progression of the thickness of the OPLL	Pre-operation and 24 months
								Signal intensity changes	Pre-operation
Highsmith et al.	2011	56	Retro	Surgeon-based	Cervical stenotic myelopathy	mJOA Nurick Odom	42 months	Cervical lordosis ROM	Pre-operation and 42 months
Lee et al.	2018	83	Retro	Cervical lordosis Neck pain Surgeon's preference	OPLL	NA	-	Cervical curvature ROM	Pre-operation and 2 years
								OPLL volume C2–7 Cobb angle T1 slope C2–7 SVA	Pre-operation
Stephens et al.	2017	137	Retro	Neck pain C2–7 sagittal angle	Cervical myelopathy	NDI mJOA	Pre-operation 6 weeks, 6 and 12 months	Forward pitch Axial canal diameter Miyazaki Spondylosis score	Pre-operation and 12 months
Yang et al.	2013	141	Retro	Surgeon-based	Cervical stenotic myelopathy	mJOA Nurick NDI	Pre- and 24 months	ROM Cervical curvature	Pre- and 24 months
								Osseous fusion	6 months post-operatively
								Area of dural sac, increase in area, spinal cord drift	Pre-operation, 6 and 24 months

NA: Not applicable; CSM: Cervical spondylotic myelopathy; mJOA: Modified Japanese orthopaedic association score; OPLL: Ossification of the posterior longitudinal ligament; NDI: Neck disability index; JOA: Japanese orthopaedic association score; SVA: Sagittal vertical axis; ROM: Range of motion.

Ajiboye et al. [28] reported that there was no difference observed in modified Japanese orthopaedic association (mJOA) score between two groups, while laminectomy with fusion was associated with larger interval regression in disc-osteophyte complex size measured on magnetic resonance imaging (MRI) compared to laminoplasty. Ha et al. [29] observed similar improvements in Health-related quality of life (HRQOL), JOA recovery, and visual analog scale (VAS) in both groups, whilst neck disability index (NDI) improved more significantly in the laminoplasty group. Laminoplasty preserved cervical lordosis, ROM and C2–C7 sagittal vertical axis (SVA) more than laminectomy with fusion group, but the progression of OPLL was suppressed by stabilization using instrumented fusion. Highsmith et al. [30] reported comparable improvements in Nurick scores, mJOA, and Odom outcomes, and comparable radiographic outcomes between groups. They also noted improved VAS neck pain in laminectomy with fusion, though at higher cost (3 times) and increased complications (2 times), compared to laminoplasty. Stephens et al. [32] found that overall pain scores and mJOA improved significantly in both groups. Improved NDI and the loss of lordosis were found in laminoplasty group. Yang et al. [33] reported that the neurological functional recovery (JOA and Nurick scores) was similar between groups. Neck function (NDI and VAS) was worse in the laminectomy and fusion group, although with the achievement of a greater extent of enlargement of the spinal canal and spinal cord drift, compared with laminoplasty. Lee et al. [31] did not report clinical outcome but demonstrated that laminectomy with fusion had the effect of reducing OPLL growth rate compared with motion-preserving laminoplasty.

3.5. Comparison between Laminoplasty and Laminectomy without Fusion

Three studies [34–36] were conducted retrospectively by comparing laminoplasty to laminectomy alone with the sample sizes ranging from of 67 to 330 (Table 3). The surgeon-based treatment was recorded in only one study (no further details provided) [35]. Two studies [34,35] included patients with CSM and the other [36] enrolled patients with OPLL only.

Table 3. Studies describing laminoplasty versus laminectomy alone.

Article	Years of Publication	Sample Size	Study Design	Allocation Basis	Cause of Myelopathy	Function Outcome	Time Point	Radiographic Outcome	Time Point
Chang et al.	2017	67	Retro	NA	CSM	JOA NDI	Pre-operation, and 12 months	C2–7 Cobb angle ROM	Pre-operation, post-operation, and 12 months
Li et al.	2019	330	Retro	Surgeon-based	CSM	Nurick	12 months	Maximal cord compression	Pre-operation
								Spinal canal expansion	Pre-operation and 6 weeks
								Cervical lordosis ROM	Pre-operation and 12 months
								Bony fusion	6 and 12 months
								Spinal cord volume	1 week
Yoo et al.	2017	73	Retro	NA	OPLL	JOA NDI	Pre-operation and >2 years	C2–7 Cobb angle SVA T1 slope	Pre-operation and >2 years

NA: Not applicable; CSM: Cervical spondylotic myelopathy; JOA: Japanese orthopaedic association score; NDI: Neck disability index; ROM: Range of motion; OPLL: Ossification of the posterior longitudinal ligament; SVA: Sagittal vertical axis.

Chang et al. [34] demonstrated similar clinical outcomes (NDI, JOA and VAS neck pain) between groups. Although shorter operation time and less blood loss was observed in the laminectomy group, Cobb angle and ROM significantly decreased at 1-year follow-up. Li et al. [35] compared laminectomy to French-door and open-door laminoplasty, and demonstrated a significantly improved Nurick score and reduced postoperative ROM in all groups at 1-year follow-up. However, French-door laminoplasty showed a higher bone union rate with smaller increased spinal cord volume compared to the other two groups. Yoo et al. [36] found no difference between laminoplasty and laminectomy in 73 patients with OPLL, neither on clinical outcomes (NDI and JOA), nor on radiographic outcomes (C2–7 Cobb angle, SVA, and T1 slope).

3.6. Comparison between Laminoplasty, Laminectomy with and without Fusion

Two retrospective studies reported comparison between laminoplasty, laminectomy with and without fusion, but none of them mentioned the allocation method (Table 4). Du et al. [37] studied 98 patients and reported that an excellent neurological improvement (JOA recovery rates $\geq$ 75 %) was achieved in patients with laminoplasty and laminectomy with fusion at 7 to 12 years follow-up, whilst a high incidence of axial symptoms (NDI) was found in the laminoplasty and laminectomy alone groups caused by loss of curvature index. In the fusion group, lateral mass screw fixation was demonstrated to effectively prevent loss of postoperative cervical curvature and therefore to reduce the incidence of axial symptoms. Lee et al. [38] investigated sagittal alignment and clinical outcome in 57 patients with CSM and OPLL, and found that cervical lordosis, C2–C7 Cobb angle, and cervical curvature index decreased gradually in all patients at minimum 2-year follow-up, with the exception of SVA which was maintained in laminectomy with fusion group. Clinical outcomes, NDI and VAS, improved in all patients. Neck pain was found to increase in laminoplasty in patients showing SVA more than 40 mm at baseline, and the progression of OPLL was observed more frequently in the laminectomy alone group than the group with fusion.

Table 4. Studies describing laminoplasty versus laminectomy with and without fusion.

Article	Years of Publication	Sample Size	Study Design	Allocation Basis	Cause of Myelopathy	Function Outcome	Time Point	Radiographic Outcome	Time Point
Du et al.	2013	98	Retro	NA	DCM and OPLL	JOA NDI	Pre-operation and 7 to 12 years	Curvature index	Pre-operation and 7 to 12 years
Lee et al.	2016	57	Retro	NA	CSM and OPLL	NDI	Pre-operation and 2 years	Curvature index C2–C7 SVA C2–C7 Cobb angle	Pre-operation and 2 years

NA: Not applicable; DCM: Degenerative cervical myelopathy; OPLL: Ossification of the posterior longitudinal ligament; JOA: Japanese orthopaedic association score; NDI: Neck disability index; CSM: Cervical spondylotic myelopathy; ROM: Range of motion; SVA: Sagittal vertical axis.

4. Discussion

4.1. Summary of Findings

DCM is a common cause of spinal cord injury, and many patients with DCM go on to develop progressive disease leading to neurological deficits and reduced quality of life.

This study has identified significant heterogeneity in the conduct and reporting of clinical research evaluating posterior surgery for multi-level DCM. This included variation in study design characteristics, such as the reporting of ethics committee approval, clear inclusion/exclusion criteria and population characteristics, such as the definition of multi-level and subtype of DCM. Most studies were conducted in Asia during recent years focusing on laminoplasty. Few studies made direct comparisons of techniques, and no high level of evidence, such as a RCT, was found. Due to the heterogeneous reporting of outcomes, it was a challenge to interpret these results and taken together this confirmed an important knowledge gap for surgeons.

4.2. Comparison between Posterior Approaches

As the most popular posterior surgical approach described in the literature, laminoplasty was compared to laminectomy with and without fusion. When compared to laminectomy with fusion, with various measurements evaluated, the clinical findings were heterogeneous and contradictory. However, two studies [29,31] reported the superiority of laminectomy with instrumented fusion at suppressing the progression of OPLL when compared with other procedures. One possible explanation is that the decrease in pulsations of the thecal sac and venous plexus after posterior fusion lead to the reduction in thickness of OPLL [39,40]. Another possibility is the removal of mechanical stimulus for cervical OPLL after posterior fusion possibly suppresses the progression of OPLL [41]. More research is still needed to draw a firm conclusion on this topic. When compared to laminectomy alone, although reported with various measurements, comparable clinical outcomes were demonstrated between groups. Cervical laminoplasty was introduced in Japan in the 1970s, with proposed advantages of protecting the spinal cord and preventing neurological deterioration by preservation of the posterior elements and stability [42,43]. However, this is still a controversial issue. In this systematic review it was not possible to show superior clinical outcomes for any particular posterior surgical procedure used to treat DCM as was the case in previous systematic reviews [44,45]. Although Du et al. [37] demonstrated laminectomy with fusion to have a JOA improvement with less incidence of axial symptoms in the comparison of three surgical approaches, this was not confirmed by Lee et al. [38]. Furthermore, a recent meta-analysis disputes this finding, which concluded that laminoplasty had fewer complications, a lower incidence of C5 palsy, better NDI scores and recovery outcomes compared to laminectomy with fusion [46]. Again, due to limited and heterogenous outcomes, no firm conclusion could be made.

Whilst the evidence base has largely focused on laminoplasty, especially in Asia, it is of note in clinical practice that the use of instrumented fusion has increased significantly. This is acknowledged by Deyo et al., who describe how the adoption of technology within spinal surgery has outstripped its rigorous evaluation [47]. More broadly, this is a recognised problem throughout surgery and underpins the IDEAL framework, and specifically the need to match innovation with evaluation [48].

Of note, CSM-S, a RCT of ventral versus dorsal surgery for DCM has recently reported [49]. In this trial, which randomised patients undergoing surgery for multi-level CSM (i.e., excluding OPLL) in the absence of kyphosis to an anterior or posterior approach in whom there was surgical equipoise, a planned subgroup analysis of laminoplasty (n = 28) vs. laminectomy and fusion (n = 69) occurred. The decision to perform a laminoplasty versus a laminectomy and fusion was at the surgeon's discretion. In this subgroup, posterior instrumented fusion was associated with significantly higher adverse events (fusion, 29.0% [95% CI, 18.7%–41.2%]; laminoplasty, 10.7% [95% CI, 2.3%–28.2%]), increased opioid use (fusion, 65.2% [95% CI, 52.8%–76.3%]; laminoplasty, 39.3% [95% CI, 21.5%–59.4%]), and worse physical function at 2 years (estimated mean 5.8; 95% CI, 1.5–10.1; p = 0.01). This difference is greater than their defined MCID. Furthermore, the rate of recovery from instrumented fusion was slower, the short-term neck disability greater and return to work delayed. In fact, these outcomes amongst the laminoplasty subgroup broadly matched anterior surgical results.

4.3. Designing a Future Comparative Study

The results of this systematic review indicate that there is no high level of evidence to guide surgeons when considering a posterior surgical approach for patients with multi-level DCM. Although improved outcomes have been reported in laminectomy with fusion, considering the significant costs, additional skill, increased operative time and reduced ROM after surgery, its superior cost-effectiveness compared to laminectomy requires evaluation. Thus, a comparative study is needed to answer this question.

Although, no firm conclusion can be drawn in this review concerning the clinical effectiveness of posterior surgical treatments, it provides useful information which will facilitate the setting up of future comparative studies. All of three posterior approaches were effective when performed for patients with multilevel DCM. However, the indications of each approach were inconsistent, and some were even contradictory [29,32], paving the way for a randomised controlled trial. The majority of previous studies have a follow-up duration within 24 months, which seems to be pragmatic. Furthermore, various outcome measures have been used in previous studies, including clinical (neurological function assessment and neck pain score) and radiological alignment (X-rays).

Ideally, a three-armed RCT would examine the effectiveness of these posterior surgical treatments. Nevertheless, some existing disputes make it difficult to conduct, such as whether a Bonferroni or similar correction factor should be employed to decrease the likelihood of a type I error in the three-armed RCT. Additionally, given that all procedures are effective to some extent and the relative differences to be detected are likely to be small, this would significantly inflate the sample size. Thus, the initial step, to examine the fundamental question of whether or not stabilisation is required after posterior decompression may be an RCT of the two extremes: laminectomy alone versus laminectomy with fusion. Such a trial has been commissioned by the National Institute for Health Research within the UK, in part owing to a very limited use of laminoplasty in UK spinal practice: The POLYFIX-DCM trial (Posterior LaminectomY and FIXation for DCM) aims to offer the first fully powered, randomised evaluation of this question and will commence recruitment in January 2022. International sites and collaborators are sought.

4.4. Limitations

Due to various definitions of 'multi-level DCM', patients who received short-range decompression may have compared to those who underwent long-range surgeries in this review. However, it is still not clear whether there is a clinical significance between them. Besides, findings in this review were generalised from studies with CSM and OPLL, which are two different pathogenic factors for DCM. Due to the paucity of comparative data, further subgroup analysis was not possible. Furthermore, the follow-up of included studies may be inadequate (mostly 1–2 years), since adjacent segment disease and bony remodelling may take years to occur and is arguably the most important difference between fusion and non-fusion surgery. This study was designed to focus on contemporary and large sample studies, and those articles with non-English language were excluded. The global representation of included studies suggests that the foreign language exclusion is unlikely to be significant. Indeed, the authors propose that assessment of 25 years of published data of large sample studies, is representative of current practice.

5. Conclusions

Studies evaluating posterior surgery for multi-level DCM demonstrate heterogeneity in the reporting of definitions, sample characteristics, as well as in clinical and radiographic outcomes. To date, no studies with a high level of evidence exist. This represents an important knowledge gap, supporting an individualised approach to DCM surgery, and a current leading research priority as identified by AO Spine RECODE DCM (aospine.org/recode).

Supplementary Materials: The following are available online at https://www.mdpi.com/article/10.3390/jcm10163653/s1, Table S1 Search strategy; Table S2 Differences in reporting characteristics and study design; Table S3 Differences in reporting clinical outcomes; Table S4 Differences in reporting radiographic outcomes.

Author Contributions: X.Y. and B.M.D. conceived and wrote the article, X.Y. and A.-A.G. selected articles and extracted data, R.S.D., E.G., E.W.D., O.M., A.B., G.W.-J., J.F., R.T., M.I., S.A., K.R., A.K.D., D.C., A.H.B., N.Q., V.K., M.T., S.M., E.A.P., G.C., M.G.F., P.J.A.H. and M.R.N.K. provided critical feedback and revised the manuscript. All authors read and approved the final manuscript.

Funding: The research was supported by the National Institute for Health Research (NIHR) Brain Injury MedTech Co-operative based at Cambridge University Hospitals NHS Foundation Trust and University of Cambridge. The views expressed are those of the author(s) and not necessarily those of the NHS, the NIHR or the Department of Health and Social Care.

Institutional Review Board Statement: Not applicable.

Informed Consent Statement: Not applicable.

Data Availability Statement: Not applicable.

Acknowledgments: X.Y. reports grant from Cultural Foundation Grant (Award number 40026482, Prins Bernhard Cultural Foundation, the Netherlands) during the conduct of the study, the grant has no role in the conduction of this research. B.M.D. is supported by a NIHR Clinical Doctoral Research Fellowship. This research aligns with the AO Spine RECODE DCM, James Lind Alliance top research priority, individualising surgery. For further information on how this process was conducted, why this question was prioritised, and on-going research activity, please visit www.aospine.org/recode/individualizing-surgery.

Conflicts of Interest: The authors declare no conflict of interest.

References

1. Davies, B.M.; Mowforth, O.D.; Smith, E.K.; Kotter, M.R. Degenerative cervical myelopathy. *BMJ* **2018**, *360*, k186. [CrossRef] [PubMed]
2. Smith, S.S.; Stewart, M.E.; Davies, B.M.; Kotter, M.R.N. The Prevalence of Asymptomatic and Symptomatic Spinal Cord Compression on Magnetic Resonance Imaging: A Systematic Review and Meta-analysis. *Glob. Spine J.* **2021**, *11*, 597–607. [CrossRef]
3. Fehlings, M.G.; Tetreault, L.A.; Riew, K.D.; Middleton, J.W.; Aarabi, B.; Arnold, P.M.; Brodke, D.S.; Burns, A.S.; Carette, S.; Chen, R.; et al. A Clinical Practice Guideline for the Management of Patients with Degenerative Cervical Myelopathy: Recommendations for Patients with Mild, Moderate, and Severe Disease and Nonmyelopathic Patients with Evidence of Cord Compression. *Glob. Spine J.* **2017**, *7*, 70s–83s. [CrossRef] [PubMed]
4. Bajamal, A.H.; Kim, S.H.; Arifianto, M.R.; Faris, M.; Subagio, E.A.; Roitberg, B.; Udo-Inyang, I.; Belding, J.; Zileli, M.; Parthiban, J. Posterior Surgical Techniques for Cervical Spondylotic Myelopathy: WFNS Spine Committee Recommendations. *Neurospine* **2019**, *16*, 421–434. [CrossRef] [PubMed]
5. Davies, B.M.; Khan, D.Z.; Mowforth, O.D.; McNair, A.G.K.; Gronlund, T.; Kolias, A.G.; Tetreault, L.; Starkey, M.L.; Sadler, I.; Sarewitz, E.; et al. RE-CODE DCM (REsearch Objectives and Common Data Elements for Degenerative Cervical Myelopathy): A Consensus Process to Improve Research Efficiency in DCM, Through Establishment of a Standardized Dataset for Clinical Research and the Definition of the Research Priorities. *Glob. Spine J.* **2019**, *9*, 65s–76s. [CrossRef]
6. Ghogawala, Z.; Benzel, E.C.; Heary, R.F.; Riew, K.D.; Albert, T.J.; Butler, W.E.; Barker, F.G., 2nd; Heller, J.G.; McCormick, P.C.; Whitmore, R.G.; et al. Cervical spondylotic myelopathy surgical trial: Randomized, controlled trial design and rationale. *Neurosurgery* **2014**, *75*, 334–346. [CrossRef] [PubMed]
7. Davies, B.M.; Francis, J.J.; Butler, M.B.; Mowforth, O.; Goacher, E.; Starkey, M.; Kolias, A.; Wynne-Jones, G.; Hutton, M.; Selvanathan, S.; et al. Current surgical practice for multi-level degenerative cervical myelopathy: Findings from an international survey of spinal surgeons. *J. Clin. Neurosci.* **2021**, *87*, 84–88. [CrossRef]
8. Ryken, T.C.; Heary, R.F.; Matz, P.G.; Anderson, P.A.; Groff, M.W.; Holly, L.T.; Kaiser, M.G.; Mummaneni, P.V.; Choudhri, T.F.; Vresilovic, E.J.; et al. Cervical laminectomy for the treatment of cervical degenerative myelopathy. *J. Neurosurg. Spine* **2009**, *11*, 142–149. [CrossRef]
9. Hale, J.J.; Gruson, K.I.; Spivak, J.M. Laminoplasty: A review of its role in compressive cervical myelopathy. *Spine J.* **2006**, *6*, 289s–298s. [CrossRef]
10. Kaptain, G.J.; Simmons, N.E.; Replogle, R.E.; Pobereskin, L. Incidence and outcome of kyphotic deformity following laminectomy for cervical spondylotic myelopathy. *J. Neurosurg.* **2000**, *93*, 199–204. [CrossRef] [PubMed]
11. Hansen-Schwartz, J.; Kruse-Larsen, C.; Nielsen, C.J. Follow-up after cervical laminectomy, with special reference to instability and deformity. *Br. J. Neurosurg.* **2003**, *17*, 301–305. [CrossRef]
12. Hyun, S.J.; Rhim, S.C.; Roh, S.W.; Kang, S.H.; Riew, K.D. The time course of range of motion loss after cervical laminoplasty: A prospective study with minimum two-year follow-up. *Spine (Phila PA 1976)* **2009**, *34*, 1134–1139. [CrossRef]
13. Houten, J.K.; Cooper, P.R. Laminectomy and posterior cervical plating for multilevel cervical spondylotic myelopathy and ossification of the posterior longitudinal ligament: Effects on cervical alignment, spinal cord compression, and neurological outcome. *Neurosurgery* **2003**, *52*, 1081–1088, discussion 1087–1088. [PubMed]
14. Anderson, P.A.; Matz, P.G.; Groff, M.W.; Heary, R.F.; Holly, L.T.; Kaiser, M.G.; Mummaneni, P.V.; Ryken, T.C.; Choudhri, T.F.; Vresilovic, E.J.; et al. Laminectomy and fusion for the treatment of cervical degenerative myelopathy. *J. Neurosurg. Spine* **2009**, *11*, 150–156. [CrossRef] [PubMed]
15. Rhee, J.M.; Basra, S. Posterior surgery for cervical myelopathy: Laminectomy, laminectomy with fusion, and laminoplasty. *Asian Spine J.* **2008**, *2*, 114–126. [CrossRef] [PubMed]
16. Hamanishi, C.; Tanaka, S. Bilateral multilevel laminectomy with or without posterolateral fusion for cervical spondylotic myelopathy: Relationship to type of onset and time until operation. *J. Neurosurg.* **1996**, *85*, 447–451. [CrossRef]
17. Guigui, P.; Benoist, M.; Deburge, A. Spinal deformity and instability after multilevel cervical laminectomy for spondylotic myelopathy. *Spine (Phila PA 1976)* **1998**, *23*, 440–447. [CrossRef] [PubMed]
18. Kim, B.S.; Dhillon, R.S. Cervical Laminectomy with or Without Lateral Mass Instrumentation: A Comparison of Outcomes. *Clin. Spine Surg.* **2019**, *32*, 226–232. [CrossRef]
19. McAllister, B.D.; Rebholz, B.J.; Wang, J.C. Is posterior fusion necessary with laminectomy in the cervical spine? *Surg. Neurol. Int.* **2012**, *3*, S225–S231. [CrossRef]
20. Abduljabbar, F.H.; Teles, A.R.; Bokhari, R.; Weber, M.; Santaguida, C. Laminectomy with or without Fusion to Manage Degenerative Cervical Myelopathy. *Neurosurg. Clin. N. Am.* **2018**, *29*, 91–105. [CrossRef]
21. Komotar, R.J.; Mocco, J.; Kaiser, M.G. Surgical management of cervical myelopathy: Indications and techniques for laminectomy and fusion. *Spine J.* **2006**, *6*, 252s–267s. [CrossRef]

22. Fehlings, M.G.; Ibrahim, A.; Tetreault, L.; Albanese, V.; Alvarado, M.; Arnold, P.; Barbagallo, G.; Bartels, R.; Bolger, C.; Defino, H.; et al. A global perspective on the outcomes of surgical decompression in patients with cervical spondylotic myelopathy: Results from the prospective multicenter AOSpine international study on 479 patients. *Spine (Phila PA 1976)* **2015**, *40*, 1322–1328. [CrossRef] [PubMed]
23. Nouri, A.; Martin, A.R.; Nater, A.; Witiw, C.D.; Kato, S.; Tetreault, L.; Reihani-Kermani, H.; Santaguida, C.; Fehlings, M.G. Influence of Magnetic Resonance Imaging Features on Surgical Decision-Making in Degenerative Cervical Myelopathy: Results from a Global Survey of AOSpine International Members. *World Neurosurg.* **2017**, *105*, 864–874. [CrossRef] [PubMed]
24. Davies, B.M.; McHugh, M.; Elgheriani, A.; Kolias, A.G.; Tetreault, L.A.; Hutchinson, P.J.A.; Fehlings, M.G.; Kotter, M.R.N. Reported Outcome Measures in Degenerative Cervical Myelopathy: A Systematic Review. *PLoS ONE* **2016**, *11*, e0157263. [CrossRef]
25. Mowforth, O.D.; Davies, B.M.; Goh, S.; O'Neill, C.P.; Kotter, M.R.N. Research Inefficiency in Degenerative Cervical Myelopathy: Findings of a Systematic Review on Research Activity Over the Past 20 Years. *Glob. Spine J.* **2020**, *10*, 476–485. [CrossRef] [PubMed]
26. Moher, D.; Liberati, A.; Tetzlaff, J.; Altman, D.G. Preferred reporting items for systematic reviews and meta-analyses: The PRISMA statement. *Preferred reporting items for systematic reviews and meta-analyses: The PRISMA statement. PLoS Med.* **2009**, *6*, e1000097. [CrossRef]
27. Campbell, M.; McKenzie, J.E.; Sowden, A.; Katikireddi, S.V.; Brennan, S.E.; Ellis, S.; Hartmann-Boyce, J.; Ryan, R.; Shepperd, S.; Thomas, J.; et al. Synthesis without meta-analysis (SWiM) in systematic reviews: Reporting guideline. *BMJ* **2020**, *368*, l6890. [CrossRef] [PubMed]
28. Ajiboye, R.M.; Zoller, S.D.; Ashana, A.A.; Sharma, A.; Sheppard, W.; Holly, L.T. Regression of Disc-Osteophyte Complexes Following Laminoplasty Versus Laminectomy with Fusion for Cervical Spondylotic Myelopathy. *Int. J. Spine Surg.* **2017**, *11*, 17. [CrossRef]
29. Ha, Y.; Shin, J.J. Comparison of clinical and radiological outcomes in cervical laminoplasty versus laminectomy with fusion in patients with ossification of the posterior longitudinal ligament. *Neurosurg. Rev.* **2019**, *43*, 1409–1421. [CrossRef]
30. Highsmith, J.M.; Dhall, S.S.; Haid, R.W., Jr.; Rodts, G.E., Jr.; Mummaneni, P.V. Treatment of cervical stenotic myelopathy: A cost and outcome comparison of laminoplasty versus laminectomy and lateral mass fusion. *J. Neurosurg. Spine* **2011**, *14*, 619–625. [CrossRef]
31. Lee, J.J.; Shin, D.A.; Yi, S.; Kim, K.N.; Yoon, D.H.; Shin, H.C.; Ha, Y. Effect of posterior instrumented fusion on three-dimensional volumetric growth of cervical ossification of the posterior longitudinal ligament: A multiple regression analysis. *Spine J.* **2018**, *18*, 1779–1786. [CrossRef] [PubMed]
32. Stephens, B.F.; Rhee, J.M.; Neustein, T.M.; Arceo, R. Laminoplasty Does not Lead to Worsening Axial Neck Pain in the Properly Selected Patient with Cervical Myelopathy: A Comparison with Laminectomy and Fusion. *Spine (Phila PA 1976)* **2017**, *42*, 1844–1850. [CrossRef] [PubMed]
33. Yang, L.; Gu, Y.; Shi, J.; Gao, R.; Liu, Y.; Li, J.; Yuan, W. Modified plate-only open-door laminoplasty versus laminectomy and fusion for the treatment of cervical stenotic myelopathy. *Orthopedics* **2013**, *36*, e79–e87. [CrossRef]
34. Chang, H.; Kim, C.; Choi, B.W. Selective laminectomy for cervical spondylotic myelopathy: A comparative analysis with laminoplasty technique. *Arch. Orthop. Trauma Surg.* **2017**, *137*, 611–616. [CrossRef] [PubMed]
35. Li, Q.; Han, X.; Wang, R.; Zhang, Y.; Liu, P.; Dong, Q. Clinical recovery after 5 level of posterior decompression spine surgeries in patients with cervical spondylotic myelopathy: A retrospective cohort study. *Asian J. Surg.* **2020**, *43*, 613–624. [CrossRef]
36. Yoo, S.; Ryu, D.; Choi, H.J.; Kuh, S.U.; Chin, D.K.; Kim, K.S.; Cho, Y.E. Ossification foci act as stabilizers in continuous-type ossification of the posterior longitudinal ligament: A comparative study between laminectomy and laminoplasty. *Acta Neurochir. (Wien.)* **2017**, *159*, 1783–1790. [CrossRef]
37. Du, W.; Wang, L.; Shen, Y.; Zhang, Y.; Ding, W.; Ren, L. Long-term impacts of different posterior operations on curvature, neurological recovery and axial symptoms for multilevel cervical degenerative myelopathy. *Eur. Spine J.* **2013**, *22*, 1594–1602. [CrossRef]
38. Lee, C.H.; Jahng, T.A.; Hyun, S.J.; Kim, K.J.; Kim, H.J. Expansive Laminoplasty Versus Laminectomy Alone Versus Laminectomy and Fusion for Cervical Ossification of the Posterior Longitudinal Ligament: Is There a Difference in the Clinical Outcome and Sagittal Alignment? *Clin. Spine Surg.* **2016**, *29*, E9–E15. [CrossRef]
39. Sjöström, L.; Jacobsson, O.; Karlström, G.; Pech, P.; Rauschning, W. Spinal canal remodelling after stabilization of thoracolumbar burst fractures. *Eur. Spine J.* **1994**, *3*, 312–317. [CrossRef]
40. Mumford, J.; Weinstein, J.N.; Spratt, K.F.; Goel, V.K. Thoracolumbar burst fractures. The clinical efficacy and outcome of nonoperative management. *Spine (Phila PA 1976)* **1993**, *18*, 955–970. [CrossRef]
41. Ota, M.; Furuya, T.; Maki, S.; Inada, T.; Kamiya, K.; Ijima, Y.; Saito, J.; Takahashi, K.; Yamazaki, M.; Aramomi, M.; et al. Addition of instrumented fusion after posterior decompression surgery suppresses thickening of ossification of the posterior longitudinal ligament of the cervical spine. *J. Clin. Neurosci.* **2016**, *34*, 162–165. [CrossRef]
42. Hirabayashi, K.; Satomi, K. Operative procedure and results of expansive open-door laminoplasty. *Spine (Phila PA 1976)* **1988**, *13*, 870–876. [CrossRef]
43. Kato, Y.; Iwasaki, M.; Fuji, T.; Yonenobu, K.; Ochi, T. Long-term follow-up results of laminectomy for cervical myelopathy caused by ossification of the posterior longitudinal ligament. *J. Neurosurg.* **1998**, *89*, 217–223. [CrossRef] [PubMed]

44. Bartels, R.H.; van Tulder, M.W.; Moojen, W.A.; Arts, M.P.; Peul, W.C. Laminoplasty and laminectomy for cervical sponydylotic myelopathy: A systematic review. *Eur. Spine J.* **2015**, *24* (Suppl. 2), 160–167. [CrossRef] [PubMed]
45. Lao, L.; Zhong, G.; Li, X.; Qian, L.; Liu, Z. Laminoplasty versus laminectomy for multi-level cervical spondylotic myelopathy: A systematic review of the literature. *J. Orthop. Surg. Res.* **2013**, *8*, 45. [CrossRef] [PubMed]
46. Wang, J.; Wo, J.; Wen, J.; Zhang, L.; Xu, W.; Wang, X. Laminoplasty versus laminectomy with fusion for treatment of multilevel cervical compressive myelopathy: An updated meta-analysis. *Postgrad. Med. J.* **2021**. [CrossRef]
47. Deyo, R.A.; Mirza, S.K. Trends and variations in the use of spine surgery. *Clin. Orthop. Relat. Res.* **2006**, *443*, 139–146. [CrossRef] [PubMed]
48. McCulloch, P.; Altman, D.G.; Campbell, W.B.; Flum, D.R.; Glasziou, P.; Marshall, J.C.; Nicholl, J.; Aronson, J.K.; Barkun, J.S.; Blazeby, J.M.; et al. No surgical innovation without evaluation: The IDEAL recommendations. *Lancet* **2009**, *374*, 1105–1112. [CrossRef]
49. Ghogawala, Z.; Terrin, N.; Dunbar, M.R.; Breeze, J.L.; Freund, K.M.; Kanter, A.S.; Mummaneni, P.V.; Bisson, E.F.; Barker, F.G., 2nd; Schwartz, J.S.; et al. Effect of Ventral vs Dorsal Spinal Surgery on Patient-Reported Physical Functioning in Patients with Cervical Spondylotic Myelopathy: A Randomized Clinical Trial. *JAMA* **2021**, *325*, 942–951. [CrossRef]

Review

Degenerative Cervical Myelopathy: Clinical Presentation, Assessment, and Natural History

Melissa Lannon and Edward Kachur *

Division of Neurosurgery, McMaster University, Hamilton, ON L8S 4L8, Canada; melissa.lannon@medportal.ca
* Correspondence: kachure@mcmaster.ca

Abstract: Degenerative cervical myelopathy (DCM) is a leading cause of spinal cord injury and a major contributor to morbidity resulting from narrowing of the spinal canal due to osteoarthritic changes. This narrowing produces chronic spinal cord compression and neurologic disability with a variety of symptoms ranging from mild numbness in the upper extremities to quadriparesis and incontinence. Clinicians from all specialties should be familiar with the early signs and symptoms of this prevalent condition to prevent gradual neurologic compromise through surgical consultation, where appropriate. The purpose of this review is to familiarize medical practitioners with the pathophysiology, common presentations, diagnosis, and management (conservative and surgical) for DCM to develop informed discussions with patients and recognize those in need of early surgical referral to prevent severe neurologic deterioration.

Keywords: degenerative cervical myelopathy; cervical spondylotic myelopathy; cervical decompression

1. Introduction

Degenerative cervical myelopathy (DCM) is now the leading cause of spinal cord injury [1,2], resulting in major disability and reduced quality of life. While precise prevalence is not well described, a 2017 Canadian study estimated a prevalence of 1120 per million [3].

DCM results from narrowing of the spinal canal due to osteoarthritic changes. This narrowing leads to chronic spinal cord compression and neurologic disability. Symptoms may range from mild dysfunction, including numbness or decreased dexterity in the upper extremities, to severe dysfunction including quadriparesis and incontinence. Importantly, clinicians should note that paresthesia in the extremities may be the first sign and is frequently overlooked by patients and providers due to its mild nature. This variable pattern of presenting symptoms may lead to a delay in diagnosis of up to 2 years [4].

Early diagnosis and surgical management may improve neurologic and overall outcomes for these patients and, importantly, prevent progressive deterioration.

2. Topics

2.1. Pathophysiology

Degenerative changes in the spine are considered a normal part of the aging process. The cervical spine is particularly prone to degenerative changes due to the mobility of this region. Typically, the degenerative process that culminates in DCM begins with deterioration of the intervertebral disk [5–7]. The intervertebral disk normally acts to distribute pressure evenly across vertebral endplates and facet joints. Normal aging leads to loss of proteoglycans and dehydration of disks, causing loss of elastic and supportive structure. As the disk collapses, it bulges posteriorly, narrowing the spinal canal and compressing the spinal cord at that level. Resultant decreased disk height produces shortening of the spinal column, ultimately producing abnormal spinal mechanics [1,7]. These altered mechanics further contribute to osteoarthritic and osteophytic changes that may worsen narrowing.

In addition to changes related to disk degeneration, the ligamentum flavum can thicken and buckle anteriorly toward the spinal cord, also resulting in compression. Finally, the posterior longitudinal ligament may contribute to degenerative cervical myelopathy by direct compression of the cord in the event of ossification of the posterior longitudinal ligament (OPLL) [5–7].

As these changes occur, stiffening of affected structures may result. To compensate, adjacent segments of the spine may develop hypermobility, which may further contribute to instability and degeneration as the process progresses.

With these mechanical changes, abnormal repetitive movement of the cervical spine may cause spinal cord irritation and compression. For example, flexion may compress the spinal cord against anterior osteophytes and intervertebral disks, while hyperextension may lead to compression between the posterior aspect of the vertebral bodies anteriorly and hypertrophied ligamentum flavum posteriorly [8].

The aforementioned compressive factors produce vascular changes within the cord, inducing ischemia and inflammation [5,7]. With these changes, chronic compression may lead to demyelination, astrogliosis, and axonal degeneration. Endothelial damage may promote further cellular injury through disruption of the blood–spinal cord barrier [5,7]. Ultimately, this histopathologic pattern leads to cell loss and the subsequent functional decline observed clinically in patients [5,7].

Interestingly, recent studies have shown an association between DCM and cerebral reorganization, seemingly to compensate for functional impairment. The majority of studies have focused on cortical reorganization, however similar changes have been observed in the brainstem [9] and the thalamus [10]. This reorganization has been seen across a number of modalities, including arterial spin labelling functional MRI (fMRI) [11], blood oxygen level dependent (BOLD) fMRI [10,12], and navigated transcranial magnetic stimulation (nTMS) [13].

Congenital cervical spinal stenosis, defined as a sagittal canal diameter less than 13 mm [14] or a Torg-Pavlov (canal diameter/vertebral body diameter) ratio less than 0.82 [15], is recognized for its significant role in predisposing patients to DCM [16–18]. Congenital narrowing of the canal produces a vulnerability in the spinal cord to even minor compression from factors described above. It has been suggested that the narrow canal seen in these patients reduces cerebrospinal fluid volume at stenosed levels, impairing the cushioning effect of kinetic energy in the setting of minor trauma and other dynamic injury mechanisms described here [19]. As such, these patients should be monitored regularly for early onset myelopathic symptoms.

2.2. Presentation

No pathognomonic sign exists for DCM. Therefore, clinicians must be cognizant of the constellation of symptoms in this variable presentation. Initially, patients with DCM most commonly present with paresthesia in one or more extremities. Patients may also report decreased dexterity, often described as "clumsiness" with buttons and zippers or changes in penmanship. Patients may note changes in mobility or frequent falls.

DCM carries a slow progressive course, so while paresthesia is commonly an early symptom, patients may present at any point along the disease course with any number of symptoms, including weakness, sensory change, decreased dexterity, and gait abnormality. Neck pain may or may not be present. Bowel and bladder symptoms may occur, however clinicians should keep in mind that these symptoms are rare and indicative of severe injury to the spinal cord [7].

Physical examination is an important aspect of diagnosis in DCM. Patients should be thoroughly assessed for weakness, particularly in the intrinsic muscles of the hands. Patients commonly exhibit hyperreflexia, clonus at the ankles and patellae, spasticity, and abnormal Babinski and Hoffmann signs, as well as loss of sensory proprioception [7].

A number of classification systems have been generated to assess severity of DCM. The most commonly utilized is the modified Japanese Orthopaedic Association (mJOA) classification, grading motor dysfunction in both upper and lower extremities as well as sensation and bladder control to characterize patients as mild (mJOA 15–17), moderate (12–14), or severe (0–11) (Table 1) [20].

Table 1. The modified Japanese Orthopaedic Association (mJOA) Score (adapted from [21]).

Category	Score	Description
Upper Extremity Motor	0	Unable to move hands
	1	Unable to eat with spoon but able to move hands
	2	Unable to button shirt but able to eat with spoon
	3	Able to button shirt with great difficulty
	4	Able to button shirt with mild difficulty OR other mild fine motor dysfunction (marked change in handwriting, frequent dropping of objects, difficulty clasping jewelry, etc.)
	5	Normal hand coordination
Lower Extremity Motor/Sensation	0	Complete loss of movement and sensation
	1	Complete loss of movement, some sensation present
	2	Unable to walk but some movement
	3	Able to walk on flat ground with walking aid
	4	Able to walk without walking aid, must hold handrail on stairs
	5	Moderate to severe gait imbalance but able to take stairs without handrail
	6	Mild imbalance standing OR walking
	7	Normal walking
Upper Extremity Sensory	0	Complete loss of hand sensation
	1	Severe loss of hand sensation OR pain
	2	Mild loss of hand sensation
	3	Normal hand sensation
Urinary function	0	Inability to voluntarily urinate (requiring catheterization)
	1	Frequent urinary incontinence (more than once monthly)
	2	Urinary urgency OR occasional stress incontinence (less than once monthly)
	3	Normal urinary function

The mJOA is a 17 point score of functional disability specific to cervical myelopathy that includes upper extremity motor, lower extremity motor/sensory, upper extremity sensory, and urinary function components. This version has been slightly modified from one previously published by Tetreault L, et al. [21].

Numerous other classification scales have been utilized in the literature, including the Myelopathy Disability Index, Prolo Scale, and Nurick Scale [22–27].

The Nurick Grading Scale focuses primarily on gait assessment, ranging from grade 0 (signs and symptoms of root involvement without evidence of spinal cord disease) to 5 (chairbound or bedridden) [26]. Although commonly utilized and frequently correlated with surgical outcome, the Nurick score is considered less sensitive than the mJOA given its focus on lower limb function. One systematic review was unable to find a conclusive association with a number of predictors of outcome for DCM, unlike the more widely utilized mJOA score [28].

The Neck Disability Index (NDI) is a ten item self-assessment measure developed to assess disability in patients with neck pain following "whiplash" injury [29]. It is now widely utilized in the evaluation of operative spine patients. The domains assessed in the NDI include pain intensity, personal care, lifting, reading, headache, concentration, work, driving, sleep, and recreation. The challenge in adapting the NDI to DCM patients is that function, not pain, is the primary concern [30].

El-Zuway et al. suggested that these myelopathic scales are inherently subjective in nature. As a result, they proposed a ten-point myelopathic scale for DCM based on myelopathic signs from clinical examination. Statistically, this scale significantly correlated with postoperative improvement in DCM patients, but was based on a small number of patients (n = 36) and further studies are needed to validate this scale [31].

Each of the proposed scales provides another aspect of assessment and means to follow patients both pre and postoperatively. However, in general, it is believed that DCM is reasonably well followed with the mJOA in conjunction with objective testing of DCM patients with examination of myelopathic signs and objective measures of grip strength, dexterity, balance, and gait [31,32]. As such, most recommendations for determining severity of DCM in patients and clinical decision making primarily utilize mJOA.

2.3. Differential Diagnoses

A number of differential diagnoses may present similarly to DCM. These conditions may be differentiated through comprehensive assessment. In addition, one systematic review identified MRI as the most valuable investigative tool to differentiate DCM from other clinical entities [33]. See Table 2.

Table 2. Approach to differential diagnoses of DCM.

Differential Diagnosis	Differentiating Findings
Amyotrophic lateral sclerosis [7,33]	Presence of cranial nerve findings (e.g., dysphagia, dysarthria) Absence of sensory findings
Brain neoplasm	Presence of cranial nerve findings Lateralizing findings (e.g., unilateral weakness/sensory changes) Headache Vomiting Altered level of consciousness
Multiple sclerosis [7,33]	Visual changes Cranial nerve findings Fatigue
Peripheral nerve entrapment (e.g., carpal tunnel syndrome, ulnar neuropathy) [33]	Absence of upper motor neuron findings
Normal pressure hydrocephalus	Cognitive disturbances Speech or swallowing difficulty
Vitamin B deficiency [7,33]	Fatigue Cognitive disturbances Glossitis Visual changes

A list of differential diagnoses for consideration in patients presenting with signs and symptoms of DCM.

2.4. Diagnosis

Thorough neurologic examination is the first step in diagnosis of DCM, followed by magnetic resonance imaging (MRI) to assess for spinal cord compression and confirm the diagnosis. It is important to consider that degenerative changes are common in asymptomatic patients, with 98% of healthy patients in their 20s showing degenerative disk disease on MRI [34]. As such, MRI findings should be carefully interpreted in the context of clinical signs and symptoms.

The absence of a cerebrospinal fluid (CSF) signal on T2-weighted images (T2WI) allows for assessment of cord compression, while cord signal change has been associated with disease severity in cervical myelopathy. Specifically, T1-weighted imaging (T1WI) hypointensity has been noted as particularly important and indicative of cord injury associated with more severe functional impairment, higher frequency of myelopathic findings, and decreased potential for recovery [35].

Another sign on MRI that has been associated with cervical myelopathy is the "snake eyes appearance" sign, whereby bilateral, symmetric, hyperintense circular foci are seen within the gray matter of the spinal cord on T2WI (Figure 1). This finding is thought to represent cystic necrosis at the junction of the central gray matter and the posterior ventrolateral column, in addition to cell loss in the anterior horn. Chronic mechanical compression and vascular insufficiency are thought to be the most significant contributors to this pathogenic process. Although the literature is sporadic and inconsistent, this finding has been associated with negative prognosis for recovery in nearly half of patients in whom it is identified [36].

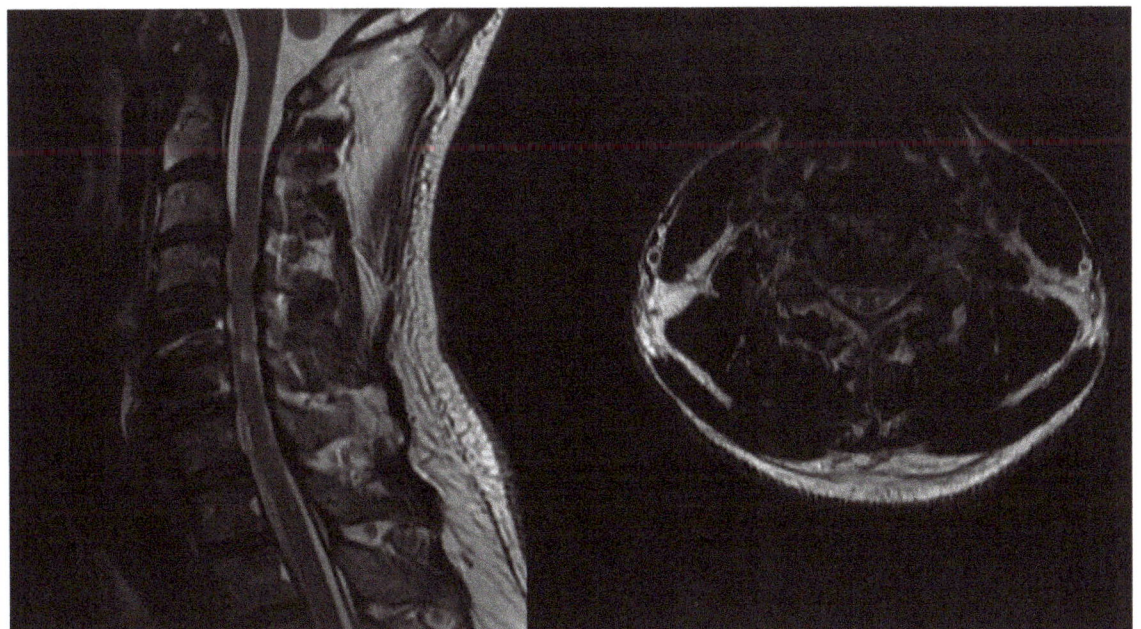

Figure 1. 'Snake eyes appearance' sign on MRI. Bilateral, circular symmetric foci can be observed within the grey matter on T2WI MRI, thought to represent cystic necrosis secondary to chronic compression and vascular insufficiency.

Martin et al. suggested that the primary purpose of MRI in DCM is to establish the diagnosis and for surgical planning. In their longitudinal study of DCM patients, MRI had a sensitivity of only 28% in detecting clinical deterioration of DCM and should not be relied upon as a measure to follow DCM patients [32].

Plain radiographs with flexion and extension views may be beneficial in these patients to rule out instability and assess the need for surgical instrumentation in planning, but for diagnostic purposes, clinical examination and MRI remain the mainstay.

Computed tomography (CT) of the cervical spine may be useful for surgical planning to detect the degree of degenerative changes, osteophytes, and for instrumentation planning. CT myelogram may be utilized in rare instances to provide information on spinal cord compression in patients with contraindication to MRI or in cases where excess artifact exists due to previous instrumentation.

Advanced imaging techniques have allowed improved investigation of microstructural and functional changes within the spinal cord as a result of DCM. In the future, these tools may provide improved diagnoses and prognostication for patients. In particular, diffusion tensor imaging (DTI) may be useful in identifying patients likely to benefit from surgical intervention. This technique uses directional diffusivity of water in each voxel to measure axonal integrity. The most reliable measure in DTI studies with DCM patients is fractional anisotropy (FA), measured from 0 (isotropic diffusion—same in all directions) to 1 (anisotropic—all in one direction). One systematic review found preoperative FA at the level of most severe spinal cord compression correlated closely with mJOA scores and postoperative mJOA changes [37]. It may also allow earlier detection of spinal cord injury in DCM [38].

Other advanced MRI techniques used in recent DCM literature include magnetization transfer (MT), myelin water fraction (MWF), and MR spectroscopy [35]. An ongoing study is investigating the role of microdiffusion imaging (MIDI) in DCM. This modality utilizes diffusion-weighted imaging (DWI) postprocessing to detect tissue alterations in each voxel [39].

Further adjuncts to diagnosis may be used, particularly in complex cases with multiple comorbidities with potential to cloud the clinical picture (e.g., patients with peripheral neuropathy or a previous peripheral nerve injury). In these cases, electromyography (EMG), electroneurography, and evoked potentials may be beneficial. Compared with healthy subjects, a number of surface EMG changes have been observed in DCM patients. Of these, prolonged duration activation of tibialis anterior was particularly useful clinically and a lack of coactivation of gastrocnemius suggested the presence in this finding may be due to impaired proprioception in DCM [40,41]. A number of studies have utilized somatosensory evoked potentials (SEPs) to illustrate dorsal column dysfunction in 24–100% of patients, depending on nerve distribution tested (lower limb, ulnar nerve, median nerve) [42–45]. However, upper limb SEPs were of no utility in patients without sensory changes and lower limb SEPs cannot provide information regarding localization. Motor evoked potentials (MEPs) have also been frequently utilized and most consistently demonstrate a prolonged central motor conduction time, with abnormalities in distal upper extremities for most DCM patients [40,46–49].

Although the sensitivity of these modalities is considered quite high, they lack specificity and are ineffective in determining disease severity. Tools such as SEPs and MEPs are most useful in ruling out peripheral neuropathies and other differential diagnoses in complicated patients. While there is a diagnostic role for a number of modalities in DCM, the gold standard at this time remains thorough clinical assessment and MRI (Figure 2).

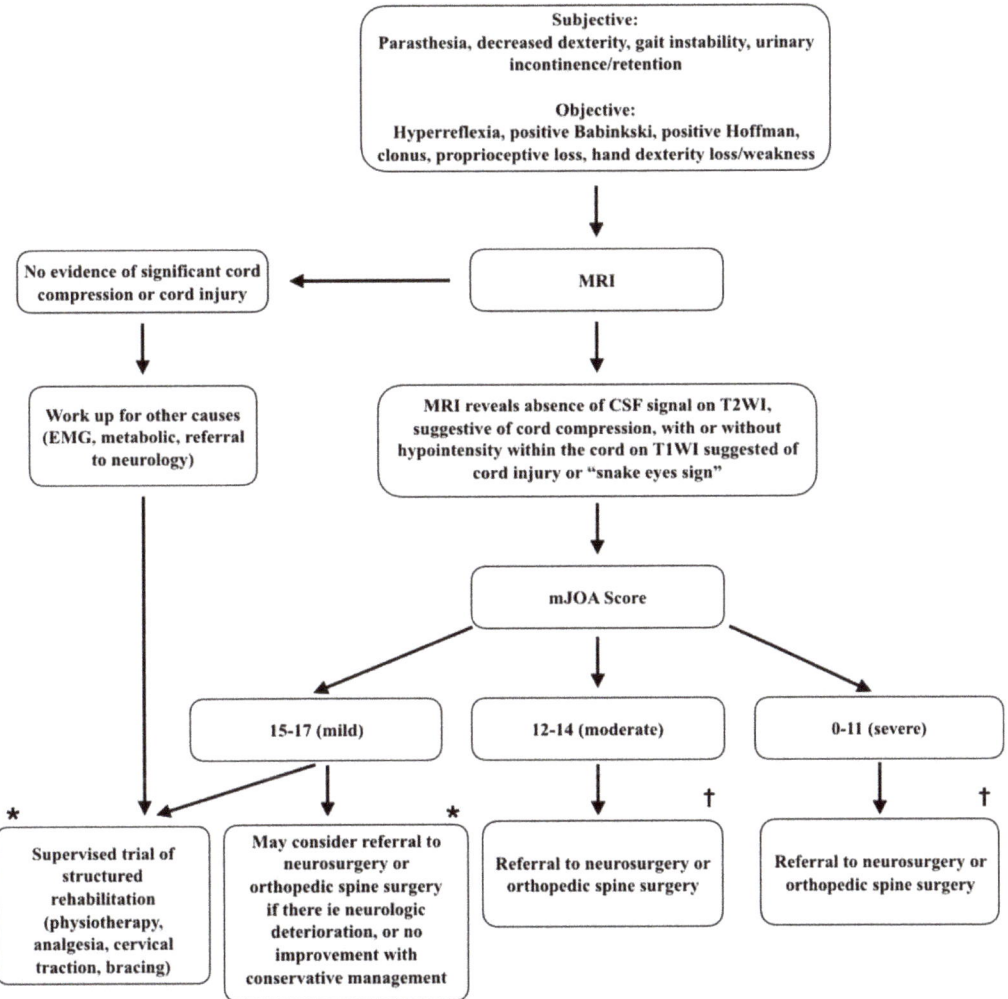

Figure 2. Approach to degenerative cervical myelopathy, summary of diagnostic and management (adapted from [50]). This summary decision tree can be used to guide decision making for medical practitioners. * denotes very low quality evidence with weak recommendation. † denotes moderate quality evidence with strong recommendation. This summary is based on Fehlings M, et al. [50].

2.5. Natural History and Conservative Management

The first description of the natural history of degenerative cervical myelopathy was provided by Lees and Turner, who followed 44 patients with clinical myelopathy at St. Bartholomew's Hospital in London. They observed a variety of durations of exacerbation, with long periods of latency interspersed. The authors noted it was common for patients to progressively decline with each exacerbation. Many patients were followed beyond five years (one patient up to 40 years) and at last follow up, 4.5% of patients had no disability, 6.8% were reported as mild disability, 47.7% moderate disability, and 40.9% of patients had severe disability. In spite of these poor outcomes, investigators concluded that a "very conservative approach" should be taken to degenerative cervical myelopathy [51].

More recent literature suggests 20–62% of patients with degenerative cervical myelopathy will have progressive neurologic deterioration within six months [52]. One randomized controlled trial compared patients undergoing anterior decompression ($n = 22$), corpectomy ($n = 6$), or laminoplasty ($n = 5$) with conservative measures including cervical collar, anti-inflammatory medications, bedrest, and avoidance of high-risk activities (e.g., heavy lifting, slippery surfaces, manipulation therapy, or prolonged neck flexion). There was no significant difference between groups in mean mJOA scores over a three year period nor the ten year period [53].

By contrast, one randomized controlled trial included functional assessments whereby blinded observers rated, by video recording, the ability of patients to perform activities of daily living, including buttoning shirts, brushing hair and teeth, putting on shoes, walking, running, and going up and down stairs. Of those patients conservatively managed, the number with declining scores increased over the course of follow-up from 6.3% at one year to 27.3% at three years. This change was not observed in operative patients, where the scores remained stable over time [54].

Similarly, a prospective study compared surgical treatment with conservative therapy including analgesia, physiotherapy, bedrest, cervical traction, and bracing. At mean follow-up at 29.8 months, surgical patients exhibited significant improvements in overall function, work, and social activities compared with conservatively treated counterparts [55].

A recent study by Martin et al. investigated the functional outcome in DCM patients treated nonoperatively in an ambispective longitudinal study. Deterioration of mJOA scores over a mean 30.3 months was observed in patients with a new diagnosis of DCM (57%, $n = 95$) and of recurrent DCM diagnosed at another level following surgery for DCM at the alternative level (73%, $n = 22$). The deterioration occurred with mild, moderate, and severe cases of DCM. The authors concluded that DCM appears to have a poor natural history and serial assessment by a battery of tests assessing for grip strength, dexterity, balance, and gait, in addition to the mJOA, in order to detect clinical deterioration where surgery would be indicated [32].

The wide variability in rate of deterioration may be related to the various methods of assessment in DCM. Further prospective studies are needed to better delineate the natural history of DCM.

One notable risk for patients with cervical myelopathy is the development of myelopathic symptoms secondary to minor trauma, particularly with neck hyperextension. There is a paucity of literature assessing the true prevalence of spinal cord injury from minor trauma in these patients, but it remains a concern for care providers nonetheless.

2.6. Surgical Management

The decision to proceed with surgery for DCM requires a comprehensive discussion between the patient and medical and surgical providers. It should be clear from the start that the objective of surgery is to prevent further neurologic deterioration, as returning the patient to baseline is sometimes an unattainable outcome. However, literature does support the possibility of improvement, with one large retrospective, multicenter study of 2156 patients showing significant improvement in 18.8% of patients (2-point improvement in mJOA scores) between baseline and 3 month follow-up, with continued improvement to 12 month follow-up in patients with severe baseline scores [56].

As described previously, indication for surgical intervention is symptomatic myelopathy, especially if progressive, in conjunction with radiologic confirmation of cord compression and exclusion of concomitant contributing pathologies [23,57].

A number of surgical approaches exist for DCM and can be performed via anterior or posterior approaches, with or without the need for spinal fusion. Anterior decompression requires removal of the intervertebral disk (diskectomy), with contemporary approaches, including anterior fusion to prevent late disk space collapse and subsequent failure with recurrent symptoms, as had historically been the case. In some cases, the vertebral body is also removed (corpectomy) and the disk or vertebral body is replaced with an intervertebral cadaveric bone graft, iliac crest autograft, fibular allograft, or polyethereterketone or titanium cages. Anterior plating is often used adjunctively to provide further stabilization. Anterior approaches are often selected for patients with ventral compression, kyphosis, and/or compression at one to three levels [23,57]. In select cases with appropriate preoperative alignment, typically in younger patients, disk arthroplasty may be used as an alternative to anterior fusion [58].

For patients with multilevel disease, significant ligamentum flavum hypertrophy, or congenital narrowing of the canal posterior approaches are more favorable. These approaches are achieved through laminectomy (with or without fusion) or laminoplasty. Laminectomy involves removing the posterior elements (bilateral laminae, spinous processes, ligamentum flavum) to increase the diameter of the spinal canal. Commonly, lateral mass screws are placed with connecting rods bilaterally to provide stabilization and allow time for bone fusion to occur. In patients with loss of lordosis or evidence of instability and listhesis on preoperative radiographs, fusion is of particular importance [23,57]. Laminoplasty can be achieved in patients without evidence of instability and with preserved lordosis. This procedure expands the diameter of the canal through hinging open the laminae, displacing them laterally or posterolaterally. The laminae are fixed in this hinged position with graft, sutures, or plates [57,59]. For complex patients, a combination of anterior and posterior approaches may be used.

Risks associated with surgical decompression for DCM must be discussed at length with the patient, including risk of permanent neurologic compromise, osteomyelitis, diskitis, meningitis, gait disturbance, quadriparesis, bowel or bladder dysfunction, C5 palsy, injury to the vertebral and/or carotid arteries resulting in stroke, cerebrospinal fluid leak, dislodgement of bone grafts and/or hardware, adjacent segment disease with need for further surgery, and anesthetic risk. Specific to anterior approaches, risk of injury to the trachea and/or esophagus, and recurrent laryngeal nerve palsy should also be discussed. Increasing patient age and comorbidities substantially increase surgical risk for patients. Again, it should be highlighted that the goal of surgery is to prevent further neurologic deterioration, but a risk of surgery is that there is no change in disease course or no improvement in symptoms [57].

Intraoperative neuromonitoring (somatosensory evoked potentials, transcranial motor evoked potentials) is frequently utilized in spinal surgery, with some uptake in both anterior and posterior decompressions for DCM. A recent systematic review reported that intraoperative monitoring may be a helpful tool in these surgical procedures given its high sensitivity and specificity for intraoperative neural damage detection. However, at this time evidence is limited, with no criteria for indications for its use [60]. An earlier systematic review made similar conclusions, noting that MEP/SEP monitoring may provide a sensitive tool for detecting neurologic injury during anterior approaches, intraoperative changes are not specific, and its recognition has not been found to prevent neurologic injury or result in improved outcome [61]. With appropriate patient selection after thorough assessment, it should be noted that these approaches are commonly performed and risk of progression of DCM should be balanced with limited surgical risk in consideration of these patients.

3. Conclusions

DCM is a common clinical entity with increasing prevalence. Patients with clinically progressive myelopathic symptoms and correlating radiographic evidence of cord compression should be referred for surgical evaluation if it is within the patient's care goals to prevent further neurologic deterioration. Discussion regarding conservative management and role for surgery in the medical setting may occur, with referral to surgical expertise where appropriate.

Author Contributions: Conceptualization, writing, original draft preparation, review and editing were contributed to equally by both authors. Supervision was provided by E.K. Both authors have read and agreed to the published version of the manuscript.

Funding: This research received no external funding.

Data Availability Statement: No additional data was utilized for the creation of this manuscript.

Conflicts of Interest: The authors declare no conflict of interest.

References

1. Kalsi-Ryan, S.; Karadimas, S.K.; Fehlings, M.G. Cervical Spondylotic Myelopathy: The Clinical Phenomenon and the Current Pathobiology of an Increasingly Prevalent and Devastating Disorder. *Neuroscientist* **2013**, *19*, 409–421. [CrossRef]
2. Witiw, C.D.; Fehlings, M.G. Degenerative cervical myelopathy. *Can. Med. Assoc. J.* **2017**, *189*, E116. [CrossRef] [PubMed]
3. Bakhsheshian, J.; Mehta, V.A.; Liu, J.C. Current Diagnosis and Management of Cervical Spondylotic Myelopathy. *Glob. Spine J.* **2017**, *7*, 572–586. [CrossRef] [PubMed]
4. Behrbalk, E.; Salame, K.; Regev, G.J.; Keynan, O.; Boszczyk, B.; Lidar, Z. Delayed diagnosis of cervical spondylotic myelopathy by primary care physicians. *Neurosurg. Focus* **2013**, *35*, E1. [CrossRef] [PubMed]
5. Baptiste, D.C.; Fehlings, M.G. Pathophysiology of cervical myelopathy. *Spine J.* **2006**, *6*, S190–S197. [CrossRef] [PubMed]
6. Fehlings, M.G.; Skaf, G. A Review of the Pathophysiology of Cervical Spondylotic Myelopathy With Insights for Potential Novel Mechanisms Drawn From Traumatic Spinal Cord Injury. *Spine* **1998**, *23*, 2730–2736. [CrossRef]
7. Vilaça, C.D.O.; Orsini, M.; Araujo Leite, M.A.; De Freitas, M.R.G.; Davidovich, E.; Fiorelli, R.; Fiorelli, S.; Fiorelli, C.; Oliveira, A.B.; Pessoa, B.L. Cervical spondylotic myelopathy: What the neurologist should know. *Neurol. Int.* **2016**, *8*, 69–73. [CrossRef]
8. Milligan, J.; Ryan, K.; Fehlings, M.; Bauman, C. Degenerative cervical myelopathy: Diagnosis and management in primary care. *Can. Fam. Physician Med. Fam. Can.* **2019**, *65*, 619–624.
9. Wang, C.; Laiwalla, A.; Salamon, N.; Ellingson, B.M.; Holly, L.T. Compensatory brainstem functional and structural connectivity in patients with degenerative cervical myelopathy by probabilistic tractography and functional MRI. *Brain Res.* **2020**, *1749*, 147129. [CrossRef]
10. Peng, X.; Tan, Y.; He, L.; Ou, Y. Alterations of functional connectivity between thalamus and cortex before and after decompression in cervical spondylotic myelopathy patients: A resting-state functional MRI study. *NeuroReport* **2020**, *31*, 365–371. [CrossRef] [PubMed]
11. Zhou, F.; Huang, M.; Wu, L.; Tan, Y.; Guo, J.; Zhang, Y.; He, L.; Gong, H. Altered perfusion of the sensorimotor cortex in patients with cervical spondylotic myelopathy: An arterial spin labeling study. *J. Pain Res.* **2018**, *11*, 181–190. [CrossRef]
12. Bhagavatula, I.D.; Shukla, D.; Sadashiva, N.; Saligoudar, P.; Prasad, C.; Bhat, D.I. Functional cortical reorganization in cases of cervical spondylotic myelopathy and changes associated with surgery. *Neurosurg. Focus* **2016**, *40*, E2. [CrossRef]
13. Zdunczyk, A.; Schwarzer, V.; Mikhailov, M.; Bagley, B.; Rosenstock, T.; Picht, T.; Vajkoczy, P. The Corticospinal Reserve Capacity: Reorganization of Motor Area and Excitability As a Novel Pathophysiological Concept in Cervical Myelopathy. *Neurosurgery* **2018**, *83*, 810–818. [CrossRef] [PubMed]
14. Bajwa, N.S.; Toy, J.O.; Young, E.Y.; Ahn, N.U. Establishment of parameters for congenital stenosis of the cervical spine: An anatomic descriptive analysis of 1066 cadaveric specimens. *Eur. Spine J.* **2012**, *21*, 2467–2474. [CrossRef] [PubMed]
15. Pavlov, H.; Torg, J.S.; Robie, B.; Jahre, C. Cervical spinal stenosis: Determination with vertebral body ratio method. *Radiology* **1987**, *164*, 771–775. [CrossRef]
16. Countee, R.W.; Vijayanathan, T. Congenital stenosis of the cervical spine: Diagnosis and management. *J. Natl. Med. Assoc.* **1979**, *71*, 257–264. [PubMed]
17. Bernhardt, M.; Hynes, R.A.; Blume, H.W.; White, A.A. Cervical spondylotic myelopathy. *J. Bone Jt. Surg. Am.* **1993**, *75*, 119–128. [CrossRef] [PubMed]
18. Singh, A.; Tetreault, L.; Fehlings, M.; Fischer, D.; Skelly, A. Risk factors for development of cervical spondylotic myelopathy: Results of a systematic review. *Evid. Based Spine Care J.* **2013**, *3*, 35–42. [CrossRef] [PubMed]
19. Nouri, A.; Tetreault, L.; Singh, A.; Karadimas, S.K.; Fehlings, M.G. Degenerative Cervical Myelopathy: Epidemiology, Genetics, and Pathogenesis. *Spine* **2015**, *40*, E675–E693. [CrossRef]
20. Kato, S.; Oshima, Y.; Oka, H.; Chikuda, H.; Takeshita, Y.; Miyoshi, K.; Kawamura, N.; Masuda, K.; Kunogi, J.; Okazaki, R.; et al. Comparison of the Japanese Orthopaedic Association (JOA) Score and Modified JOA (mJOA) Score for the Assessment of Cervical Myelopathy: A Multicenter Observational Study. *PLoS ONE* **2015**, *10*, e0123022. [CrossRef]
21. Tetreault, L.; Kopjar, B.; Nouri, A.; Arnold, P.; Barbagallo, G.; Bartels, R.; Qiang, Z.; Singh, A.; Zileli, M.; Vaccaro, A.; et al. The modified Japanese Orthopaedic Association scale: Establishing criteria for mild, moderate and severe impairment in patients with degenerative cervical myelopathy. *Eur. Spine J.* **2017**, *26*, 78–84. [CrossRef]
22. Chiles, B.W.; Leonard, M.A.; Choudhri, H.F.; Cooper, P.R. Cervical spondylotic myelopathy: Patterns of neurological deficit and recovery after anterior cervical decompression. *Neurosurgery* **1999**, *44*, 762–769. [CrossRef]
23. Hukuda, S.; Mochizuki, T.; Ogata, M.; Shichikawa, K.; Shimomura, Y. Operations for cervical spondylotic myelopathy. A comparison of the results of anterior and posterior procedures. *J. Bone Jt. Surg. Br. Vol.* **1985**, *67*, 609–615. [CrossRef]
24. Herdmann, J.; Linzbach, M.; Krzan, M.; Dvorak, J.; Bock, W.J.; Bauer, B.L.; Brock, M.; Klinger, M. *The European Myelopathy Score*; Springer: Berlin/Heidelberg, Germany, 1994; p. 268.
25. Keller, A.; Von Ammon, K.; Klaiber, R.; Waespe, W. [Spondylogenic cervical myelopathy: Conservative and surgical therapy]. *Schweiz. Med. Wochenschr.* **1993**, *123*, 1682–1691.

26. Nurjck, S. The pathogenesis of the spinal cord disorder associated with cervical spondylosis. *Brain* **1972**, *95*, 87–100. [CrossRef]
27. Prolo, D.J.; Oklund, S.A.; Butcher, M. Toward uniformity in evaluating results of lumbar spine operations. A paradigm applied to posterior lumbar interbody fusions. *Spine* **1986**, *11*, 601–606. [CrossRef] [PubMed]
28. Tetreault, L.A.; Karpova, A.; Fehlings, M.G. Predictors of outcome in patients with degenerative cervical spondylotic myelopathy undergoing surgical treatment: Results of a systematic review. *Eur. Spine J.* **2015**, *24*, 236–251. [CrossRef]
29. Vernon, H.; Mior, S. The Neck Disability Index: A study of reliability and validity. *J. Manip. Physiol. Ther.* **1991**, *14*, 409–415.
30. Goyal, D.K.C.; Murphy, H.A.; Hollern, D.A.; Divi, S.N.; Nicholson, K.; Stawicki, C.; Kaye, I.D.; Schroeder, G.D.; Woods, B.I.; Kurd, M.F.; et al. Is the Neck Disability Index an Appropriate Measure for Changes in Physical Function After Surgery for Cervical Spondylotic Myelopathy? *Int. J. Spine Surg.* **2020**, *14*, 53–58. [CrossRef] [PubMed]
31. El-Zuway, S.; Farrokhyar, F.; Kachur, E. Myelopathic signs and functional outcome following cervical decompression surgery: A proposed myelopathy scale. *J. Neurosurg. Spine* **2016**, *24*, 871–877. [CrossRef]
32. Martin, A.R.; Kalsi-Ryan, S.; Akbar, M.A.; Rienmueller, A.C.; Badhiwala, J.H.; Wilson, J.R.; Tetreault, L.A.; Nouri, A.; Massicotte, E.M.; Fehlings, M.G. Clinical outcomes of nonoperatively managed degenerative cervical myelopathy: An ambispective longitudinal cohort study in 117 patients. *J. Neurosurg. Spine* **2021**, *34*, 821–829. [CrossRef]
33. Kim, H.J.; Tetreault, L.A.; Massicotte, E.M.; Arnold, P.M.; Skelly, A.C.; Brodt, E.D.; Riew, K.D. Differential Diagnosis for Cervical Spondylotic Myelopathy: Literature Review. *Spine* **2013**, *38*, S78–S88. [CrossRef]
34. Nakashima, H.; Yukawa, Y.; Suda, K.; Yamagata, M.; Ueta, T.; Kato, F. Cervical Disc Protrusion Correlates With the Severity of Cervical Disc Degeneration: A Cross-Sectional Study of 1211 Relatively Healthy Volunteers. *Spine* **2015**, *40*, E774–E779. [CrossRef] [PubMed]
35. Nouri, A.; Martin, A.R.; Kato, S.; Reihani-Kermani, H.; Riehm, L.E.; Fehlings, M.G. The Relationship Between MRI Signal Intensity Changes, Clinical Presentation, and Surgical Outcome in Degenerative Cervical Myelopathy: Analysis of a Global Cohort. *Spine* **2017**, *42*, 1851–1858. [CrossRef] [PubMed]
36. Fontanella, M.M.; Zanin, L.; Bergomi, R.; Fazio, M.; Zattra, C.M.; Agosti, E.; Saraceno, G.; Schembari, S.; De Maria, L.; Quartini, L.; et al. Snake-Eye Myelopathy and Surgical Prognosis: Case Series and Systematic Literature Review. *J. Clin. Med.* **2020**, *9*, 2197. [CrossRef]
37. Rindler, R.S.; Chokshi, F.H.; Malcolm, J.G.; Eshraghi, S.R.; Mossa-Basha, M.; Chu, J.K.; Kurpad, S.N.; Ahmad, F.U. Spinal Diffusion Tensor Imaging in Evaluation of Preoperative and Postoperative Severity of Cervical Spondylotic Myelopathy: Systematic Review of Literature. *World Neurosurg.* **2017**, *99*, 150–158. [CrossRef] [PubMed]
38. D'Avanzo, S.; Ciavarro, M.; Pavone, L.; Pasqua, G.; Ricciardi, F.; Bartolo, M.; Solari, D.; Somma, T.; de Divitiis, O.; Cappabianca, P.; et al. The Functional Relevance of Diffusion Tensor Imaging in Patients with Degenerative Cervical Myelopathy. *J. Clin. Med.* **2020**, *9*, 1828. [CrossRef] [PubMed]
39. Hohenhaus, M.; Egger, K.; Klingler, J.-H.; Hubbe, U.; Reisert, M.; Wolf, K. Is microdiffusion imaging able to improve the detection of cervical myelopathy? Study protocol of a prospective observational trial (MIDICAM-Trial). *BMJ Open* **2019**, *9*, e029153. [CrossRef] [PubMed]
40. Nardone, R.; Höller, Y.; Brigo, F.; Frey, V.N.; Lochner, P.; Leis, S.; Golaszewski, S.; Trinka, E. The contribution of neurophysiology in the diagnosis and management of cervical spondylotic myelopathy: A review. *Spinal Cord* **2016**, *54*, 756–766. [CrossRef]
41. Malone, A.; Meldrum, D.; Gleeson, J.; Bolger, C. Electromyographic characteristics of gait impairment in cervical spondylotic myelopathy. *Eur. Spine J.* **2013**, *22*, 2538–2544. [CrossRef]
42. El Negamy, E.; Sedgwick, E.M. Delayed cervical somatosensory potentials in cervical spondylosis. *J. Neurol. Neurosurg. Psychiatry* **1979**, *42*, 238–241. [CrossRef]
43. Ganes, T. Somatosensory conduction times and peripheral, cervical and cortical evoked potentials in patients with cervical spondylosis. *J. Neurol. Neurosurg. Psychiatry* **1980**, *43*, 683–689. [CrossRef]
44. Yu, Y.L.; Jones, S.J. Somatosensory evoked potentials in cervical spondylosis: Correlation of median, ulnar and posterior tibial nerve responses with clinical and radiological findings. *Brain* **1985**, *108*, 273–300. [CrossRef] [PubMed]
45. Veilleux, M.; Daube, J.R. The value of ulnar somatosensory evoked potentials (SEPs) in cervical myelopathy. *Electroencephalogr. Clin. Neurophysiol. Potentials Sect.* **1987**, *68*, 415–423. [CrossRef]
46. Abbruzzese, G.; Dall'Agata, D.; Morena, M.; Simonetti, S.; Spadavecchia, L.; Severi, P.; Andrioli, G.C.; Favale, E. Electrical stimulation of the motor tracts in cervical spondylosis. *J. Neurol. Neurosurg. Psychiatry* **1988**, *51*, 796–802. [CrossRef]
47. Chan, Y.-C.; Yeh, I.-B.; Kannan, T.A.; Wilder-Smith, E. Trapezius motor evoked potential in evaluations of corticospinal tract lesions. *Eur. J. Neurol.* **2009**, *16*, 540–543. [CrossRef]
48. Bednařík, J.; Kadaňka, Z.; Voháňka, S.; Novotný, O.; Šurelová, D.; Filipovičová, D.; Prokeš, B. The value of somatosensory and motor evoked potentials in pre-clinical spondylotic cervical cord compression. *Eur. Spine J.* **1998**, *7*, 493–500. [CrossRef] [PubMed]
49. Kalupahana, N.S.; Weerasinghe, V.S.; Dangahadeniya, U.; Senanayake, N. Abnormal parameters of magnetically evoked motor-evoked potentials in patients with cervical spondylotic myelopathy. *Spine J.* **2008**, *8*, 645–649. [CrossRef] [PubMed]
50. Fehlings, M.G.; Tetreault, L.A.; Riew, K.D.; Middleton, J.W.; Aarabi, B.; Arnold, P.M.; Brodke, D.S.; Burns, A.S.; Carette, S.; Chen, R.; et al. A Clinical Practice Guideline for the Management of Patients With Degenerative Cervical Myelopathy: Recommendations for Patients With Mild, Moderate, and Severe Disease and Nonmyelopathic Patients With Evidence of Cord Compression. *Glob. Spine J.* **2017**, *7*, 70S–83S. [CrossRef]
51. Lees, F.; Turner, J.W.A. Natural History and Prognosis of Cervical Spondylosis. *BMJ* **1963**, *2*, 1607–1610. [CrossRef] [PubMed]

52. Karadimas, S.K.; Erwin, W.M.; Ely, C.G.; Dettori, J.R.; Fehlings, M.G. Pathophysiology and Natural History of Cervical Spondylotic Myelopathy. *Spine* **2013**, *38*, S21–S36. [CrossRef]
53. Kadaňka, Z.; Bednařík, J.; Novotný, O.; Urbánek, I.; Dušek, L. Cervical spondylotic myelopathy: Conservative versus surgical treatment after 10 years. *Eur. Spine J.* **2011**, *20*, 1533–1538. [CrossRef] [PubMed]
54. Kadanka, Z.; Mares, M.; Bednarik, J.; Smrcka, V.; Krbec, M.; Stejskal, L.; Chaloupka, R.; Surelova, D.; Novotny, O.; Urbanek, I.; et al. Approaches to spondylotic cervical myelopathy: Conservative versus surgical results in a 3-year follow-up study. *Spine* **2002**, *27*, 2205–2210. [CrossRef] [PubMed]
55. Sampath, P.; Bendebba, M.; Davis, J.D.; Ducker, T.B. Outcome of Patients Treated for Cervical Myelopathy: A Prospective, Multicenter Study With Independent Clinical Review. *Spine* **2000**, *25*, 670–676. [CrossRef]
56. Khan, I.; Archer, K.R.; Wanner, J.P.; Bydon, M.; Pennings, J.S.; Sivaganesan, A.; Knightly, J.J.; Foley, K.T.; Bisson, E.F.; Shaffrey, C.; et al. Trajectory of Improvement in Myelopathic Symptoms From 3 to 12 Months Following Surgery for Degenerative Cervical Myelopathy. *Neurosurgery* **2020**, *86*, 763–768. [CrossRef]
57. SaterenZoller, E.; Cannella, D.; Chyatte, D.; Fogelson, J.; Sharma, M. Diagnosis and medical and surgical management of cervical spondylotic myelopathy. *JAAPA J. Am. Acad. Physician Assist. Lippincott Williams Wilkins* **2015**, *28*, 29–36. [CrossRef]
58. Samuel, A.M.; Moore, H.G.; Vaishnav, A.S.; McAnany, S.; Albert, T.; Iyer, S.; Katsuura, Y.; Gang, C.H.; Qureshi, S.A. Effect of Myelopathy on Early Clinical Improvement After Cervical Disc Replacement: A Study of a Local Patient Cohort and a Large National Cohort. *Neurospine* **2019**, *16*, 563–573. [CrossRef] [PubMed]
59. Heller, J.G.; Edwards, C.C.; Murakami, H.; Rodts, G.E. Laminoplasty Versus Laminectomy and Fusion for Multilevel Cervical Myelopathy: An Independent Matched Cohort Analysis. *Spine* **2001**, *26*, 1330–1336. [CrossRef]
60. Di Martino, A.; Papalia, R.; Caldaria, A.; Torre, G.; Denaro, L.; Denaro, V. Should evoked potential monitoring be used in degenerative cervical spine surgery? A systematic review. *J. Orthop. Traumatol.* **2019**, *20*, 19. [CrossRef] [PubMed]
61. Resnick, D.K.; Anderson, P.A.; Kaiser, M.G.; Groff, M.W.; Heary, R.F.; Holly, L.T.; Mummaneni, P.V.; Ryken, T.C.; Choudhri, T.F.; Vresilovic, E.J.; et al. Electrophysiological monitoring during surgery for cervical degenerative myelopathy and radiculopathy. *J. Neurosurg. Spine* **2009**, *11*, 245–252. [CrossRef]

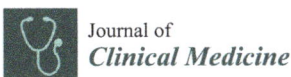

Journal of
Clinical Medicine

Review

Degenerative Cervical Myelopathy: Insights into Its Pathobiology and Molecular Mechanisms

Ji Tu [1,†], Jose Vargas Castillo [2,†], Abhirup Das [1,2,*] and Ashish D. Diwan [1,2]

1. Spine Labs, St. George and Sutherland Clinical School, University of New South Wales, Kogarah, NSW 2217, Australia; ji.tu@student.unsw.edu.au (J.T.); A.Diwan@spine-service.org (A.D.D.)
2. Spine Service, St. George Hospital, Kogarah, NSW 2217, Australia; fellow@spine-service.org
* Correspondence: abhirupdas@unsw.edu.au
† These authors have made an equal contribution.

Abstract: Degenerative cervical myelopathy (DCM), earlier referred to as cervical spondylotic myelopathy (CSM), is the most common and serious neurological disorder in the elderly population caused by chronic progressive compression or irritation of the spinal cord in the neck. The clinical features of DCM include localised neck pain and functional impairment of motor function in the arms, fingers and hands. If left untreated, this can lead to significant and permanent nerve damage including paralysis and death. Despite recent advancements in understanding the DCM pathology, prognosis remains poor and little is known about the molecular mechanisms underlying its pathogenesis. Moreover, there is scant evidence for the best treatment suitable for DCM patients. Decompressive surgery remains the most effective long-term treatment for this pathology, although the decision of when to perform such a procedure remains challenging. Given the fact that the aged population in the world is continuously increasing, DCM is posing a formidable challenge that needs urgent attention. Here, in this comprehensive review, we discuss the current knowledge of DCM pathology, including epidemiology, diagnosis, natural history, pathophysiology, risk factors, molecular features and treatment options. In addition to describing different scoring and classification systems used by clinicians in diagnosing DCM, we also highlight how advanced imaging techniques are being used to study the disease process. Last but not the least, we discuss several molecular underpinnings of DCM aetiology, including the cells involved and the pathways and molecules that are hallmarks of this disease.

Keywords: degenerative cervical myelopathy (DCM); cervical spondylotic myelopathy (CSM); spinal cord disorder; spinal cord compression; neck pain; blood-spinal cord barrier; microbes

Citation: Tu, J.; Vargas Castillo, J.; Das, A.; Diwan, A.D. Degenerative Cervical Myelopathy: Insights into Its Pathobiology and Molecular Mechanisms. *J. Clin. Med.* **2021**, *10*, 1214. https://doi.org/10.3390/jcm10061214

Academic Editor: Allan R. Martin

Received: 16 February 2021
Accepted: 9 March 2021
Published: 15 March 2021

Publisher's Note: MDPI stays neutral with regard to jurisdictional claims in published maps and institutional affiliations.

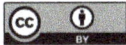

Copyright: © 2021 by the authors. Licensee MDPI, Basel, Switzerland. This article is an open access article distributed under the terms and conditions of the Creative Commons Attribution (CC BY) license (https://creativecommons.org/licenses/by/4.0/).

1. Introduction

Degenerative cervical myelopathy (DCM), also known as cervical spondylotic myelopathy (CSM), is the commonest cause of chronic spinal cord dysfunction worldwide. It is a significant cause of functional disability and leads to a significant ongoing economic burden to those affected by it, their families and their community [1]. DCM is a chronic, primarily non-traumatic and progressive condition. Structures involved in its pathogenesis include the intervertebral discs, vertebral endplates, osteophytes, zygapophyseal and uncovertebral joints and ligaments such as the ligamentum flavum or the posterior longitudinal ligament [2,3]. Although a few papers have been written about its natural history, pathophysiology and treatment, little is known about the molecular mechanisms underlying this condition.

2. Epidemiology

The prevalence of DCM in the general population is unknown. A magnetic resonance imaging (MRI) study of asymptomatic individuals showed that up to 25% of the subjects who were less than 40 years old had radiological findings compatible with cervical spondylosis. The incidence of such findings was 60% amongst people older than forty [4]. A cervical disc bulge was present in 88% of 1211 healthy volunteers in another study [5]. With aging, the frequency, size and number of bulging discs increases, while the sagittal diameter and axial area of the dural sac and spinal cord decrease, making this condition a formidable problem in the aging population [6,7].

It has been estimated that degenerative conditions of the spine account for more than 50% of all non-traumatic spinal cord injuries in the United Stated and Japan, and 22% in Australia [8]. The regional incidence for DCM is estimated to be 76 per million in North America, 26 per million in Europe and 6 per million in Australia [8]. This number does not include the patients who may have radiological findings of DCM without symptoms or with very mild symptoms.

The proportion of patients with DCM who underwent surgical treatment was estimated as 1.6 per 100,000 inhabitants [9]. Predicting a patient's potential for functional recovery before and after surgical decompression remains elusive largely due to the uncertain natural progression of spinal cord pathophysiology [10,11]. This lack of understanding makes the timing and type of treatment offered to patients vary greatly among clinicians.

3. Diagnosis

DCM can present clinically as localised neck pain, radiculopathy, myelopathy or a combination of these. Other features of cervical degeneration can include cervicogenic headaches, vertebrobasilar symptoms and precordial pain. All of these makes DCM a part of the differential diagnostic for a diverse number of conditions. This paper focuses on the myelopathy as a consequence of spondylosis; therefore, other conditions like radiculopathy or vertebrobasilar symptoms mentioned prior will not be thoroughly explored, although they are often intertwined with DCM. Despite technological advances, DCM remains a clinical diagnosis [12]. Components needed to make this diagnosis include a history of myelopathic complaints, findings in the physical examination suggestive of myelopathy and this is corroborated by advanced imaging studies showing compression of the spinal cord. However, patients with this condition may have very subtle clinical findings and often, these are not picked up by the unsuspecting clinician.

Diagnosis of DCM is not only difficult due to unsuspecting clinicians, but also because of an overlap in symptoms that may present with other conditions frequently found in the aged population. Regardless, the diagnosis of DCM begins with a thorough history. Clinical symptoms related to DCM include pain or stiffness in the neck, upper extremity clumsiness, gait instability, non-dermatomal numbness or weakness, loss of dexterity, poor coordination, lower extremity weakness, urgency of urination and defecation [13]. Physical examination includes assessment of the cervical spine range of motion (Table 1 and Supplementary Table S1) [14]. A limited neck extension should be taken into consideration should surgical treatment be offered, to prevent any iatrogenic hyperextension injury of the neck [15]. Myelopathic signs to be looked for include hyperreflexia, a positive Hoffmann test, a positive Babinski test, clonus and inverted brachioradialis reflex (IBR) [16]. Other possible findings on the physical examination include lower limb spasticity, atrophy of intrinsic hand muscles and corticospinal distribution motor deficits [17]. Furthermore, radiculopathy symptoms can be present as a confounding factor in DCM. A recent study found that over 50% of the patients with DCM had associated radiculopathy [8]. This can complicate the findings in the physical examination, as myelopathy usually presents with hyperreflexia and radiculopathy with hyporeflexia.

Patients with DCM more often than not present with positive clinical findings. Seventy nine percent of DCM patients have a positive myelopathic sign and 69% have a positive nerve provocative sign [12]. These numbers are higher in patients with spinal cord changes on an MRI where 95% of patients will have a positive myelopathic sign, especially Hoffmann's sign (80%). However, patients with cord signal changes can show no signs or symptoms. Close to 20% show no myelopathic sign at the time of presentation and almost

30% lacked hyperreflexia in any reflex arc tested [12]. The absence of these clinical signs should not be a source of doubt for establishing the diagnosis as that may be a cause for delay when offering surgical treatment.

Table 1. Common findings in the physical examination of patients with degenerative cervical myelopathy (DCM). Each symptom is described separately with a proposed mechanism, as well as their sensitivity and specificity.

Sign/Symptom	Description	Explanation	Sensitivity	Specificity
Hyperreflexia	Reflex greater than 3 on a 0 to 4 scale. (0: absent, 1: hypoactive, 2: normal, 3: hyperactive without clonus, 4: very hyperactive often with clonus.	Interruption of corticospinal and other descending pathways that influence the two-neuron reflex arc due to a suprasegmental lesion. Normally, the cerebral cortex or a number of brainstem nuclei influence the sensory input of the muscle by inhibiting the motor neuron in the anterior horn of the spinal cord. If a descending tract carrying these inhibitory signals is lost, the reflex is augmented.	72%	43%
Hyperreflexia Biceps	Percussion or tapping of the biceps tendon, close to its insertion in the ulna. Greater than 3 on a 0–4 scale.	Mainly C5. Small C6 component.	62%	49%
Hyperreflexia Brachioradialis (BR)	Percussion of the BR tendon distally. Greater than 3 on a 0–4 scale.	Evaluates neurologic integrity of C6.	21%	89%
Hyperreflexia Triceps	Percussion on the distal tendon of the triceps muscle.	Evaluates C7 neurologic integrity.	36%	78%
Hyperreflexia Patella	Percussion on the patellar tendon, with quadriceps relaxed.	Evaluates L4 neurologic integrity.	33%	76%
Hyperreflexia Achilles	Percussion in the Achilles tendon, with a relaxed gastro-soleus muscle.	Evaluates S1 neurologic integrity.	26%	81%
Hoffman	Hand in neutral position, flicking of the distal phalanx of the middle finger causes flexion of the distal phalanx of the thumb and second and third phalanx of the second finger.	Thought to represent a lesion in the corticospinal tracts [18].	59%	84%
Inverted Brachioradialis reflex (IBR)	When eliciting a BR reflex, there is contraction of the finger flexors with diminished BR reflex.	Thought to be caused by a lesion at C5-C6 (damage to the alpha motoneurons) and hyper-active response levels below (C8) [19].	51%	81%
Clonus	Forcefully dorsiflexing the ankle and maintaining pressure on the sole of the foot while observing for rhythmic beats of ankle flexion and extension. More than 3 beats required.	Hyper-active stretch reflexes in clonus are believed to be caused by self- excitation, which is not inhibited by the corticospinal tract (if there is an injury in the spinal cord) [20].	13%	100%
Babinski	Firmly run a pointy instrument, on the lateral part of the sole of the foot, from the heel to the base of the toes. Positive if extension of the Hallux occurs.	The normal response to plantar stimuli is abolished by an upper motor neuron lesion. It is replaced by Babinski's reflex, where the upward going toe (although anatomically it looks like extension) is part of a flexor reflex, disinhibited by loss of upper motor neurone control, and its receptive field may extend in some instances to the leg or thigh [21].	13%	100%

Somatosensory-evoked potentials (SSEPs) and motor evoked potentials (MEPs) are often used to find objective evidence of functional abnormalities of the spinal cord. Often used during surgeries to monitor the well-being of the spinal cord in real time [22], they can also be useful for neurophysiological study for patients with equivocal clinical findings for myelopathy [23]. Some authors have suggested the use of median nerve SSEPs, others, tibial nerve or ulnar nerve SSEPs, and some have found no difference between leg and arms SSEPs.

The predictive value of MEPs and SSEPs for surgical outcomes has not been studied systematically although there are several reports of clinical-electrophysiological correlation. It has been reported that MEPs are more sensitive than SSEPs in detecting chronic myelopathy [24]. SSEPs, however, may have a stronger correlation with surgical outcomes. Due to the anatomical location of the motor pathways and sensory pathways in the spinal cord, the SSEPs usually remain untouched after MEPs may have been affected by anteriorly compressing elements (herniated discs or osteophytes). Once the SSEPs are affected, the potential for a complete recovery after surgery appears to diminish, although this hasn´t been completely proven. Altogether, the role of electrophysiological studies in the diagnosis, follow-up and during treatment for DCM remains to be better defined [25].

The assessment of DCM often includes plain radiographs. Lateral views help evaluate spinal canal narrowing, disc height, the presence of ossification of the posterior longitudinal ligament (OPLL), cervical sagittal alignment and subluxation [26]. Parameters in cervical plain radiographs that are usually measured for assessing DCM are listed in Table 2 and shown in Figure 1A. Patients with DCM often exhibit increased C2–C7 Cobb angles, upper C7 slopes, lower C7 slopes and upper T1 slopes [27].

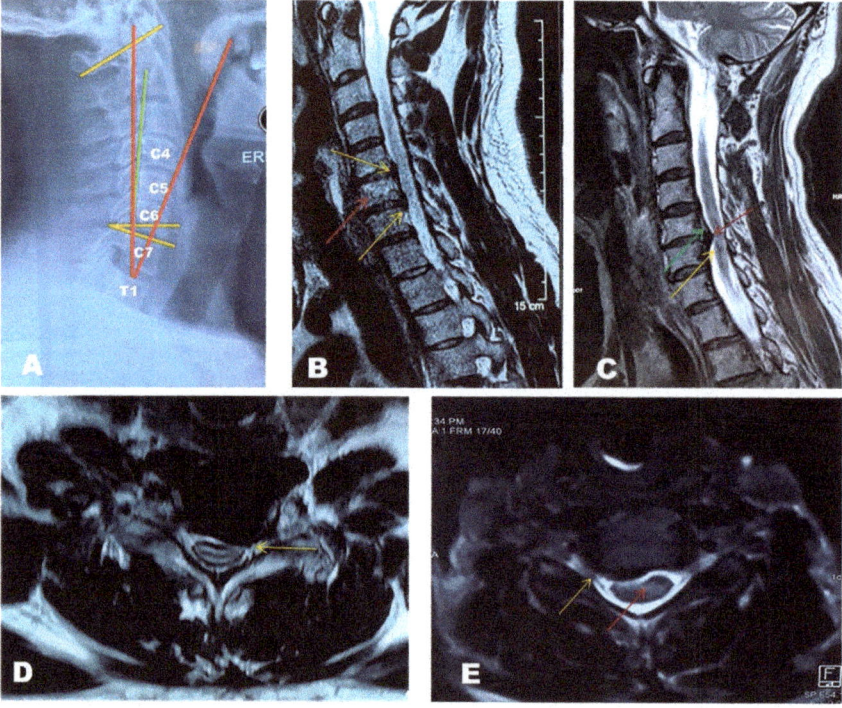

Figure 1. Radiological features of degenerative cervical myelopathy (DCM). (**A**) Standing, lateral X-ray image of a DCM patient showing a normal sagittal balance. In this case, the degeneration did not arise from a severe mal-alignment but rather from degeneration of the structures in the spinal canal. Red: Cervical tilt; Green: cervical sagittal vertical alignment (SVA); Yellow: Cobb angle C1–7 and C7 slope angle. (**B**) T2 weighted sequence of a cervical spine MRI. Sagittal cuts showing C5–C6, C6–C7 and C7–T1 degenerative disc disease with posterior osteophytes compressing the spinal cord at C5–C6 (yellow arrow up) and C6–C7 (yellow arrow down). Type 1 Modic endplate changes at the inferior endplate of C5 and superior endplate of C6 indicate low grade inflammation at this level (red arrow). The relationship between inflammation at the endplates and discs and the presence of bacteria here is unclear. (**C**) Sagittal cuts showing multilevel disc disease with a protruding disc at C5–C6 indenting the spinal cord at this level. Hyper-intensity of the cord can be noticed or a white colour on the cord that under normal circumstances appears as black surrounded by a white signal (the cerebrospinal fluid), demonstrating evidence of myelomalacia (yellow arrow). T2 mapping also showing stenosis of the cervical vertebral canal cause by ossification of the posterior longitudinal ligament (OPLL) (green arrow) with a large osteophyte complex at this level (red arrow). The only symptoms showcased by this patient were mild axial neck pain and bilateral plantar paresthesias. (**D**) Axial cut through the C5–C6 disc showing a left sided disc bulge compressing the exiting nerve root at this level (yellow arrow). (**E**) Axial cut at the C4–C5 level showing a posterior osteophyte complex (yellow arrow) abutting the spinal cord and indenting it. A hyperintense signal can be seen in the cord at this level which could indicate myelomalacia (red arrow).

Table 2. Common measurements obtained from standard cervical spine plain radiographs. These measurements are not always performed unless an important sagittal deformity of the spine is deemed responsible for the myelopathy. Some variation exists amongst different authors or according to the position of the patient at the time the radiograph was taken [28].

Radiologic Measures	Normal Values	Explanation
Cobb C1–7/C2–7 angle	18 degrees +/− 12 degrees	The angle between the line parallel to the inferior endplate of C1/C2 to parallel to the inferior endplate of C7.
C7 slope	Normal values vary according to the individual cervical lordosis	Angle between a horizontal line and the superior endplate of C7
T1 slope	Normal values vary according to the individual cervical lordosis	Angle between horizontal plane at T1 endplate
Cervical sagittal vertical alignment (SVA)	15 mm +/− 11 mm	The distance from the posterior, superior corner of C7 to the plumbline from the centroid of C2
Cervical tilt	43 degrees +/− 6 degrees	The angle between two lines, both originating from the centre of the T1 upper end plate; one is vertical to the T1 upper end plate and the other passes through the tip of the dens

A recent report on the correlation between preoperative computed tomography (CT) myelograms and clinical outcomes following surgery showed that patients with greater transverse area of spinal cord at the level of maximum compression had better results [29]. Other investigations such as kinematic CTs have shown limited potential in either demonstrating myelopathy or correlating the findings with clinical outcomes for DCM. CT based investigations have an important role in diagnosing conditions such as OPLL [30].

Table 3. Modic type endplate changes represent a classification for vertebral body endplate MRI, first described in 1988 [31]. Often used in the clinical context, these changes are situated in both the body of the vertebrae and in the endplate of the neighbouring disc. It is important to understand that Modic changes do not represent an illness but are a simple descriptive term for radiological findings in MRI.

Modic Type	T1 Findings	T2 Findings	Clinical Correlation
1	Hypointense	Hyperintense	Represent bone marrow oedema and inflammation
2	Hyperintense	Isointense	Conversion of normal hemopoietic bone marrow into fatty marrow as a result of ischemia
3	Hypointense	Hypointense	Represent subchondral bone sclerosis

MRI can provide direct proof of spinal cord compression and should often be the initial investigation; it also plays a role in choosing the right treatment and possibly predicting outcomes. MRI scans allow visualisation of soft tissue structures like intervertebral discs; therefore, early signs of degeneration in them can be detected, as well as in spinal ligaments and other structures not easily seen in other scans. It is unclear whether a direct relationship exists between the quantum of degeneration and cord signal changes independent of canal stenosis.

MRI scans can also detect changes in the signal intensity of the vertebral endplates. When associated with disc degeneration, these are called Modic endplate changes (MECs, Figure 1B) [31]. Three subtypes have been described according to MRI (Table 3). A study found type 2 changes were the most common, especially at the C5–6 and C6–7 levels [32]. However, MECs are a dynamic phenomenon. Mann et al. evaluated the natural course of MECs in 426 patients with neck pain and observed that the prevalence of type 1 MECs increased from 7.4% to 8.2% after 2.5 years follow-up [33]. Similarly, the prevalence of type

2 increased from 14.5% to 22.3%. Twelve segments with type 1 converted to type 2 during the follow-up, while no conversions from type 2 to type 1 were observed.

MRI also offers an opportunity to evaluate spinal canal stenosis (Figure 1C–E). Measuring the anterior–posterior diameter at the region of interest (ROI) is the simplest way that was used in previous studies [34]. However, what is considered a "normal value" for size of the canal varies among individuals. Fehlings et al. developed a method to assess the maximum canal compromise (MCC) after a traumatic cervical spine injury [35]. They evaluated canal size at the ROI by comparing it to the average canal size at the levels above and below it. Although designed for traumatic spinal injury, it has been used for degenerative conditions. Similar to MCC, they also developed the maximum spinal cord compression (MSCC) index to measure the spinal cord compression [36]. Our retrospective study showed that the ratio of the canal diameter to the average of mid-vertebral cephalic and caudal canal diameters is the most sensitive mid-sagittal plane metric for assessing spinal canal stenosis, whereas the ratio of the anteroposterior diameter to the transverse diameter of the cord is the most sensitive axial plane metric [37]. MRI had a role in predicting outcomes in one study: spinal cord atrophy, multilevel T2 hyperintensity, T1 focal hypointensity combined with T2 focal hyperintensity were indicators of poor prognosis for DCM [38].

Certain studies suggest that some spinal cord signal changes can only become evident when a dynamic MRI (flexion/extension MRI) is utilised. A study with 50 patients showed that intensity changes on the spinal cord were made evident with a flexion MRI in 40% of the patients, whereas a neutral MRI only showed these changes in 26% of the patients and an extension MRI only did so in 14% of them [39]. These findings may explain why some MRIs could return negative findings for typical cervical myelopathy, and why these findings might be apparent after surgery in a new MRI. Other authors have reported extension MRIs as helpful to make spinal cord changes evident in patients with DCM, although the relationship between these findings and clinical outcomes is yet to be proven [40].

In addition to conventional MRI, novel techniques have been applied to investigate central nervous system (CNS) pathology, including Diffusion Tensor Imaging (DTI), Diffusion Tensor Tractography (DTT) and Diffusion Basis Spectrum Imaging (DBSI). DTI can estimate the integrity of the tissue microstructure by modelling the diffusion of water within the tissue [41]. DTI is used in brain tumour surgery and has been extrapolated to spinal conditions (Figure 2) [42]. DTI parameters include the Fractional Anisotropy (FA) and Apparent Diffusion Coefficient (ADC). A prospective study found that DTI ratios were more valuable than absolute DTI parameters for the evaluation of DCM, as the latter can be confounded by age and cervical level [43]. DTT is a functional imaging technique, which allows tracking of the nerve fibres based on their FA values and can be demonstrated when the nerve fibres get distorted, disoriented or even interrupted as the severity of the spinal compression varies. DTT and DTI are more valuable than routine MRI scans for diagnosis and predicting outcomes in DCM patients [44,45]. DBSI allows for the quantification of axonal injury, demyelination and inflammation in DCM patients.

Several score systems have been used throughout the years to study DCM. Based mostly on signs or symptoms, their importance relies on the prognostic value they may have and to facilitate comparison of different treatment methods. An overview of the most common ones is detailed in Table 4, including their advantages and shortcomings [46,47].

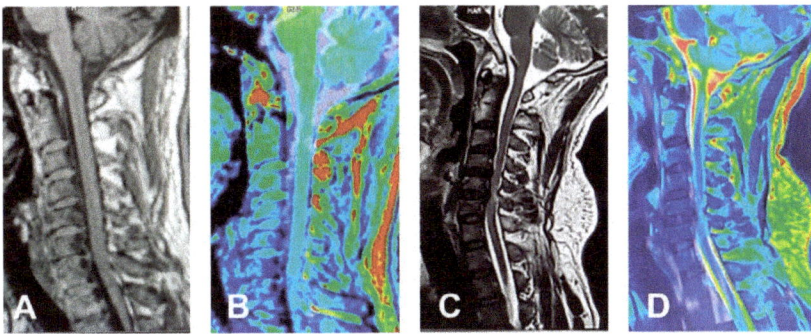

Figure 2. A 38-year-old female presented with history of chronic neck pain: (**A**) No disc herniation and spinal cord compression was showed on sagittal T1 weighted MRI. (**B**) The diffusion tensor imaging (DTI) maps do not show obvious change as well. A 43-year-old female with right brachialgia: (**C**) Sagittal T2 weighted MRI shows spinal cord compression with hyperintense cord signals at C4/5 and C5/6 levels. (**D**) DTI image shows loss of blue colour of the normal cord.

Table 4. Clinicians use scoring systems to categorise the severity of different conditions. Often different classifications arise as different groups come up with their own systems; however, international consensus groups usually choose one system to standardise publications and treatments across the board. This has not been the case with DCM. Several different systems are still been used by different authors based on their preference. The following are the most common classification systems currently in use, along with a guide to their score meaning, presence of radiologic features, short-comings and advantages. Showcasing the complete classifications is beyond the scope of this review. To obtain the complete scoring systems, please follow the link to the reference [15,47–49].

Name	Scoring Method	Radiologic Findings	Correlation to Symptoms	Limitations	Advantages
Nurick	0–5. The higher the grade, the more severe the deficit.	No	Affected by gait function (++), lower limbs paresis and paraesthesia and vegetative symptoms (+).	Less accurate post-op scoring; Does not pick up upper extremity disfunction	Evaluates economic situation in connection to gait function.
mJOA	0–17. The lower the score, the more severe the deficits. Normal: 16–17, grade 1: 12–15, grade 2: 8–11, grade 3: 0–7. Upper extremity 23.5%; lower extremity 23.5%; sensory 35.4%; bladder and bowel 17.6%	No	Affected by paraesthesia of lower limbs and paresis of upper limbs (++) and dysdiadochokinesia and vegetative symptoms (+).	Does not take economic factors into consideration	Good for assessing outcomes (post-intervention).
CMS	Upper and lower extremity are analysed separately. 0–5 each. The higher the grade, the more severe the deficit.	Weak correlation between low severity in the lower limb score and C-Spine mal-alignment	Affected by dysdiadochokinesia, gait function and paresis of upper extremity (++) and vegetative symptoms (+)	Does not take economic factors into consideration	Good for assessing function/symptoms of upper/lower extremities/as it evaluates them individually. Good at assessing clinical state and grade of severity of CSM.
EMS	5–18. The lower the score the more severe the deficits. Normal function: 17+, grade 1: 13–16, grade 2: 9–12, grade 3: 5–8. Upper extremity 27.8%, lower extremity 22.2%, coordination 16.7%, paraesthesia/pain 16.0%, bladder and bowel function 16.7%	No	Affected by dysdiadochokinesia (++) and paresis of the upper extremity and vegetative symptoms (+)		Good at assessing clinical state and grade of severity of CSM. Better sensitivity to reveal functional deficit (by assessing proprioception/coordination).
Prolo scale	2–10. The lower the score the more severe the deficits. Normal function: 9+, grade 1: 7 + 8, grade 2: 5 + 6, grade 3: 2–4. Economic status 50%; functional status 50%.	No	Mildly affected by vegetative symptoms (+)	Does not reflect clinical symptoms significantly -Not good for pre-op assessing the grade of severity	Good correlation between high pre-op scores and better outcomes. Good for assessing normalisation" and rehabilitation (regained ability for work or for leisure time).

mJOA: modified Japanese Orthopaedic Association; CMS: Cervical Myelopathy Scale; EMS: European Myelopathy Scale.

4. Natural History

The natural history of DCM is still not clear. While the nature of the injury and ultimate consequences share similarities with acute spinal cord injuries, the pathophysiology differs [10]. An old descriptive study from 1956 described the average age for the appearance of symptoms to be at around 50 years of age and 70% of the patients were between 40 to 59 years. Out of 120 patients with DCM, 5% of them had a rapid onset of symptoms followed by long periods of remission, 20% had a slow progressive worsening of neurofunction and 75% had a stepwise decline of neurofunction [50]. The progression of symptoms in patients with DCM has been studied. In 1963, a retrospective study of DCM to understand its natural history, found that a majority of patients had a poor prognosis, with more than 87% progressing to moderate or severe disability at the last follow-up [51].

A prospective research in 199 asymptomatic patients with cervical spinal cord encroachment detected by radiology was conducted to find out the effects of traumatic episodes (head, spine, trunk or shoulders) on these patients. A total of 14 episodes were recorded during a median 44 months follow-up, and only one patient developed myelopathy. Meanwhile, 44 patients without a history of trauma developed myelopathic symptoms. It can be inferred that the risk of developing myelopathy in asymptomatic patients with cervical spinal cord encroachment after minor trauma is low [52]. However, another study in patients with OPLL showed that minor trauma is of importance in the development or deterioration of myelopathy in said patients [53].

5. Pathophysiology

5.1. Spinal Cord Compression and Ischemic Injury

Mechanical compression is the corner stone of spinal cord dysfunction in DCM. Studies on bovine cervical spinal cords showed a different stress distribution between white and grey matter, which varied with strain rate, compression volume and the position of compression. These differences may explain the diverse signs and symptoms found in DCM [54]. In an animal model of chronically compressed spinal cord (tiptoe-walking Yoshimura (twy) mice), *p62* and autophagy markers (autolysosomes and autophagic vesicles) were found to accumulate in neurons, axons, astrocytes and oligodendrocytes. These molecules are linked to neuronal cell death [55]. Fas-mediated apoptosis of neurons and oligodendrocytes and an increase in inflammatory cells were also observed in twy mice and post-mortem human spinal cords samples of DCM patients in a different study [56]. Mechanical compression can also lead to ischemia and hypoxia, which would result in spinal cord dysfunction, similar to that found in acute traumatic spinal cord injuries. The compression can be caused by static and/or dynamic factors. The static factors refer to structural spondylotic abnormalities such as disc degeneration, which result in cervical canal stenosis. The dynamic factors include changes to the normal cervical spine biomechanics and tensile stresses transmitted to the spinal cord from the dentate ligaments, which attach the lateral pia to the lateral dura [57,58].

Ischemic injury was first described in the pathophysiology of degenerative spondylitis in 1948 [59]. Further studies confirmed the observation with human and animal evidence. Ischemia related tissue changes, including flattening of the cord, swelling of myelin and axons, demyelination in the posterolateral and anterolateral columns and neuronal loss in the anterior horns have been observed in the spinal cord of DCM patients. The chronic compression can obstruct branches of the anterior spinal artery with the ensuing ischemic damage, as shown in a series of post-mortem case reports [60]. Researchers found motor disturbances were worsened by induced exacerbated spinal cord hypoperfusion. They proved this by exsanguination plus ligation of the carotid and vertebral arteries in a cervical chronic compression dog model [61,62]. Rodent experiments have also proved that chronic compression of the cervical spinal cord leads to architectural changes of the microvessel network and altered distribution of spinal cord blood flow [63].

5.2. Spine Deformity and Instability

Cervical sagittal malalignment is a contributing factor to DCM [27]. The cervical spine has a lordotic disposition, that can be first seen as early as the 9th week of gestation [14]. As mentioned earlier, with aging and the ensuing degeneration, several alignment abnormalities may arise, such as increased lordosis, scoliosis and kyphosis. These changes can compromise the volume of the vertebral canal, reducing the space available for the spinal cord. A study conducted in North America showed moderate negative correlation between cord cross-sectional area and modified Japanese Orthopaedic Association (mJOA) scores in patients with kyphotic deformities in the cervical spine [64]. Kyphotic deformities may lead to spinal cord tethering and stretching, resulting in increased intramedullary pressure and impaired microcirculation, leading to demyelination, neuronal loss and myelopathy [65]. Atlantoaxial joint instability is also believed to be associated with subaxial cervical instability and the appearance of DCM [66,67].

5.3. Ossification of the Ligaments

Ossification of the posterior longitudinal ligament (OPLL), anterior longitudinal ligament (OALL) and/or of the ligamentum flavum (OLF) can affect the space available for the spinal cord and subsequently cause DCM [68]. Its incidence in the Japanese population is estimated as between 1.9 and 4.3%, averaging 3.0% in other Asian countries [69]. However, it's only 0.1 to 1.7% among Caucasian cohorts [70]. Although the mechanism of OPLL remains poorly understood, it shares similarities with diffuse idiopathic skeletal hyperostosis (DISH). Some systemic hormones are considered to play a role in the initiation and development of OPLL, such as 1,25-dihydroxyvitamin D, parathyroid hormone, insulin and leptin, as well as local growth factors, such as transforming growth factor-β (TGF-β) and bone morphogenetic protein (BMP) [71].

5.4. Biomechanical Changes

The increased association of DCM with aging raises the issue whether anchoring of the cervical spinal cord by dentate ligaments provides tensile friction to cause microtrauma of the spinal cord, or whether the changing stiffness of the neural tissue and extracellular matrix (ECM) in the spinal cord can possibly make the spinal cord stiffer and susceptible to repetitive micro-injury with progressive age. Such biomechanical non-compressive mechanisms have been explored. Finite element analysis (FEA) showed that intramedullary stress contributes to DCM pathogenesis [54,72]. One study has indicated that a threshold of intramedullary stress to present symptoms of myelopathy actually existed and is related to neurological dysfunction [73]. A 3D finite element model showed that cervical flexion-induced spinal cord stress results in muscle atrophy and weakness [74].

6. Risk Factors

6.1. Aging

Aging is associated with tissue degeneration and a change in the chemical properties of tissues. Not surprisingly, the prevalence of cervical cord compression increases with increasing age [75]. DCM is uncommon in patients under 40 years of age. Most patients are diagnosed with DCM in their fifth decade of life [76]. A prospective longitudinal study in healthy volunteers revealed that the incidence of foraminal stenosis, posterior disc protrusion and disc space narrowing in MRI was higher in elderly subjects [77]. Aging is also associated with changes in the sagittal alignment of the cervical spine, namely, loss of the physiologic lordosis [78].

6.2. Genetic Polymorphism

It has long been speculated that DCM has genetic predisposition [79]. In 2012, a retrospective study based on over 2 million Utah residents showed a relative risk of 5.21 and 1.95 for first degree and third degree DCM patients' relatives, respectively [80].

Polymorphisms in a number of genes that have been identified as contributing to the development of DCM are listed in Table 5.

Table 5. List of genes associated with DCM pathology.

Gene	DCM Features	Reference
Brain-derived neurotrophic factor (BDNF)	Worse mJOA and Nurick scores	[81]
Osteoprotegerin (OPG)	Worse mJOA score	[82]
Osteopontin (OPN)	Worse mJOA score	[83]
Hypoxia inducible factor-1α (HIF-1α)	Worse mJOA score	[84]
Apolipoprotein E (APOE)	Worse mJOA score	[85,86]
BMPs (BMP4, BMP9, BMPR1A)	Radiographic severity of DCM	[87,88]
RUNX2	Responsible for OPLL	[89]
BMP2	Responsible for OPLL	[90]
Vitamin D receptor (VDR)	Radiologic changes and mJOA scores	[89,91]
Vitamin D binding protein (VDBP)	Radiologic changes and mJOA scores	[91]
Collagen IX	Radiologic changes and mJOA scores	[92]
Collagen α2(XI)	Radiographic severity of DCM	[93]

6.3. Microbes

One of the emerging risk factors for DCM that has been coming to the fore recently is bacterial infection. Low virulence bacterial infections have been observed in degenerate cervical discs of DCM patients undergoing surgery; however, it is not yet clear if these infections play a role in the development of clinical symptoms [94,95]. *Propionibacterium acnes* and coagulase-negative *Staphylococci* were the most commonly identified bacteria. Interestingly, a recent study indicated that the lumbar intervertebral discs harbour their own unique bacterial population (disc microbiome), and alterations in bacterial diversity (dysbiosis), both in the disc and gut, strongly correlate with disc disorders in back pain patients [96]. Further study is warranted to verify if similar disc microbiome exists in the cervical disc and whether dysbiosis plays any role in DCM pathogenesis and surgery outcomes.

7. Molecular Features
7.1. Cervical Intervertebral Disc Degeneration

Intervertebral disc (IVD) degeneration is a common finding; 98% of healthy adults show IVD degeneration in their 20s [97]. It is pivotal for the development of cervical spondylosis. The IVD consists of three specialised tissues: the central nucleus pulposus (NP), the outer fibrillar annulus fibrosus (AF) and the cartilage end plates (CEP) that anchor the disc to the adjacent vertebral bones. Most of the molecular studies of IVD degeneration focus on lumbar IVDs, and while it is true that they share similar biologic characteristics, there are several differences between cervical and lumbar IVDs. In human, collagen content is highest in cervical IVD, whereas polyanion concentration is highest in lumbar discs [98]. Compared to the lumbar AF, the fibres of the cervical AF are more perpendicular to the endplates in orientation [99].

IVD degeneration leads to an increased biomechanical stress on the rest of the cervical spine (Figure 3A). It has been shown to increase the shear stress on the vertebral cortical bone which leads to remodelling of this bone and to the formation of osteophytes. These abnormal bony formations can cause DCM and radiculopathy [100,101]. An in vivo study showed that neurotrophins, BDNF and Nerve Growth Factor (NGF) are increased in painful cervical discs and correlated with clinical findings [102]. Revascularisation into the disc is also a feature in DCM [103]. Disrupted disc microenvironment and senescence of IVD cells induce the imbalance between their ECM anabolism and catabolism. The degradation of ECM components and deterioration of the major structural proteoglycan aggrecan result in reduced hydration, loss of disc height and an overall inability to absorb compressive load [104]. During this process, inflammation, cell apoptosis and mitochondrial dysfunction are widely prevalent [105,106].

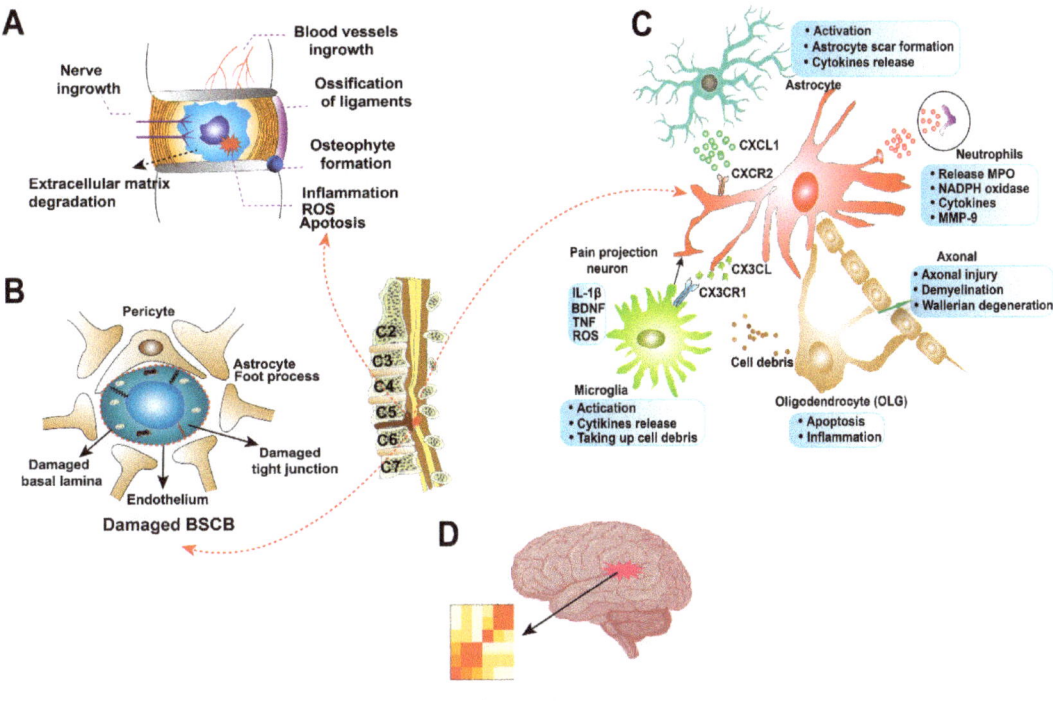

Figure 3. Molecular features of degenerative cervical myelopathy (DCM). (**A**) The hallmarks of cervical disc degeneration. Compared to healthy intervertebral disc, the degenerative disc has increased blood vessel and neuronal ingrowth. Increased inflammation, reactive oxygen species (ROS) and cell apoptosis result in extracellular matrix degradation. The cartilage endplate may be calcified, and osteophytes form on the adjacent vertebral bones. Ossification of the posterior longitudinal ligament (OPLL) can also be found in degenerative cervical spines. (**B**) Blood–spinal cord barrier (BSCB) is disrupted in DCM, with the features of damaged basal lamina and tight junction. (**C**) The roles of cells types in spinal cord during DCM. Astrocyte participates in scar formation in spinal cord; and activated astrocytes can release CXCL1 to interact with CXCR2 receptor on neurons, inducing descending neuron degeneration in spinal cord. CX3CL/CX3CR1 interaction between microglia and neuron regulates neuroinflammation in DCM. Microglia can also take up cell debris from other cells, such as apoptosis oligodendrocytes (OLG). Infiltrating neutrophils release myeloperoxidase (MPO), nicotinamide adenine dinucleotide phosphate oxidase (NADPH oxidase) and other cytokines in the microenvironment. Neutrophils can also express Matrix metalloproteinase (MMP)-9 as a strong pro-inflammatory molecule. (**D**) The brain metabolic profile was found to change in DCM patients.

7.2. Blood-Spinal Cord Barrier Dysfunction

The local environment around the blood–spinal cord barrier (BSCB) undergoes profound biochemical and cellular changes with DCM (Figure 3B). The different pathways and interactions involved in this process are not quite completely understood. BSCB is the continuation of the blood–brain barrier (BBB); however, a few morphological and functional differences exist between them [107]. BSCB provides a special immune-privileged environment to the spinal cord, protecting the CNS from neurotoxic insults. These insults may include peripheral immune cell invasion, cytokines and reactive oxygen species (ROS).

The presence of these elements leads to neuroinflammation and neurodegeneration [108]. There is evidence that spinal cord trauma leads to dysfunction of the BSCB [107]. Three markers of different size (fluorescently labelled hydrazide, fluorescently labelled bovine serum albumin and immunohistochemically labelled red blood cells) showed greater concentrations in the grey matter than in white matter, and correlated better to the rate of spinal cord compression than to the depth of compression [109]. Longitudinal dynamic contrast-enhanced MRI (DCE-MRI) studies revealed that the BSCB remained compromised even 56 days after moderately severe injury to the spinal cord in an animal model. A significant correlation between decreased BSCB permeability and improved motor recovery was also observed [110].

Endothelial cells are responsible for the integrity of the BSCB. Quantitative loss and dysfunction of these cells can induce impairments in the BSCB, resulting in spinal cord oedema and inflammation [107]. Oestrogens are thought to have an effect on the overall health of the structure, as it has been shown that tamoxifen, an oestrogen-receptor inhibitor, bolsters the BSCB, by means of decreasing tissue oedema and IL-1β production and decreasing myelin loss in spinal cord injury (SCI) [111]. A prospective non-randomised controlled study revealed increased BSCB permeability in DCM patients, as evident from the increased levels on Albumin Q, IgG, and IgA into intrathecal space [112]. The severity of BSCB disruption and the diffusion of IgG were also found to be related to the clinical status. Swelling of the spinal cord can also be seen after BSCB disruption, and it has been found in roughly 8% of patients with DCM [113]. Radiologically, a disruption of BSCB can be seen in the form of positive intramedullary Gadolinium enhancement around the white matter vessels in an MRI sequence [114].

7.3. Axonal Injury

An important feature of DCM, axonal injury (Figure 3C), can be evaluated using FA obtained from DTI MRI. The concept underpinning this technology is that water molecules diffuse differently along the tissues depending on the type of tissue, their integrity, architecture and presence of barriers, providing information about its orientation and quantitative anisotropy. Analyses of the FA values of different neural elements provide information about the relative indemnity of said structure. Differences in the FA ratios of DCM patients from different mJOA score subgroups were observed in a recent study [44]. This could mean that the severity of DCM is related to axonal integrity. Decompression of spinal cord was also found to correlate with axonal sprouting in another imaging study, although the clinical implications are not clear [115]. Axonal degeneration can be activated by different stimuli including mechanical injury, axonal transport defects or drugs [116]. Some studies indicate that axonal degeneration may be an early event in neurodegenerative diseases and may precede any radiological findings of compression [117,118]. This observation suggests that there may be other catalysts for axonal injury, besides the aforementioned. The presence of microbial and/or inflammatory metabolites, or potentially micro-trauma, could be one or more of them.

7.4. Astrocytes

In 1895, Michael von Lenhossék used the word astrocyte to describe the star-shaped glial cells in vertebrates. They are the most abundant, constituting nearly 1/3 of the cells in the human CNS. Astrocytes perform many important functions in the CNS. They are involved in maintaining homeostasis at the synapse and regulating neuronal signalling. They act as an essential part of BSCB, protecting neurons from oxidative damage by controlling the access of peripheral cells to the spinal cord. They also take part in forming the glial scar after an injury, along with microglia/macrophages and ECM molecules [119]. Astrocytes increase their number and migrate to the damaged site. In severe injuries, they surround the SCI lesions and form a glial scar, acting as a physical barrier to contain the injured area [120,121].

Astrocytes alter the composition of the ECM following an injury. Several ECM components like chondroitin sulphate proteoglycans and tenascins are markedly upregulated in astrocytes after being stimulated [122]. Astrogliosis is the proliferation and hypertrophy of astrocytes, resulting in scar formation via the activation of signalling pathways such as STAT3 and TGF-β. A histological study of horses with chronic compressive myelopathy found astrogliosis a prominent and persistent finding in their spinal cords [123]. Researchers have demonstrated that chronic mechanical compression of the cervical spinal cord leads to astrogliosis in the dorsal horns of the spinal cord [124]. Activated astrocytes express intermediate pro-inflammatory filaments in their membrane, such as glial fibrillary acidic proteins (GFAP), nestin and vimentin. In a rabbit model of unilateral spinal cord compression, the density of GFAP-positive astrocytes was significantly increased, providing evidence they play a role in compressive pathology of the spinal cord [125].

Reactive astrocytes also contribute to the release of both pro- and anti-inflammatory cytokines such as interleukins (IL-1 and IL-6), TGF-β, interferon γ (IFN-γ) and tumour necrosis factor-α (TNF-α). These cytokines modulate inflammation and play a role in secondary injury mechanisms [126]. The release of the chemokine CXCL1 from astrocytes and the subsequent activation of its CXCR2 receptor on neurons is evidence of the crosstalk between the two cell types (Figure 3C). This particular interaction induces descending neuron degeneration in spinal cord [127]. Astrocytes are also involved in neuropathic pain modulation and processing. Toll-like receptor 4 (TLR-4) pathway contributes to astrocyte activation and astrogliosis during chronic pain sensitization in the spinal cord [128]. Animal experiments proved cervical contusion-induced neuropathic pain is associated with persistent astrocyte activation in the superficial dorsal horn [129].

7.5. Microglia and Neutrophils

As the resident macrophage cells, microglia are central players in the innate immune response following injury to the CNS (Figure 3C). Under normal circumstances, they patrol their micro-environment in search for abnormal epitopes to trigger a defence response. However, after an injury, they take part in the production of harmful ROS and pro-inflammatory cytokines. They also contribute to the glial scar found around damaged tissue in the CNS [130]. Neutrophils and activated microglia appear in the first few days of SCI and are loaded with destructive oxidative and proteolytic enzymes. Oxidative activity related to myeloperoxidase (MPO) and nicotinamide adenine dinucleotide phosphate oxidase (NADPH oxidase) released by neutrophils are mainly associated with neutrophils and activated microglia, while phagocytic macrophages have weak or no enzyme expression. Matrix metalloproteinase (MMP) 9 is only expressed by neutrophils and is a strong pro-inflammatory molecule [131]. Neutrophils are only detectable for up to ten days after the initial injury, with activated microglia, a few monocytes/macrophages and numerous phagocytic macrophages lingering for weeks to months afterwards.

The main biochemical difference between SCI and DCM is that the latter, being a chronic process, is driven by chronic inflammation, and thus, the molecular markers and characteristic cell types are different to those seen in acute responses. It has been shown that activated macrophages/microglia are the predominant cell types in both the early and late phases of DCM [56]. A chemokine often involved in the chemotaxis of monocytes and leucocytes called fractalkine (CX3CL1) was found to be widely expressed in the membrane of neurons, while its receptor (CX3CR1) is highly expressed on microglia [132]. Animal experiments on ischemic mice shed some light on the role of CX3CR1 during ischemia in the CNS [133,134]. Under ischemic conditions (common in DCM), the development of activated microglia in CX3CR1 knockout mice was significantly impaired. Post-mortem immunohistochemistry revealed CX3CR1 depletion led to a decrease in the activation of microglia/macrophages, while leukocyte recruitment increased. This suggests that CX3CR1 plays a role in the regulation of microglia and neuroinflammation in conditions like DCM [134,135].

Microglia has also been involved in mechanisms for neuropathic pain. It has been shown that inhibiting the function or expression of microglial-produced molecules, such as activated protein-kinases, p38 and other extracellular signal-regulated protein kinase, suppresses the abnormal excitability of dorsal horn neurons found in neuropathic pain [136,137].

7.6. Oligodendrocytes

Oligodendrocytes (OLG) support and insulate the axons of neurons (Figure 3C). Abnormalities in OLG are associated with neurological symptoms and are a common finding in acute and chronic spinal cord injuries. An immuno-histochemical study of patients with DCM showed that the distribution of apoptotic OLG was analogous to the degeneration of the long tracts in cervical spinal cord [133]. The relatively low reduced glutathione and high iron concentration in OLG renders them vulnerable to oxidative stress (present in inflammatory conditions of the spinal cord) [138]. The pro-inflammatory cytokines, IL-1β and TNF-α, were found to inhibit the expression of myelin genes in human OLG through the alteration of the cellular redox system [108].

The dysfunction of OLG is deeply related to demyelination. Demyelinated corticospinal tracts are a constant finding in DCM [139–141]. However, whether primary demyelination appears as a result of damage to OLG or myelin loss comes secondary to axonal degeneration remains unclear. Demyelination has been identified in compressed spinal cord samples [142,143] and successfully reproduced using toxin-induced models, virus-induced and autoimmune models [144]. This explains the myriad of causes that may lead to this condition. Evidence shows that neuronal and OLG apoptosis contribute to demyelination and Wallerian degeneration, resulting in neurological deficit [145,146]. Decreased myelin content in the spinal cord was shown to be associated with impaired spinal cord conduction [147]. A study using surgery-induced spinal cord compression in a horse model showed that OLG apoptosis immediately occurred after the injury and was consistent with the extent of demyelination. This indicates that OLG apoptosis induced by compression contributes to demyelination [142]. At least two different pathways have been proposed to explain the apoptosis of OLG in DCM: (1) via Endoplasmic Reticulum (ER)–mitochondria interaction (increased caspase-12 and cytochrome c) and (2) upregulation of E1F2 (a pro-apoptotic transcription factor associated with the p53 protein in its apoptotic pathway) (Figure 4) [148]. Between ER and mitochondria, mitochondrial fission protein Fission 1 homologue (Fis1) and Bap31 at the ER can combine to form Fis1-Bap31 complex (ARCosome), serving as a platform for caspase-8 activation, leading to apoptosis [149]. E1F2 phosphorylation can enhance CHOP translation, leading to inflammasome activation and cytokines release [150,151].

Fas ligand mediated OLG apoptosis has been shown to contribute to cell death and inflammation in a model of DCM [56]. TNF-α is also a known inducer of apoptosis of neurons and OLG. In the early phases of SCI, TNF-α serves as an external signal triggering apoptosis in OLG, but its role has not been determined in DCM [152]. Apoptosis signal-regulating kinase 1 (ASK1), Jun N-terminal kinase (JNK) and p38 signal pathways were found to be activated in OLG in an animal model of chronic spinal cord compression [153]. Notably, ASK1 can be activated by TNF-α or Fas and act as a mediator of JNK activation. Some counterbalances have also been seen in the spinal cord against apoptotic cascades. Insulin-like growth factor-1 (IGF-1) can protect myelin and oligodendrocytes from TNF-α induced apoptosis [154].

Inflammasome, a cytosolic multiprotein oligomer of the innate immune system responsible for the activation of inflammatory responses, has been detected during inflammatory states in multiple cell types of the CNS, including OLG [155]. Increased intracellular calcium (Ca^{2+}) leads to the release of ROS and NLRP3 inflammasome complex activation, which itself facilitates caspase-1 autoactivation and the subsequent proteolytic cleavage and release of IL-1β [156].

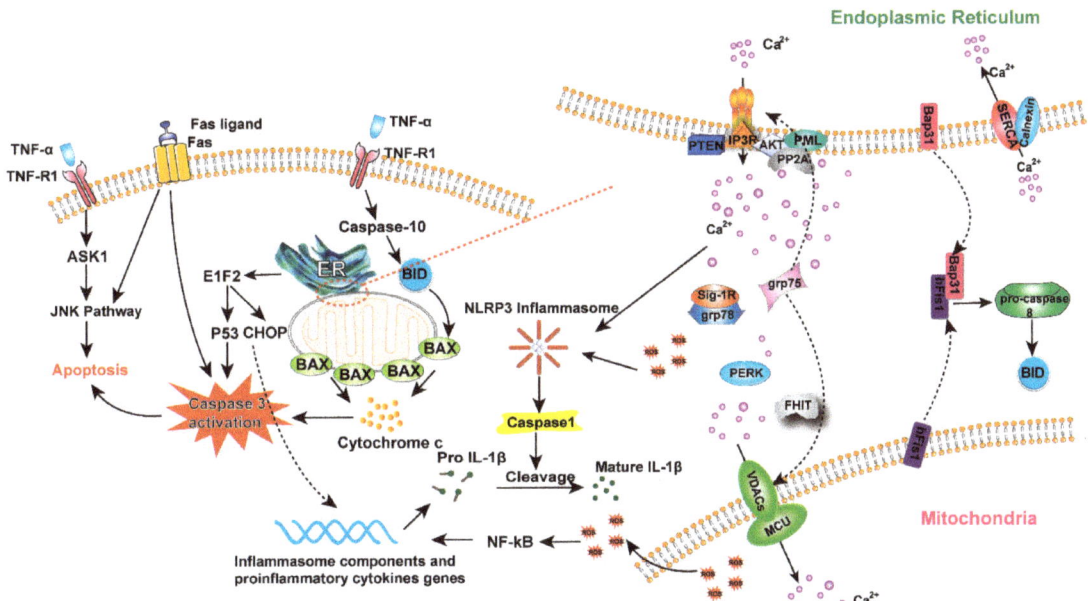

Figure 4. Apoptosis and inflammation regulation in oligodendrocytes (OLG) during DCM. (**Left**) Pathways for apoptosis and inflammation regulation in OLG. In DCM, TNF-α and Fas/FasL pathway and downstream caspase-3 induced apoptosis pathways can be activated. Inflammasome components and proinflammatory cytokines are elevated during the process. (**Right**) Magnification of the ER–mitochondria interactions. Several molecules in contact sites can regulate inflammasome activation, ROS accumulation, Ca^{2+} transfer and apoptosis.

A key regulator, phosphatase and tensin homolog (PTEN), regulates Ca^{2+} release from the ER. PTEN can counteract the inositol-1,4,5-trisphosphate receptors (IP3Rs)-induced Ca^{2+} release mediated by AKT phosphorylation [157]. Other chaperone proteins, like sigma-1 receptor (SIG1R)/GRP78, GRP75, fragile histidine triad diadenosine triphosphatase (FHIT) and protein kinase R (PKR)-like endoplasmic reticulum kinase (PERK) also participate in regulating the Ca^{2+} movement between cell members [158]. PTEN is considered to be a major negative regulator of neuronal regeneration in SCI [159]. The role of PTEN in DCM is still elusive, although studies in chronic demyelinating diseases show that PTEN is required during OLG development and repair and its inactivation may lead to loss of myelin and axon integrity [160].

7.7. Brain Reorganization

DCM not only displays an array of changes in the cervical spine, but also in the brain. Cortical and cerebellar abnormalities have been found in DCM patient [161–163]. The relationship between DCM and brain reorganisation has been shown by blood oxygenation level dependent functional MRI (fMRI) analysis. A study analysing changes in the volume of activation (VOA) between patients with DCM and healthy controls showed changes in VOA are associated with neurological status and can change after surgical decompression [164]. Metabolic profiles in brains were measured by proton MR spectroscopy in 21 DCM patients and 16 healthy volunteers and metabolite levels in the cerebellum were found to be significantly different between these cohorts (Figure 3D). Some of these metabolites, myo-inositol and choline across primary motor cortices, N-acetylaspartate (NAA; marker of neuronal integrity) and glutamate–glutamine in the left motor cortex, and myo-inositol and glutamate–glutamine in the cerebellum, were found to be significantly associated with postoperative clinical status [165]. These metabolic profile changes may arise due to brain reorganization in DCM.

8. Treatment

There is a lack of evidence to support a best treatment for patients with DCM. Often, the therapeutic options offered to a patient, regardless if they are surgical or not, depend more on their doctor's preference instead of strong scientific evidence to support one or another approach [166].

8.1. Non-Surgical Treatment

Classic papers described a poor prognosis for DCM (regardless of the type of treatment applied), and thus recommended a non-operative approach [51]. This includes physical therapy with strengthening of the muscles in the neck, back and pelvic girdle to improve gait and pain. Exercises aimed at improving proprioception and balance take a central place when it comes to non-operative measures to assist patients with this condition. Other methods such as heat packs and acupuncture are often used to alleviate the symptoms [51]. A 10-year prospective randomised study found there was no significant difference in outcomes or survival between a conservative and an operative treatment in patients with mild and moderate DCM [166]. A recent systematic review found lack of sufficient evidence to adequately assess the role of non-operative treatment in DCM and a clinically significant gain of function was not observed in the majority of patients following a structured non-operative treatment program [167].

In recent years, neuroactive drugs have shown a potential value for the treatment of DCM. Oestrogens have been found to inhibit glutamate induced apoptosis, by suppressing caspase-3 in neuronal cells [168]. However, some studies showed that tamoxifen, an oestrogen-receptor blocker, can inhibit ROS and lipid peroxidation after ischemia/hypoxia and has been used to treat SCI [169,170]. Riluzole has been demonstrated to alleviate neuropathic pain in DCM rodent model [124]. Pregabalin is a drug commonly used to control chronic neurogenic pain in various conditions. It was found to have a protective effect in OLG from glutamate-induced apoptosis [171]. Other molecules with well-known antioxidant effects like pyrrolidine dithiocarbamate and vitamin E have also shown to have protective effects in OLG against apoptosis [108]. Among them, pregabalin are most well studied in relieving DCM and showed low to moderate evidence for beneficial effects on some neuropathic symptoms [172].

8.2. Surgical Treatment

A posterior approach to decompress the spinal canal was the first procedure described in spine surgery. The relative ease of the approach and its reported clinical success made it a common surgery for pathologies such as disc herniations, abscesses and spinal tuberculosis. Eventually, it was used to decompress the cervical spinal cord. Often multilevel, it has shown mixed results over time, and importantly it has been shown to be associated with important complications. Post-laminectomy kyphosis has been described at high rates up to 47% according to some series [173]. The cervical spine transmits close to 1/3 of compressive loads through the vertebral bodies and 2/3 through the posterior elements [174]. Acknowledging this has led to a shift in surgeon's preference from decompression alone to decompression plus fusion [175]. Recent studies, including a small randomised controlled trial (RCT) have shown that in certain patients, i.e., those with preserved cervical lordosis, decompression alone could be as effective as decompression with fusion [176,177].

A common procedure used to treat DCM is the Anterior Cervical Decompression and Fusion (ACDF) surgery. This procedure has its roots in the realisation by surgeons that disc herniations needed to be removed for the neurological symptoms to improve. Several techniques described the debulking of a herniated disc from a posterior approach but often they would sacrifice nerve roots or require important mobilisation of the spinal cord, which carried severe consequences. With the first anterior approaches described during the second half of the 20th Century, decompression of the cervical spine from the front became a more suitable option and opened possibilities to address issues that were before impossible to take care of like sagittal alignment, cervical spondylosis and segmental instability. The first anterior discectomy/fusion surgeries were described in 1955 and 1958. The first series of cervical arthroplasties was reported in 1966, falling out of favour for some decades until regaining popularity in the 1990's. Although with modern techniques, the success rate has improved and risks have decreased, some series still report non-union at around 10% and ongoing pain in the same values, if not higher. Another issue with the anterior approach is its ineffectiveness to successfully address multilevel (more than 3) disease in DCM [178]. Advantages of the anterior approach are lower rates of surgical site infection, less postoperative pain and the possibility to address sagittal alignment. The rate of complications such as adjacent segment degeneration and subsidence are still unclear [179].

Laminoplasty is another popular technique, in which the laminae are cut and then moved and fixed in a new position to increase the space of the spinal cord. Proposed advantages of this technique include preservation of the native bone, and movement of the cervical spine and slower progression of myelopathy compared to laminectomy. These advantages, however, have not been shown unequivocally [180,181].

The goal with these procedures is to decompress the encroached spine. However, some issues related with these decompressions have been noticed. Nearly 10% of patients have shown worsening of neurological symptoms and almost half do not show neurologic improvement even six months after the decompression surgery [182]. Ischemia-reperfusion injury (IRI) has been identified as an important mechanism to explain these findings [183]. After blood flow returns to an ischemic spinal cord, a major cytokine release occurs. Cytokines released include TNF-α, CCL-2, CCL-3, CCL-5, CXCL1, IL-1β and IL-6; all of them are associated with a strong local immune response, with the oxidative and apoptotic damage that comes with it [184,185]. Although the exact mechanism remains unclear, several processes play a role, including leucocyte recruitment, cytokine cascades, microvessel endothelial damage and apoptosis [186]. Reperfusion to the site of compression and oxidative damage would explain acute and subacute neurological decline after surgery.

9. Future Directions

The lack of diagnostic tools that would enable the detection of DCM from its early stages indicates the need for new research in this area. fMRI and DTI are promising techniques, providing evidence of metabolic changes and microstructural tissue lesions that are impossible to detect with conventional MRI. There is also need for novel imaging techniques, such as diffusion MRI (dMRI), that can provide more information about microstructure. Further research into the molecular mechanisms of DCM is a must. Understanding the mechanisms seen in cervical IVD with those seen in the lumbar spine would be of great value to direct future therapies. The role of previously unsuspected components in the pathophysiology of the disease is just beginning to be elucidated. For instance, the effect of a person's unique microbiome profile and the inflammatory response it may have locally around the cervical spine and systemically may explain, at least partly, degenerative changes that could lead to DCM. Moreover, as a chronic condition, the profile of DCM biomarkers could help predict flare-ups of the disease, which could assist in choosing therapeutic alternatives better suited to each patient.

10. Conclusions

With an aging population, the incidence and prevalence of DCM will continue to increase. The economic burden will soar too, because DCM is a common cause of disability in the aged population. Surgical decompression, although unpredictable, continues to be a common treatment, even though it sometimes leads to worsening of symptoms. The pathophysiology of the disease is not completely understood, and several mechanisms have been postulated to explain it. The key for successfully treating DCM could be partly hidden in the huge array of interactions that take place and have been mentioned in our review. Understanding all the factors associated with this condition will undoubtedly shed some light on future treatment alternatives, not only for this condition, but for many other neurodegenerative conditions that may share similar pathways in their physiopathology.

Supplementary Materials: The following are available online at https://www.mdpi.com/2077-0383/10/6/1214/s1, Table S1: Normal range of motion of the cervical spine.

Author Contributions: J.T., J.V.C., A.D. and A.D.D. conceived and wrote the article. J.T. drew the figures. J.T. and J.V.C. created the tables. A.D. and A.D.D. provided critical feedback and revised the manuscript. J.T. and J.V.C. made an equal contribution. All authors read and approved the final manuscript.

Funding: The investigators are supported by grants from UNSW Sydney University International Postgraduate Award (UIPA) to J.T.; internal research funds from Spine Service (St. George Hospital Campus) to A.D.D. and A.D.; an unrestricted education and research donation form Nuvasive Australia to UNSW Spine Labs; fellowship training support from Globus Medical to J.V.C.

Institutional Review Board Statement: Not applicable.

Informed Consent Statement: Not applicable.

Data Availability Statement: Not applicable.

Acknowledgments: We would like to thank Zhaomin Zheng (Sun Yat-sen University) and Wentian Li (UNSW Sydney) for their feedback.

Conflicts of Interest: The authors declare no conflict of interest.

References

1. Tracy, J.A.; Bartleson, J.D. Cervical Spondylotic Myelopathy. *Neurologist* **2010**, *16*, 176–187. [CrossRef]
2. Emery, S.E.; Bohlman, H.H.; Bolesta, M.J.; Jones, P.K. Anterior Cervical Decompression and Arthrodesis for the Treatment of Cervical Spondylotic Myelopathy. Two to Seventeen-Year Follow-up. *J. Bone Jt. Surg. Am.* **1998**, *80*, 941–951. [CrossRef]
3. Badhiwala, J.H.; Ahuja, C.S.; Akbar, M.A.; Witiw, C.D.; Nassiri, F.; Furlan, J.C.; Curt, A.; Wilson, J.R.; Fehlings, M.G. Degenerative cervical myelopathy—Update and future directions. *Nat. Rev. Neurol.* **2020**, *16*, 108–124. [CrossRef]
4. Boden, S.D.; McCowin, P.R.; Davis, D.; Dina, T.S.; Mark, A.S.; Wiesel, S. Abnormal magnetic-resonance scans of the cervical spine in asymptomatic subjects. A prospective investigation. *J. Bone Jt. Surg. Am.* **1990**, *72*, 1178–1184. [CrossRef]
5. Nakashima, H.; Yukawa, Y.; Suda, K.; Yamagata, M.; Ueta, T.; Kato, F. Abnormal Findings on Magnetic Resonance Images of the Cervical Spines in 1211 Asymptomatic Subjects. *Spine* **2015**, *40*, 392–398. [CrossRef]
6. Fontes, R.B.D.V.; Baptista, J.S.; Rabbani, S.R.; Traynelis, V.C.; Liberti, E.A. Structural and Ultrastructural Analysis of the Cervical Discs of Young and Elderly Humans. *PLoS ONE* **2015**, *10*, e0139283. [CrossRef] [PubMed]
7. Kato, F.; Yukawa, Y.; Suda, K.; Yamagata, M.; Ueta, T. Normal morphology, age-related changes and abnormal findings of the cervical spine. Part II: Magnetic resonance imaging of over 1200 asymptomatic subjects. *Eur. Spine J.* **2012**, *21*, 1499–1507. [CrossRef] [PubMed]
8. Gibson, J.; Nouri, A.; Krueger, B.; Lakomkin, N.; Nasser, R.; Gimbel, D.; Cheng, J. Degenerative Cervical Myelopathy: A Clinical Review. *Yale J. Biol. Med.* **2018**, *91*, 43–48. [PubMed]
9. Boogaarts, H.D.; Bartels, R.H.M.A. Prevalence of cervical spondylotic myelopathy. *Eur. Spine J.* **2015**, *24* (Suppl. 2), 139–141. [CrossRef]
10. Jiang, H.; Wang, J.; Xu, B.; Yang, H.; Zhu, Q. A model of acute central cervical spinal cord injury syndrome combined with chronic injury in goats. *Eur. Spine J.* **2017**, *26*, 56–63. [CrossRef]
11. Tan, L.A.; Riew, K.D.; Traynelis, V.C. Cervical Spine Deformity—Part 2: Management Algorithm and Anterior Techniques. *Neurosurgery* **2017**, *81*, 561–567. [CrossRef] [PubMed]
12. Rhee, J.; Hamasaki, T.; Heflin, J.; Freedman, B. Prevalence of Physical Signs in Cervical Myelopathy: A Prospective Controlled Study. *Spine* **2009**, *34*, 890–895. [CrossRef] [PubMed]
13. Harrop, J.S.; Naroji, S.; Maltenfort, M.; Anderson, D.G.; Albert, T.; Ratliff, J.K.; Ponnappan, R.K.; Rihn, J.A.; Smith, H.E.; Hilibrand, A.; et al. Cervical myelopathy: A clinical and radiographic evaluation and correlation to cervical spondylotic myelopathy. *Spine* **2010**, *35*, 620–624. [CrossRef]
14. Tan, L.A.; Riew, K.D.; Traynelis, V.C. Cervical Spine Deformity—Part 1: Biomechanics, Radiographic Parameters, and Classification. *Neurosurgery* **2017**, *81*, 197–203. [CrossRef]
15. Lebl, D.R.; Hughes, A.; Cammisa, F.P., Jr.; O'Leary, P.F. Cervical Spondylotic Myelopathy: Pathophysiology, Clinical Presentation, and Treatment. *HSS J.* **2011**, *7*, 170–178. [CrossRef] [PubMed]

16. Acharya, S.; Srivastava, A.; Virmani, S.; Tandon, R. Resolution of Physical Signs and Recovery in Severe Cervical Spondylotic Myelopathy After Cervical Laminoplasty. *Spine* **2010**, *35*, E1083–E1087. [CrossRef] [PubMed]
17. Kalsi-Ryan, S.; Karadimas, S.K.; Fehlings, M.G. Cervical spondylotic myelopathy: The clinical phenomenon and the current pathobiology of an increasingly prevalent and devastating disorder. *Neuroscientist* **2013**, *19*, 409–421. [CrossRef]
18. Glaser, J.A.; Curé, J.K.; Bailey, K.L.; Morrow, D.L. Cervical spinal cord compression and the Hoffmann sign. *Iowa Orthop. J.* **2001**, *21*, 49–52.
19. Estanol, B.V.; Marin, O.S. Mechanism of the inverted supinator reflex. A clinical and neurophysiological study. *J. Neurol. Neurosurg. Psychiatry* **1976**, *39*, 905–908. [CrossRef]
20. Boyraz, I.; Uysal, H.; Koc, B.; Sarman, H. Clonus: Definition, mechanism, treatment. *Med. Glas. Zenica* **2015**, *12*, 19–26.
21. Lance, J.W. The Babinski sign. *J. Neurol. Neurosurg. Psychiatry* **2002**, *73*, 360–362. [CrossRef]
22. Bydon, A.; Ritzl, E.K.; Sciubba, D.M.; Witham, T.F.; Xu, R.; Sait, M.; Wolinsky, J.-P.; Gokaslan, Z.L. A role for motor and somatosensory evoked potentials during anterior cervical discectomy and fusion for patients without myelopathy: Analysis of 57 consecutive cases. *Surg. Neurol. Int.* **2011**, *2*, 133. [CrossRef] [PubMed]
23. Morishita, Y.; Hida, S.; Naito, M.; Matsushima, U. Evaluation of cervical spondylotic myelopathy using somatosensory-evoked potentials. *Int. Orthop.* **2005**, *29*, 343–346. [CrossRef]
24. Lyu, R.K.; Tang, L.M.; Chen, C.; Chang, H.S.; Wu, Y.R. The use of evoked potentials for clinical correlation and surgical outcome in cervical spondylotic myelopathy with intramedullary high signal intensity on MRI. *J. Neurol. Neurosurg. Psychiatry* **2004**, *75*, 256–261. [PubMed]
25. Lo, Y.L. How has electrophysiology changed the management of cervical spondylotic myelopathy? *Eur. J. Neurol.* **2008**, *15*, 781–786. [CrossRef] [PubMed]
26. Xing, R.; Zhou, G.; Chen, Q.; Liang, Y.; Dong, J. MRI to measure cervical sagittal parameters: A comparison with plain radiographs. *Arch. Orthop. Trauma Surg.* **2017**, *137*, 451–455. [CrossRef] [PubMed]
27. Scheer, J.K.; Tang, J.A.; Smith, J.S.; Acosta, F.L., Jr.; Protopsaltis, T.S.; Blondel, B.; Bess, S.; Shaffrey, C.I.; Deviren, V.; Lafage, V.; et al. Cervical spine alignment, sagittal deformity, and clinical implications: A review. *J. Neurosurg. Spine* **2013**, *19*, 141–159. [CrossRef] [PubMed]
28. Park, J.H.; Cho, C.B.; Song, J.H.; Kim, S.W.; Ha, Y.; Oh, J.K. T1 Slope and Cervical Sagittal Alignment on Cervical CT Radiographs of Asymptomatic Persons. *J. Korean Neurosurg. Soc.* **2013**, *53*, 356–359. [CrossRef] [PubMed]
29. Blease Graham, C.; Wippold, F.J.; Bae, K.T.; Pilgram, T.K.; Shaibani, A.; Kido, D.K. Comparison of CT myelography performed in the prone and supine positions in the detection of cervical spinal stenosis. *Clin. Radiol.* **2001**, *56*, 35–39. [CrossRef]
30. Abiola, R.; Rubery, P.; Mesfin, A. Ossification of the Posterior Longitudinal Ligament: Etiology, Diagnosis, and Outcomes of Nonoperative and Operative Management. *Glob. Spine J.* **2016**, *6*, 195–204. [CrossRef] [PubMed]
31. Modic, M.T.; Steinberg, P.M.; Ross, J.S.; Masaryk, T.J.; Carter, J.R. Degenerative disk disease: Assessment of changes in vertebral body marrow with MR imaging. *Radiology* **1988**, *166 (Pt 1)*, 193–199. [CrossRef]
32. Gao, X.; Li, J.; Shi, Y.; Li, S.; Shen, Y. Asymmetrical degenerative marrow (Modic) changes in cervical spine: Prevalence, correlative factors, and surgical outcomes. *J. Orthop. Surg. Res.* **2018**, *13*, 85. [CrossRef] [PubMed]
33. Mann, E.; Peterson, C.K.; Hodler, J.; Pfirrmann, C.W.A. The evolution of degenerative marrow (Modic) changes in the cervical spine in neck pain patients. *Eur. Spine J.* **2014**, *23*, 584–589. [CrossRef] [PubMed]
34. Yoshimatsu, H.; Nagata, K.; Goto, H.; Sonoda, K.; Ando, N.; Imoto, H.; Mashima, T.; Takamiya, Y. Conservative treatment for cervical spondylotic myelopathy. prediction of treatment effects by multivariate analysis. *Spine J.* **2001**, *1*, 269–273. [CrossRef]
35. Fehlings, M.G.; Rao, S.C.; Tator, C.H.; Skaf, G.; Arnold, P.; Benzel, E.; Dickman, C.; Cuddy, B.; Green, B.; Hitchon, P.; et al. The optimal radiologic method for assessing spinal canal compromise and cord compression in patients with cervical spinal cord injury. Part II: Results of a multicenter study. *Spine* **1999**, *24*, 605–613. [CrossRef]
36. Furlan, J.C.; Kailaya-Vasan, A.; Aarabi, B.; Fehlings, M.G. A Novel Approach to Quantitatively Assess Posttraumatic Cervical Spinal Canal Compromise and Spinal Cord Compression: A Multicenter Responsiveness Study. *Spine* **2011**, *36*, 784–793. [CrossRef] [PubMed]
37. Sritharan, K.; Chamoli, U.; Kuan, J.; Diwan, A.D. Assessment of degenerative cervical stenosis on T2-weighted MR imaging: Sensitivity to change and reliability of mid-sagittal and axial plane metrics. *Spinal Cord* **2020**, *58*, 238–246. [CrossRef] [PubMed]
38. Nouri, A.; Tetreault, L.; Côté, P.; Zamorano, J.J.; Dalzell, K.; Fehlings, M.G. Does Magnetic Resonance Imaging Improve the Predictive Performance of a Validated Clinical Prediction Rule Developed to Evaluate Surgical Outcome in Patients With Degenerative Cervical Myelopathy? *Spine* **2015**, *40*, 1092–1100. [CrossRef] [PubMed]
39. Zhang, L.; Zeitoun, D.; Rangel, A.; Lazennec, J.Y.; Catonné, Y.; Pascal-Moussellard, H. Preoperative evaluation of the cervical spondylotic myelopathy with flexion-extension magnetic resonance imaging: About a prospective study of fifty patients. *Spine* **2011**, *36*, E1134–E1139. [CrossRef]
40. Dalbayrak, S.; Yaman, O.; Firidin, M.N.; Yilmaz, T.; Yilmaz, M. The contribution of cervical dynamic magnetic resonance imaging to the surgical treatment of cervical spondylotic myelopathy. *Turk. Neurosurg.* **2015**, *25*, 36–42.
41. Rutman, A.M.; Peterson, D.J.; Cohen, W.A.; Mossa-Basha, M. Diffusion Tensor Imaging of the Spinal Cord: Clinical Value, Investigational Applications, and Technical Limitations. *Curr. Probl. Diagn. Radiol.* **2018**, *47*, 257–269. [CrossRef] [PubMed]

42. D'Avanzo, S.; Ciavarro, M.; Pavone, L.; Pasqua, G.; Ricciardi, F.; Bartolo, M.; Solari, D.; Somma, T.; De Divitiis, O.; Cappabianca, P.; et al. The Functional Relevance of Diffusion Tensor Imaging in Patients with Degenerative Cervical Myelopathy. *J. Clin. Med.* **2020**, *9*, 1828. [CrossRef]
43. Wang, K.; Zhu, S.; Mueller, B.; Lim, K.; Liu, Z.; He, B. A New Method to Derive White Matter Conductivity From Diffusion Tensor MRI. *IEEE Trans. Biomed. Eng.* **2008**, *55*, 2481–2486. [CrossRef]
44. Wang, K.; Chen, Z.; Zhang, F.; Song, Q.; Hou, C.; Tang, Y.; Wang, J.; Chen, S.; Bian, Y.; Hao, Q.; et al. Evaluation of DTI Parameter Ratios and Diffusion Tensor Tractography Grading in the Diagnosis and Prognosis Prediction of Cervical Spondylotic Myelopathy. *Spine* **2017**, *42*, E202–E210. [CrossRef] [PubMed]
45. Zhang, H.; Guan, L.; Hai, Y.; Liu, Y.; Ding, H.; Chen, X. Multi-shot echo-planar diffusion tensor imaging in cervical spondylotic myelopathy. *Bone Jt. J.* **2020**, *102-B*, 1210–1218. [CrossRef] [PubMed]
46. Dalitz, K.; Vitzthum, H.-E. Evaluation of five scoring systems for cervical spondylogenic myelopathy. *Spine J.* **2019**, *19*, e41–e46. [CrossRef]
47. Herdmann, J.; Linzbach, M.; Krzan, M. The European Myelopathy Score. In *Advances in Neurosurgery*; Baucher, B.L., Brock, M., Klinger, M., Eds.; Springer: Berlin, Germany, 1994.
48. Vitzthum, H.-E.; Dalitz, K. Analysis of five specific scores for cervical spondylogenic myelopathy. *Eur. Spine J.* **2007**, *16*, 2096–2103. [CrossRef]
49. Revanappa, K.K.; Rajshekhar, V. Comparison of Nurick grading system and modified Japanese Orthopaedic Association scoring system in evaluation of patients with cervical spondylotic myelopathy. *Eur. Spine J.* **2011**, *20*, 1545–1551. [CrossRef]
50. Clarke, E.; Robinson, P.K. Cervical myelopathy: A complication of cervical spondylosis. *Brain* **1956**, *79*, 483–510. [CrossRef]
51. Lees, F.; Turner, J.W. Natural history and prognosis of cervical spondylosis. *Br. Med. J.* **1963**, *2*, 1607–1610. [CrossRef]
52. Bednarik, J.; Sládková, D.; Kadaňka, Z.; Dušek, L.; Keřkovský, M.; Voháňka, S.; Novotný, O.; Urbánek, I.; Němec, M. Are subjects with spondylotic cervical cord encroachment at increased risk of cervical spinal cord injury after minor trauma? *J. Neurol. Neurosurg. Psychiatry* **2011**, *82*, 779–781. [CrossRef]
53. Katoh, S.; Ikata, T.; Hirai, N.; Okada, Y.; Nakauchi, K. Influence of minor trauma to the neck on the neurological outcome in patients with ossification of the posterior longitudinal ligament (OPLL) of the cervical spine. *Spinal Cord* **1995**, *33*, 330–333. [CrossRef] [PubMed]
54. Ichihara, K.; Taguchi, T.; Sakuramoto, I.; Kawano, S.; Kawai, S. Mechanism of the spinal cord injury and the cervical spondylotic myelopathy: New approach based on the mechanical features of the spinal cord white and gray matter. *J. Neurosurg.* **2003**, *99* (Suppl. 3), 278–285. [CrossRef]
55. Tanabe, F.; Yone, K.; Kawabata, N.; Sakakima, H.; Matsuda, F.; Ishidou, Y.; Maeda, S.; Abematsu, M.; Komiya, S.; Setoguchi, T. Accumulation of p62 in degenerated spinal cord under chronic mechanical compression: Functional analysis of p62 and autophagy in hypoxic neuronal cells. *Autophagy* **2011**, *7*, 1462–1471. [CrossRef] [PubMed]
56. Yu, W.R.; Liu, T.; Kiehl, T.-R.; Fehlings, M.G. Human neuropathological and animal model evidence supporting a role for Fas-mediated apoptosis and inflammation in cervical spondylotic myelopathy. *Brain* **2011**, *134 (Pt 5)*, 1277–1292. [CrossRef]
57. Morishita, Y.; Naito, M.; Hymanson, H.; Miyazaki, M.; Wu, G.; Wang, J.C. The relationship between the cervical spinal canal diameter and the pathological changes in the cervical spine. *Eur. Spine J.* **2009**, *18*, 877–883. [CrossRef] [PubMed]
58. Levine, D.N. Pathogenesis of cervical spondylotic myelopathy. *J. Neurol. Neurosurg. Psychiatry* **1997**, *62*, 334–340. [CrossRef] [PubMed]
59. Brain, W.R.; Knight, G.C.; Bull, J.W.D. Discussion on rupture of the intervertebral disc in the cervical region. *Proc. R. Soc. Med.* **1948**, *41*, 509–516. [PubMed]
60. Mair, W.G.P.; Druckman, R. The pathology of spinal cord lesions and their relation to the clinical features in protrusion of cervical intervertebral discs: A Report of Four Cases. *Brain* **1953**, *76*, 70–91. [CrossRef] [PubMed]
61. Gooding, M.R.; Wilson, C.B.; Hoff, J.T. Experimental cervical myelopathy. Effects of ischemia and compression of the canine cervical spinal cord. *J. Neurosurg.* **1975**, *43*, 9–17. [CrossRef]
62. Gooding, M.R.; Wilson, C.B.; Hoff, J.T. Experimental cervical myelopathy: Autoradiographic studies of spinal cord blood flow patterns. *Surg. Neurol.* **1976**, *5*, 233–239. [PubMed]
63. Kurokawa, R.; Murata, H.; Ogino, M.; Ueki, K.; Kim, P. Altered Blood Flow Distribution in the Rat Spinal Cord under Chronic Compression. *Spine* **2011**, *36*, 1006–1009. [CrossRef]
64. Smith, J.S.; Lafage, V.; Ryan, D.J.; Shaffrey, C.I.; Schwab, F.J.; Patel, A.A.; Brodke, D.S.; Arnold, P.M.; Riew, K.D.; Traynelis, V.C.; et al. Association of myelopathy scores with cervical sagittal balance and normalized spinal cord volume: Analysis of 56 preoperative cases from the AOSpine North America Myelopathy study. *Spine* **2013**, *38* (Suppl. 1), S161–S70. [CrossRef]
65. Ames, C.P.; Blondel, B.; Scheer, J.K.; Schwab, F.J.; Le Huec, J.C.; Massicotte, E.M.; Patel, A.A.; Traynelis, V.C.; Kim, H.J.; Shaffrey, C.I.; et al. Cervical radiographical alignment: Comprehensive assessment techniques and potential importance in cervical myelopathy. *Spine* **2013**, *38* (Suppl. 1), S149–S60. [CrossRef] [PubMed]
66. Goel, A. Role of Subaxial Spinal and Atlantoaxial Instability in Multisegmental Cervical Spondylotic Myelopathy. *Acta Neurochir. Suppl.* **2019**, *125*, 71–78. [CrossRef] [PubMed]
67. Goel, A.; Dhar, A.; Shah, A.; Jadhav, D.; Bakale, N.; Vaja, T.; Jadhav, N. Central or Axial Atlantoaxial Dislocation as a Cause of Cervical Myelopathy: A Report of Outcome of 5 Cases Treated by Atlantoaxial Stabilization. *World Neurosurg.* **2019**, *121*, e908–e916. [CrossRef]

68. Ohara, Y. Ossification of the Ligaments in the Cervical Spine, Including Ossification of the Anterior Longitudinal Ligament, Ossification of the Posterior Longitudinal Ligament, and Ossification of the Ligamentum Flavum. *Neurosurg. Clin. N. Am.* **2018**, *29*, 63–68. [CrossRef]
69. Matsunaga, S.; Sakou, T. Ossification of the posterior longitudinal ligament of the cervical spine: Etiology and natural history. *Spine* **2012**, *37*, E309–E314. [CrossRef]
70. McAfee, P.C.; Regan, J.J.; Bohlman, H.H. Cervical cord compression from ossification of the posterior longitudinal ligament in non-orientals. *J. Bone Jt. Surg. Br.* **1987**, *69*, 569–575. [CrossRef]
71. Li, H.; Jiang, L.S.; Dai, L.Y. Hormones and growth factors in the pathogenesis of spinal ligament ossification. *Eur. Spine J.* **2007**, *16*, 1075–1084. [CrossRef]
72. Kato, Y.; Kanchiku, T.; Imajo, Y.; Kimura, K.; Ichihara, K.; Kawano, S.; Hamanaka, D.; Yaji, K.; Taguchi, T. Biomechanical study of the effect of degree of static compression of the spinal cord in ossification of the posterior longitudinal ligament. *J. Neurosurg. Spine* **2010**, *12*, 301–305. [CrossRef]
73. Takahashi, K.; Ozawa, H.; Sakamoto, N.; Minegishi, Y.; Sato, M.; Itoi, E. Influence of intramedullary stress on cervical spondylotic myelopathy. *Spinal Cord* **2013**, *51*, 761–764. [CrossRef]
74. Kato, Y.; Kataoka, H.; Ichihara, K.; Imajo, Y.; Kojima, T.; Kawano, S.; Hamanaka, D.; Yaji, K.; Taguchi, T. Biomechanical study of cervical flexion myelopathy using a three-dimensional finite element method. *J. Neurosurg. Spine* **2008**, *8*, 436–441. [CrossRef]
75. Nagata, K.; Yoshimura, N.; Muraki, S.; Hashizume, H.; Ishimoto, Y.; Yamada, H.; Takiguchi, N.; Nakagawa, Y.; Oka, H.; Kawaguchi, H.; et al. Prevalence of cervical cord compression and its association with physical performance in a population-based cohort in Japan: The Wakayama Spine Study. *Spine* **2012**, *37*, 1892–1898. [CrossRef]
76. Davies, B.M.; Mowforth, O.D.; Smith, E.K.; Kotter, M.R. Degenerative cervical myelopathy. *BMJ* **2018**, *360*, k186. [CrossRef]
77. Okada, E.; Matsumoto, M.; Ichihara, D.; Chiba, K.; Toyama, Y.; Fujiwara, H.; Momoshima, S.; Nishiwaki, Y.; Hashimoto, T.; Ogawa, J.; et al. Aging of the cervical spine in healthy volunteers: A 10-year longitudinal magnetic resonance imaging study. *Spine* **2009**, *34*, 706–712. [CrossRef] [PubMed]
78. Tang, R.; Ye, I.B.; Cheung, Z.B.; Kim, J.S.; Cho, S.K. Age-related Changes in Cervical Sagittal Alignment: A Radiographic Analysis. *Spine* **2019**, *44*, E1144–E1150. [CrossRef] [PubMed]
79. Bull, J.; El Gammal, T.; Popham, M. A possible genetic factor in cervical spondylosis. *Br. J. Radiol.* **1969**, *42*, 9–16. [CrossRef] [PubMed]
80. Patel, A.A.; Spiker, W.R.; Daubs, M.; Brodke, D.S.; Cannon-Albright, L.A. Evidence of an Inherited Predisposition for Cervical Spondylotic Myelopathy. *Spine* **2012**, *37*, 26–29. [CrossRef] [PubMed]
81. Abode-Iyamah, K.O.; Stoner, K.E.; Grossbach, A.J.; Viljoen, S.V.; McHenry, C.L.; Petrie, M.A.; Dahdaleh, N.S.; Grosland, N.M.; Shields, R.K.; Howard, M.A.; et al. Effects of brain derived neurotrophic factor Val66Met polymorphism in patients with cervical spondylotic myelopathy. *J. Clin. Neurosci.* **2016**, *24*, 117–121. [CrossRef]
82. Yu, H.-M.; Chen, X.-L.; Wei, W.; Yao, X.-D.; Sun, J.-Q.; Su, X.-T.; Lin, S.-F. Effect of osteoprotegerin gene polymorphisms on the risk of cervical spondylotic myelopathy in a Chinese population. *Clin. Neurol. Neurosurg.* **2018**, *175*, 149–154. [CrossRef] [PubMed]
83. Wu, J.; Wu, N.; Guo, K.; Yuan, F.; Ran, B. OPN Polymorphism is Associated with the Susceptibility to Cervical Spondylotic Myelopathy and its Outcome After Anterior Cervical Corpectomy and Fusion. *Cell. Physiol. Biochem.* **2014**, *34*, 565–574. [CrossRef] [PubMed]
84. Wang, Z.-C.; Hou, X.-W.; Shao, J.; Ji, Y.-J.; Li, L.; Zhou, Q.; Yu, S.-M.; Mao, Y.-L.; Zhang, H.-J.; Zhang, P.-C.; et al. HIF-1α Polymorphism in the Susceptibility of Cervical Spondylotic Myelopathy and Its Outcome after Anterior Cervical Corpectomy and Fusion Treatment. *PLoS ONE* **2014**, *9*, e110862. [CrossRef]
85. Setzer, M.; Hermann, E.; Seifert, V.; Marquardt, G. Apolipoprotein E Gene Polymorphism and the Risk of Cervical Myelopathy in Patients With Chronic Spinal Cord Compression. *Spine* **2008**, *33*, 497–502. [CrossRef]
86. Setzer, M.; Vrionis, F.D.; Hermann, E.J.; Seifert, V.; Marquardt, G. Effect of apolipoprotein E genotype on the outcome after anterior cervical decompression and fusion in patients with cervical spondylotic myelopathy. *J. Neurosurg. Spine* **2009**, *11*, 659–666. [CrossRef] [PubMed]
87. Ren, Y.; Feng, J.; Liu, Z.-Z.; Wan, H.; Li, J.-H.; Lin, X. A new haplotype in BMP4 implicated in ossification of the posterior longitudinal ligament (OPLL) in a Chinese population. *J. Orthop. Res.* **2012**, *30*, 748–756. [CrossRef]
88. Ren, Y.; Liu, Z.-Z.; Feng, J.; Wan, H.; Li, J.-H.; Wang, H.; Lin, X. Association of a BMP9 Haplotype with Ossification of the Posterior Longitudinal Ligament (OPLL) in a Chinese Population. *PLoS ONE* **2012**, *7*, e40587. [CrossRef]
89. Liu, Y.; Zhao, Y.; Chen, Y.; Shi, G.; Yuan, W. RUNX2 Polymorphisms Associated with OPLL and OLF in the Han Population. *Clin. Orthop. Relat. Res.* **2010**, *468*, 3333–3341. [CrossRef] [PubMed]
90. Wang, H.; Liu, D.; Yang, Z.; Tian, B.; Li, J.; Meng, X.; Wang, Z.; Yang, H.; Lin, X. Association of bone morphogenetic protein-2 gene polymorphisms with susceptibility to ossification of the posterior longitudinal ligament of the spine and its severity in Chinese patients. *Eur. Spine J.* **2008**, *17*, 956–964. [CrossRef] [PubMed]
91. Song, D.W.; Wu, Y.D.; Tian, D.D. Association of VDR-FokI and VDBP-Thr420Lys polymorphisms with cervical spondylotic myelopathy: A case-control study in the population of China. *J. Clin. Lab. Anal.* **2019**, *33*, e22669. [CrossRef] [PubMed]
92. Wang, Z.; Shi, J.; Chen, X.; Xu, G.; Li, L.; Jia, L. The role of smoking status and collagen IX polymorphisms in the susceptibility to cervical spondylotic myelopathy. *Genet. Mol. Res.* **2012**, *11*, 1238–1244. [CrossRef] [PubMed]

93. Maeda, S.; Ishidou, Y.; Koga, H.; Taketomi, E.; Ikari, K.; Komiya, S.; Takeda, J.; Sakou, T.; Inoue, I. Functional Impact of Human Collagen α2(XI) Gene Polymorphism in Pathogenesis of Ossification of the Posterior Longitudinal Ligament of the Spine. *J. Bone Miner. Res.* **2001**, *16*, 948–957. [CrossRef]
94. Chen, Y.; Wang, X.; Zhang, X.; Ren, H.; Huang, B.; Chen, J.; Liu, J.; Shan, Z.; Zhu, Z.; Zhao, F. Low virulence bacterial infections in cervical intervertebral discs: A prospective case series. *Eur. Spine J.* **2018**, *27*, 2496–2505. [CrossRef] [PubMed]
95. Bivona, L.J.; Camacho, J.E.; Usmani, F.; Nash, A.; Bruckner, J.J.; Hughes, M.; Bhandutia, A.K.; Koh, E.Y.; Banagan, K.E.; Gelb, D.E.; et al. The Prevalence of Bacterial Infection in Patients Undergoing Elective ACDF for Degenerative Cervical Spine Conditions: A Prospective Cohort Study With Contaminant Control. *Glob. Spine J.* **2021**, *11*, 13–20. [CrossRef] [PubMed]
96. Rajasekaran, S.; Soundararajan, D.C.R.; Tangavel, C.; Muthurajan, R.; Anand, K.S.S.V.; Matchado, M.S.; Nayagam, S.M.; Shetty, A.P.; Kanna, R.M.; Dharmalingam, K. Human intervertebral discs harbour a unique microbiome and dysbiosis determines health and disease. *Eur. Spine J.* **2020**, *29*, 1621–1640. [CrossRef]
97. Nakashima, H.; Yukawa, Y.; Suda, K.; Yamagata, M.; Ueta, T.; Kato, F. Cervical Disc Protrusion Correlates With the Severity of Cervical Disc Degeneration: A Cross-Sectional Study of 1211 Relatively Healthy Volunteers. *Spine* **2015**, *40*, E774-9. [CrossRef] [PubMed]
98. Scott, J.E.; Bosworth, T.R.; Cribb, A.M.; Taylor, J.R. The chemical morphology of age-related changes in human intervertebral disc glycosaminoglycans from cervical, thoracic and lumbar nucleus pulposus and annulus fibrosus. *J. Anat.* **1994**, *184 (Pt 1)*, 73–82.
99. Zhu, W.; Sha, S.; Liu, Z.; Li, Y.; Xu, L.; Zhang, W.; Qiu, Y.; Zhu, Z. Influence of the Occipital Orientation on Cervical Sagittal Alignment: A Prospective Radiographic Study on 335 Normal Subjects. *Sci. Rep.* **2018**, *8*, 15336. [CrossRef]
100. Kumaresan, S.; Yoganandan, N.; Pintar, F.A.; Maiman, D.J.; Goel, V.K. Contribution of disc degeneration to osteophyte formation in the cervical spine: A biomechanical investigation. *J. Orthop. Res.* **2001**, *19*, 977–984. [CrossRef]
101. Friedenberg, Z.B.; Miller, W.T. Degenerative disc disease of the cervical spine. *J. Bone Jt. Surg. Am.* **1963**, *45*, 1171–1178. [CrossRef]
102. Kartha, S.; Zeeman, M.E.; Baig, H.A.; Guarino, B.B.; Winkelstein, B.A. Upregulation of BDNF and NGF in Cervical Intervertebral Discs Exposed to Painful Whole-Body Vibration. *Spine* **2014**, *39*, 1542–1548. [CrossRef] [PubMed]
103. Sitte, I.; Klosterhuber, M.; Lindtner, R.A.; Freund, M.C.; Neururer, S.B.; Pfaller, K.; Kathrein, A. Morphological changes in the human cervical intervertebral disc post trauma: Response to fracture-type and degeneration grade over time. *Eur. Spine J.* **2016**, *25*, 80–95. [CrossRef]
104. Kepler, C.K.; Ponnappan, R.K.; Tannoury, C.A.; Risbud, M.V.; Anderson, D.G. The molecular basis of intervertebral disc degeneration. *Spine J.* **2013**, *13*, 318–330. [CrossRef] [PubMed]
105. Song, Y.; Li, S.; Geng, W.; Luo, R.; Liu, W.; Tu, J.; Wang, K.; Kang, L.; Yin, H.; Wu, X.; et al. Sirtuin 3-dependent mitochondrial redox homeostasis protects against AGEs-induced intervertebral disc degeneration. *Redox Biol.* **2018**, *19*, 339–353. [CrossRef] [PubMed]
106. Molinos, M.; Almeida, C.R.; Caldeira, J.; Cunha, C.; Gonçalves, R.M.; Barbosa, M.A. Inflammation in intervertebral disc degeneration and regeneration. *J. R. Soc. Interface* **2015**, *12*, 20141191. [CrossRef]
107. Bartanusz, V.; Jezova, D.; Alajajian, B.; Digicaylioglu, M. The blood-spinal cord barrier: Morphology and Clinical Implications. *Ann. Neurol.* **2011**, *70*, 194–206. [CrossRef]
108. Lev, N.; Gilgun-Sherki, Y.; Offen, D.; Melamed, E. Chapter 13—The Role of Oxidative Stress in the Pathogenesis of Multiple Sclerosis: Current State. In *Oxidative Stress and Neurodegenerative Disorders*; Qureshi, G.A., Parvez, S.H., Eds.; Elsevier Science B.V.: Amsterdam, The Netherlands, 2007; pp. 283–295.
109. Maikos, J.T.; Shreiber, D.I. Immediate Damage to The Blood-Spinal Cord Barrier Due to Mechanical Trauma. *J. Neurotrauma* **2007**, *24*, 492–507. [CrossRef]
110. Cohen, D.M.; Patel, C.B.; Ahobila-Vajjula, P.; Sundberg, L.M.; Chacko, T.; Liu, S.-J.; Narayana, P.A. Blood-spinal cord barrier permeability in experimental spinal cord injury: Dynamic contrast-enhanced MRI. *NMR Biomed.* **2009**, *22*, 332–341. [CrossRef]
111. Tian, D.-S.; Liu, J.-L.; Xie, M.-J.; Zhan, Y.; Qu, W.-S.; Yu, Z.-Y.; Tang, Z.-P.; Pan, D.-J.; Wang, W. Tamoxifen attenuates inflammatory-mediated damage and improves functional outcome after spinal cord injury in rats. *J. Neurochem.* **2009**, *109*, 1658–1667. [CrossRef] [PubMed]
112. Blume, C.; Geiger, M.F.; Brandenburg, L.O.; Müller, M.; Mainz, V.; Kalder, J.; Albanna, W.; Clusmann, H.; Mueller, C.A. Patients with degenerative cervical myelopathy have signs of blood spinal cord barrier disruption, and its magnitude correlates with myelopathy severity: A prospective comparative cohort study. *Eur. Spine J.* **2020**, *29*, 986–993. [CrossRef] [PubMed]
113. Tachibana, N.; Oichi, T.; Kato, S.; Sato, D.; Hasebe, H.; Hirai, S.; Taniguchi, Y.; Matsubayashi, Y.; Mori, H.; Tanaka, S.; et al. Spinal cord swelling in patients with cervical compression myelopathy. *BMC Musculoskelet. Disord.* **2019**, *20*, 284. [CrossRef]
114. Oklinski, M.K.; Lim, J.-S.; Choi, H.-J.; Oklinska, P.; Skowronski, M.T.; Kwon, T.-H. Immunolocalization of Water Channel Proteins AQP1 and AQP4 in Rat Spinal Cord. *J. Histochem. Cytochem.* **2014**, *62*, 598–611. [CrossRef] [PubMed]
115. Dhillon, R.S.; Parker, J.; Syed, Y.A.; Edgley, S.A.; Young, A.; Fawcett, J.W.; Jeffery, N.D.; Franklin, R.J.M.; Kotter, M.R. Axonal plasticity underpins the functional recovery following surgical decompression in a rat model of cervical spondylotic myelopathy. *Acta Neuropathol. Commun.* **2016**, *4*, 89. [CrossRef] [PubMed]
116. Salvadores, N.; Sanhueza, M.; Manque, P.; Court, F.A. Axonal Degeneration during Aging and Its Functional Role in Neurodegenerative Disorders. *Front. Neurosci.* **2017**, *11*, 451. [CrossRef]
117. Adalbert, R.; Coleman, M.P. Review: Axon pathology in age-related neurodegenerative disorders. *Neuropathol. Appl. Neurobiol.* **2013**, *39*, 90–108. [CrossRef]

118. Deckwerth, T.L.; Johnson, E.M. Neurites Can Remain Viable after Destruction of the Neuronal Soma by Programmed Cell Death (Apoptosis). *Dev. Biol.* **1994**, *165*, 63–72. [CrossRef] [PubMed]
119. Blackburn, D.; Sargsyan, S.; Monk, P.N.; Shaw, P.J. Astrocyte function and role in motor neuron disease: A future therapeutic target? *Glia* **2009**, *57*, 1251–1264. [CrossRef]
120. Anderson, M.A.; Burda, J.E.; Ren, Y.; Ao, Y.; O'Shea, T.M.; Kawaguchi, R.; Coppola, R.K.G.; Khakh, B.S.; Deming, T.J. Astrocyte scar formation aids central nervous system axon regeneration. *Nature* **2016**, *532*, 195–200. [CrossRef]
121. Chung, W.-S.; Clarke, L.E.; Wang, G.X.; Stafford, B.K.; Sher, A.; Chakraborty, C.; Joung, J.; Foo, L.C.; Thompson, A.; Chen, C.; et al. Astrocytes mediate synapse elimination through MEGF10 and MERTK pathways. *Nature* **2013**, *504*, 394–400. [CrossRef]
122. Song, I.; Dityatev, A. Crosstalk between glia, extracellular matrix and neurons. *Brain Res. Bull.* **2018**, *136*, 101–108. [CrossRef]
123. Yovich, J.V.; Gould, D.H.; LeCouteur, R. Chronic cervical compressive myelopathy in horses: Patterns of astrocytosis in the spinal cord. *Aust. Vet. J.* **1991**, *68*, 334. [CrossRef]
124. Moon, E.S.; Karadimas, S.K.; Yu, W.-R.; Austin, J.W.; Fehlings, M.G. Riluzole attenuates neuropathic pain and enhances functional recovery in a rodent model of cervical spondylotic myelopathy. *Neurobiol. Dis.* **2014**, *62*, 394–406. [CrossRef]
125. Ozawa, H.; Wu, Z.J.; Tanaka, Y.; Kokubun, S. Morphologic Change and Astrocyte Response to Unilateral Spinal Cord Compression in Rabbits. *J. Neurotrauma* **2004**, *21*, 944–955. [CrossRef]
126. Liddelow, S.A.; Barres, B.A. Reactive Astrocytes: Production, Function, and Therapeutic Potential. *Immunity* **2017**, *46*, 957–967. [CrossRef] [PubMed]
127. Vidal, P.M.; Karadimas, S.K.; Ulndreaj, A.; Laliberte, A.M.; Tetreault, L.; Forner, S.; Wang, J.; Foltz, W.D.; Fehlings, M.G. Delayed decompression exacerbates ischemia-reperfusion injury in cervical compressive myelopathy. *JCI Insight* **2017**, *2*, 11. [CrossRef] [PubMed]
128. Liu, T.; Han, Q.; Chen, G.; Huang, Y.; Zhao, L.-X.; Berta, T.; Gao, Y.-J.; Qingjian, H. Toll-like receptor 4 contributes to chronic itch, alloknesis, and spinal astrocyte activation in male mice. *Pain* **2016**, *157*, 806–817. [CrossRef]
129. Putatunda, R.; Hala, T.J.; Chin, J.; Lepore, A.C. Chronic at-level thermal hyperalgesia following rat cervical contusion spinal cord injury is accompanied by neuronal and astrocyte activation and loss of the astrocyte glutamate transporter, GLT1, in superficial dorsal horn. *Brain Res.* **2014**, *1581*, 64–79. [CrossRef] [PubMed]
130. David, S.; Kroner, A. Repertoire of microglial and macrophage responses after spinal cord injury. *Nat. Rev. Neurosci.* **2011**, *12*, 388–399. [CrossRef]
131. Fleming, J.C.; Norenberg, M.D.; Ramsay, D.A.; Dekaban, G.A.; Marcillo, A.E.; Saenz, A.D.; Pasquale-Styles, M.; Dietrich, W.D.; Weaver, L.C. The cellular inflammatory response in human spinal cords after injury. *Brain* **2006**, *129*, 3249–3269. [CrossRef]
132. Harrison, J.K.; Jiang, Y.; Chen, S.; Xia, Y.; Maciejewski, D.; McNamara, R.K.; Streit, W.J.; Salafranca, M.N.; Adhikari, S.; Thompson, D.A.; et al. Role for neuronally derived fractalkine in mediating interactions between neurons and CX3CR1-expressing microglia. *Proc. Natl. Acad. Sci. USA* **1998**, *95*, 10896–10901. [CrossRef]
133. Yamaura, I.; Yone, K.; Nakahara, S.; Nagamine, T.; Baba, H.; Uchida, K.; Komiya, S. Mechanism of Destructive Pathologic Changes in the Spinal Cord Under Chronic Mechanical Compression. *Spine* **2002**, *27*, 21–26. [CrossRef] [PubMed]
134. Fumagalli, S.; Perego, C.; Ortolano, F.; De Simoni, M.-G. CX3CR1 deficiency induces an early protective inflammatory environment in ischemic mice. *Glia* **2013**, *61*, 827–842. [CrossRef] [PubMed]
135. Tang, Z.; Gan, Y.; Liu, Q.; Yin, J.-X.; Liu, Q.; Shi, J.; Shi, F.-D. CX3CR1 deficiency suppresses activation and neurotoxicity of microglia/macrophage in experimental ischemic stroke. *J. Neuroinflamm.* **2014**, *11*, 26. [CrossRef] [PubMed]
136. Tsuda, M. Microglia in the spinal cord and neuropathic pain. *J. Diabetes Investig.* **2016**, *7*, 17–26. [CrossRef] [PubMed]
137. Gwak, Y.S.; Hulsebosch, C.E. Remote astrocytic and microglial activation modulates neuronal hyperexcitability and below-level neuropathic pain after spinal injury in rat. *Neuroscience* **2009**, *161*, 895–903. [CrossRef]
138. Juurlink, B.H.J.; Thorburne, S.K.; Hertz, L. Peroxide-scavenging deficit underlies oligodendrocyte susceptibility to oxidative stress. *Glia* **1998**, *22*, 371–378. [CrossRef]
139. Bai, L.; Lennon, D.P.; Caplan, A.I.; DeChant, A.; Hecker, J.; Kranso, J.; Zaremba, A.; Miller, R.H. Hepatocyte growth factor mediates mesenchymal stem cell–induced recovery in multiple sclerosis models. *Nat. Neurosci.* **2012**, *15*, 862–870. [CrossRef]
140. Kim, B.S.; Jin, Y.-H.; Meng, L.; Hou, W.; Kang, H.S.; Park, H.S.; Koh, C.-S. IL-1 signal affects both protection and pathogenesis of virus-induced chronic CNS demyelinating disease. *J. Neuroinflamm.* **2012**, *9*, 217. [CrossRef] [PubMed]
141. Giacoppo, S.; Galuppo, M.; Iori, R.; De Nicola, G.R.; Cassata, G.; Bramanti, P.; Mazzon, E. Protective Role of (RS)-glucoraphanin Bioactivated with Myrosinase in an Experimental Model of Multiple Sclerosis. *CNS Neurosci. Ther.* **2013**, *19*, 577–584. [CrossRef] [PubMed]
142. Huang, S.-Q.; Tang, C.-L.; Sun, S.-Q.; Yang, C.; Xu, J.; Wang, K.-J.; Lu, W.-T.; Huang, J.; Zhuo, F.; Qiu, G.-P.; et al. Demyelination Initiated by Oligodendrocyte Apoptosis through Enhancing Endoplasmic Reticulum–Mitochondria Interactions and Id2 Expression after Compressed Spinal Cord Injury in Rats. *CNS Neurosci. Ther.* **2014**, *20*, 20–31. [CrossRef]
143. McGavern, D.B.; Murray, P.D.; Rodriguez, M. Quantitation of spinal cord demyelination, remyelination, atrophy, and axonal loss in a model of progressive neurologic injury. *J. Neurosci. Res.* **1999**, *58*, 492–504. [CrossRef]
144. Lassmann, H.; Bradl, M. Multiple sclerosis: Experimental models and reality. *Acta Neuropathol.* **2017**, *133*, 223–244. [CrossRef] [PubMed]

145. Ackery, A.; Robins, S.; Fehlings, M.G. Inhibition of Fas-Mediated Apoptosis through Administration of Soluble Fas Receptor Improves Functional Outcome and Reduces Posttraumatic Axonal Degeneration after Acute Spinal Cord Injury. *J. Neurotrauma* **2006**, *23*, 604–616. [CrossRef] [PubMed]
146. Emery, E.; Aldana, P.; Bunge, M.B.; Puckett, W.; Srinivasan, A.; Keane, R.W.; Bethea, J.; Levi, A.D.O. Apoptosis after traumatic human spinal cord injury. *J. Neurosurg.* **1998**, *89*, 911–920. [CrossRef]
147. Liu, H.; MacMillian, E.L.; Jutzeler, C.R.; Ljungberg, E.; MacKay, A.L.; Kolind, S.H.; Mädler, B.; Li, D.K.B.; Dvorak, M.F.; Curt, A.; et al. Assessing structure and function of myelin in cervical spondylotic myelopathy: Evidence of demyelination. *Neurology* **2017**, *89*, 602–610. [CrossRef] [PubMed]
148. Ma, L.; Yu, H.-J.; Gan, S.-W.; Gong, R.; Mou, K.-J.; Xue, J.; Sun, S.-Q. p53-Mediated oligodendrocyte apoptosis initiates demyelination after compressed spinal cord injury by enhancing ER-mitochondria interaction and E2F1 expression. *Neurosci. Lett.* **2017**, *644*, 55–61. [CrossRef] [PubMed]
149. Iwasawa, R.; Mahul-Mellier, A.-L.; Datler, C.; Pazarentzos, E.; Grimm, S. Fis1 and Bap31 bridge the mitochondria-ER interface to establish a platform for apoptosis induction. *EMBO J.* **2011**, *30*, 556–568. [CrossRef]
150. Palam, L.R.; Baird, T.D.; Wek, R.C. Phosphorylation of eIF2 Facilitates Ribosomal Bypass of an Inhibitory Upstream ORF to Enhance CHOP Translation. *J. Biol. Chem.* **2011**, *286*, 10939–10949. [CrossRef]
151. Lebeaupin, C.; Proics, E.; De Bieville, C.H.D.; Rousseau, D.; Bonnafous, S.; Patouraux, S.; Adam, G.; Lavallard, V.J.; Rovere, C.; Le Thuc, O.; et al. ER stress induces NLRP3 inflammasome activation and hepatocyte death. *Cell Death Dis.* **2015**, *6*, e1879. [CrossRef]
152. Lee, Y.B.; Yune, T.Y.; Baik, S.Y.; Shin, Y.H.; Dua, S.; Rhimb, H.; Lee, E.B.; Kim, Y.C.; Shin, M.L.; Markelonis, G.J.; et al. Role of Tumor Necrosis Factor-α in Neuronal and Glial Apoptosis after Spinal Cord Injury. *Exp. Neurol.* **2000**, *166*, 190–195. [CrossRef]
153. Takenouchi, T.; Setoguchi, T.; Yone, K.; Komiya, S. Expression of apoptosis signal-regulating kinase 1 in mouse spinal cord under chronic mechanical compression: Possible involvement of the stress-activated mitogen-activated protein kinase pathways in spinal cord cell apoptosis. *Spine* **2008**, *33*, 1943–1950. [CrossRef]
154. Ye, P.; Kollias, G.; D'Ercole, A.J. Insulin-like growth factor-I ameliorates demyelination induced by tumor necrosis factor-α in transgenic mice. *J. Neurosci. Res.* **2007**, *85*, 712–722. [CrossRef] [PubMed]
155. Walsh, J.G.; Muruve, D.A.; Power, C. Inflammasomes in the CNS. *Nat. Rev. Neurosci.* **2014**, *15*, 84–97. [CrossRef]
156. Abais, J.M.; Xia, M.; Zhang, Y.; Boini, K.M.; Li, P.-L. Redox Regulation of NLRP3 Inflammasomes: ROS as Trigger or Effector? *Antioxid. Redox Signal.* **2015**, *22*, 1111–1129. [CrossRef]
157. Bononi, A.; Pinton, P. Study of PTEN subcellular localization. *Methods* **2015**, *77–78*, 92–103. [CrossRef] [PubMed]
158. Ouyang, Y.-B.; Giffard, R.G. ER-Mitochondria Crosstalk during Cerebral Ischemia: Molecular Chaperones and ER-Mitochondrial Calcium Transfer. *Int. J. Cell Biol.* **2012**, *2012*, 493934. [CrossRef] [PubMed]
159. Goncalves, M.B.; Malmqvist, T.; Clarke, E.; Hubens, C.J.; Grist, J.; Hobbs, C.; Trigo, D.; Risling, M.; Angeria, M.; Damberg, P.; et al. Neuronal RARβ Signaling Modulates PTEN Activity Directly in Neurons and via Exosome Transfer in Astrocytes to Prevent Glial Scar Formation and Induce Spinal Cord Regeneration. *J. Neurosci.* **2015**, *35*, 15731–15745. [CrossRef]
160. Harrington, E.P.; Zhao, C.; Fancy, S.P.; Kaing, S.; Franklin, R.J.; Rowitch, D.H. Oligodendrocyte PTEN is required for myelin and axonal integrity, not remyelination. *Ann. Neurol.* **2010**, *68*, 703–716. [CrossRef] [PubMed]
161. Dong, Y.; Holly, L.T.; Albistegui-DuBois, R.; Yan, X.; Marehbian, J.; Newton, J.M.; Dobkin, B.H. Compensatory cerebral adaptations before and evolving changes after surgical decompression in cervical spondylotic myelopathy. *J. Neurosurg. Spine* **2008**, *9*, 538–551. [CrossRef]
162. Tam, S.; Barry, R.L.; Bartha, R.; Duggal, N. Changes in functional magnetic resonance imaging cortical activation after decompression of cervical spondylosis: Case report. *Neurosurgery* **2010**, *67*, E863-4, Discussion E864. [CrossRef]
163. Holly, L.T.; Dong, Y.; Albistegui-DuBois, R.; Marehbian, J.; Dobkin, B. Cortical reorganization in patients with cervical spondylotic myelopathy. *J. Neurosurg. Spine* **2007**, *6*, 544–551. [CrossRef]
164. Duggal, N.; Rabin, D.; Bartha, R.; Barry, R.L.; Gati, J.S.; Kowalczyk, I.; Fink, M. Brain reorganization in patients with spinal cord compression evaluated using fMRI. *Neurology* **2010**, *74*, 1048–1054. [CrossRef] [PubMed]
165. Craciunas, S.C.; Gorgan, M.R.; Ianosi, B.; Lee, P.; Burris, J.; Cirstea, C.M. Remote motor system metabolic profile and surgery outcome in cervical spondylotic myelopathy. *J. Neurosurg. Spine* **2017**, *26*, 668–678. [CrossRef]
166. Kadaňka, Z.; Bednarik, J.; Novotný, O.; Urbánek, I.; Dušek, L. Cervical spondylotic myelopathy: Conservative versus surgical treatment after 10 years. *Eur. Spine J.* **2011**, *20*, 1533–1538. [CrossRef] [PubMed]
167. Tetreault, L.A.; Rhee, J.; Prather, H.; Kwon, B.K.; Wilson, J.R.; Martin, A.R.; Andersson, I.B.; Dembek, A.H.; Pagarigan, K.T.; Dettori, J.R.; et al. Change in Function, Pain, and Quality of Life Following Structured Nonoperative Treatment in Patients With Degenerative Cervical Myelopathy: A Systematic Review. *Glob. Spine J.* **2017**, *7* (Suppl. 3), 42S–52S. [CrossRef]
168. Zhang, Y.; Bhavnani, B.R. Glutamate-induced apoptosis in neuronal cells is mediated via caspase-dependent and independent mechanisms involving calpain and caspase-3 proteases as well as apoptosis inducing factor (AIF) and this process is inhibited by equine estrogens. *BMC Neurosci.* **2006**, *7*, 49. [CrossRef] [PubMed]
169. Perez, E.; Wang, X.; Simpkins, J.W. Chapter 22—Role of Antioxidant Activity of Estrogens in their Potent Neuroprotection. In *Oxidative Stress and Neurodegenerative Disorders*; Qureshi, G.A., Parvez, S.H., Eds.; Elsevier Science B.V.: Amsterdam, The Netherlands, 2007; pp. 503–524.
170. Miranda, J.D.; Colón, J.M. Tamoxifen: An FDA approved drug with neuroprotective effects for spinal cord injury recovery. *Neural Regen. Res.* **2016**, *11*, 1208–1211. [CrossRef] [PubMed]

171. Ha, K.-Y.; Kim, Y.-H.; Rhyu, K.-W.; Kwon, S.-E. Pregabalin as a neuroprotector after spinal cord injury in rats. *Eur. Spine J.* **2008**, *17*, 864–872. [CrossRef] [PubMed]
172. Onakpoya, I.J.; Thomas, E.T.; Lee, J.J.; Goldacre, B.; Heneghan, C.J. Benefits and harms of pregabalin in the management of neuropathic pain: A rapid review and meta-analysis of randomised clinical trials. *BMJ Open* **2019**, *9*, e023600. [CrossRef] [PubMed]
173. Abduljabbar, F.H.; Teles, A.R.; Bokhari, R.; Weber, M.; Santaguida, C. Laminectomy with or Without Fusion to Manage Degenerative Cervical Myelopathy. *Neurosurg. Clin. N. Am.* **2018**, *29*, 91–105. [CrossRef] [PubMed]
174. Pal, G.P.; Sherk, H.H. The Vertical Stability of the Cervical Spine. *Spine* **1988**, *13*, 447–449. [CrossRef] [PubMed]
175. Manzano, G.R.; Casella, G.; Wang, M.Y.; Vanni, S.; Levi, A.D. A Prospective, Randomized Trial Comparing Expansile Cervical Laminoplasty and Cervical Laminectomy and Fusion for Multilevel Cervical Myelopathy. *Neurosurgery* **2012**, *70*, 264–277. [CrossRef] [PubMed]
176. Bartels, R.H.; Groenewoud, H.; Peul, W.C.; Arts, M.P. Lamifuse: Results of a randomized controlled trial comparing laminectomy without and with fusion for cervical spondylotic myelopathy. *J. Neurosurg. Sci.* **2017**, *61*, 134–139. [PubMed]
177. Chiaki, H.; Seisuke, T. Bilateral multilevel laminectomy with or without posterolateral fusion for cervical spondylotic myelopathy: Relationship to type of onset and time until operation. *J. Neurosurg.* **1996**, *85*, 447–451.
178. Denaro, V.; Di Martino, A. Cervical Spine Surgery: An Historical Perspective. *Clin. Orthop. Relat. Res.* **2011**, *469*, 639–648. [CrossRef]
179. Wilson, J.R.; Tetreault, L.A.; Kim, J.; Shamji, M.F.; Harrop, J.S.; Mroz, T.; Cho, S.; Fehlings, M.G. State of the Art in Degenerative Cervical Myelopathy: An Update on Current Clinical Evidence. *Neurosurgery* **2017**, *80*, S33–S45. [CrossRef]
180. Hirano, Y.; Ohara, Y.; Mizuno, J.; Itoh, Y. History and Evolution of Laminoplasty. *Neurosurg. Clin. N. Am.* **2018**, *29*, 107–113. [CrossRef]
181. Fehlings, M.G.; Santaguida, C.; Tetreault, L.; Arnold, P.; Barbagallo, G.; Defino, H.; Kale, S.; Zhou, Q.; Yoon, T.S.; Kopjar, B. Laminectomy and fusion versus laminoplasty for the treatment of degenerative cervical myelopathy: Results from the AOSpine North America and International prospective multicenter studies. *Spine J.* **2017**, *17*, 102–108. [CrossRef]
182. Cheung, W.Y.; Arvinte, D.; Wong, Y.W.; Luk, K.D.K.; Cheung, K.M.C. Neurological recovery after surgical decompression in patients with cervical spondylotic myelopathy—A prospective study. *Int. Orthop.* **2008**, *32*, 273–278. [CrossRef]
183. Karadimas, S.K.; Laliberte, A.M.; Tetreault, L.; Chung, Y.S.; Arnold, P.; Foltz, W.D.; Fehlings, M.G. Riluzole blocks perioperative ischemia-reperfusion injury and enhances postdecompression outcomes in cervical spondylotic myelopathy. *Sci. Transl. Med.* **2015**, *7*, 316ra194. [CrossRef]
184. Smith, P.D.; Puskas, F.; Meng, X.; Lee, J.H.; Cleveland, J.C.; Weyant, M.J.; Fullerton, D.; Reece, T.B. The Evolution of Chemokine Release Supports a Bimodal Mechanism of Spinal Cord Ischemia and Reperfusion Injury. *Circulation* **2012**, *126* (Suppl. 1), S110–S117. [CrossRef] [PubMed]
185. Chen, Y.; Hallenbeck, J.M.; Ruetzler, C.; Bol, D.; Thomas, K.; Berman, N.E.J.; Vogel, S.N. Overexpression of Monocyte Chemoattractant Protein 1 in the Brain Exacerbates Ischemic Brain Injury and is Associated with Recruitment of Inflammatory Cells. *J. Cereb. Blood Flow Metab.* **2003**, *23*, 748–755. [CrossRef] [PubMed]
186. Ma, Z.; Dong, Q.; Lyu, B.; Wang, J.; Quan, Y.; Gong, S. The expression of bradykinin and its receptors in spinal cord ischemia-reperfusion injury rat model. *Life Sci.* **2019**, *218*, 340–345. [CrossRef] [PubMed]

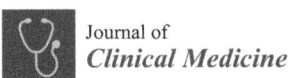

Systematic Review

How Is Spinal Cord Function Measured in Degenerative Cervical Myelopathy? A Systematic Review

Khadija H. Soufi, Tess M. Perez, Alexis O. Umoye, Jamie Yang, Maria Burgos and Allan R. Martin *

Department of Neurological Surgery, University of California, Davis, Sacramento, CA 95817, USA; khsoufi@ucdavis.edu (K.H.S.); tmperez@ucdavis.edu (T.M.P.); aoumoye@ucdavis.edu (A.O.U.); jmmyang@ucdavis.edu (J.Y.); mdburgos@ucdavis.edu (M.B.)
* Correspondence: armartin@ucdavis.edu

Citation: Soufi, K.H.; Perez, T.M.; Umoye, A.O.; Yang, J.; Burgos, M.; Martin, A.R. How Is Spinal Cord Function Measured in Degenerative Cervical Myelopathy? A Systematic Review. *J. Clin. Med.* **2022**, *11*, 1441. https://doi.org/10.3390/jcm11051441

Academic Editor: Maria A. Poca

Received: 19 January 2022
Accepted: 23 February 2022
Published: 5 March 2022

Publisher's Note: MDPI stays neutral with regard to jurisdictional claims in published maps and institutional affiliations.

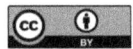

Copyright: © 2022 by the authors. Licensee MDPI, Basel, Switzerland. This article is an open access article distributed under the terms and conditions of the Creative Commons Attribution (CC BY) license (https://creativecommons.org/licenses/by/4.0/).

Abstract: Degenerative cervical myelopathy (DCM) is a prevalent condition in which spinal degeneration causes cord compression and neurological dysfunction. The spinal cord is anatomically complex and operates in conjunction with the brain, the musculoskeletal system, and numerous organs to control numerous functions, including simple and coordinated movement, sensation, and autonomic functions. As a result, accurate and comprehensive measurement of spinal cord function in patients with DCM and other spinal pathologies is challenging. This project aimed to summarize the neurological, functional, and quality of life (QoL) outcome measures currently in use to quantify impairment in DCM. A systematic review of the literature was performed to identify prospective studies with at least 100 DCM subjects that utilized one or more quantitative neurological, functional, or QoL outcome measures. A total of 148 studies were identified. The most commonly used instruments were subjective functional scales including the Japanese Orthopedic Association (JOA) (71 studies), modified JOA (mJOA) (66 studies), Neck Disability Index (NDI) (54 studies), and Nurick (39 studies), in addition to the QoL measure Short-Form-36 (SF-36, 52 studies). A total of 92% (320/349) of all outcome measures were questionnaires, whereas objective physical testing of neurological function (strength, gait, balance, dexterity, or sensation) made up 8% (29/349). Studies utilized an average of 2.36 outcomes measures, while 58 studies (39%) utilized only a single outcome measure. No studies were identified that specifically assessed the dorsal column sensory pathway or respiratory, bowel, or sexual function. In the past five years, there were no significant differences in the number of total, functional, or QoL outcome measures used, but physical testing of neurological function has increased ($p = 0.005$). Prior to 2017, cervical spondylotic myelopathy (CSM) was the most frequently used term to describe the study population, whereas in the last five years, DCM has become the preferred terminology. In conclusion, clinical studies of DCM typically utilize limited data to characterize impairment, often relying on subjective, simplistic, and non-specific measures that do not reflect the complexity of the spinal cord. Although accurate measurement of impairment in DCM is challenging, it is necessary for early diagnosis, monitoring for deterioration, and quantifying recovery after therapeutic interventions. Clinical decision-making and future clinical studies in DCM should employ a combination of subjective and objective assessments to capture the multitude of spinal cord functions to improve clinical management and inform practice guidelines.

Keywords: degenerative cervical myelopathy; cervical spondylotic myelopathy; ossified posterior longitudinal ligament; spinal cord injury

1. Introduction

The most common cause of spinal cord dysfunction is age-related degeneration of the discs, ligaments, and vertebrae of the cervical spine causing spinal cord compression and neurological impairment, collectively known as degenerative cervical myelopathy (DCM) [1]. The term DCM encompasses cervical spondylotic myelopathy (CSM), ossification of the posterior longitudinal ligament (OPLL), ossification of the ligamentum flavum (OLF), and degenerative disc disease [1]. Symptoms typically include numbness, paresthesias, impaired hand dexterity, weakness, unsteady gait, and sphincter dysfunction. In addition, neck pain, cervicogenic headaches, and neuropathic pain have also been associated with DCM, but the relationship of these entities with myelopathy is complex, potentially indirect, and not fully elucidated. DCM is often progressive and can manifest into severe symptoms, such as frank incontinence or quadriparesis requiring a walker or wheelchair, potentially causing affected individuals to lose their independence [1].

A number of outcome measures have been historically employed to measure the degree of neurological impairment in DCM. In 1972, Nurick proposed a popular grading system for cervical myelopathy based only on gait impairment [2]. The Japanese Orthopedic Association (JOA) score was proposed in 1985 and was later revised in several versions (most recently 1994) and has been widely adopted in Japan and East Asian countries. In 1991, Benzel et al. proposed a modified JOA (mJOA) score that replaced assessment of the "use of chopsticks" with cultural references that were more appropriate for Western countries, including "buttoning a shirt" and "eating with a spoon". The use of the mJOA has subsequently increased, including several clinical trials and as the basis of the categorization of DCM into mild (mJOA $\geq$ 15), moderate (mJOA 12–14), and severe (mJOA < 12) [3]. The reliance on these outcome measures has increased to the point that clinical practice guidelines (CPGs) published by AOSpine are based on the mJOA alone, recommending surgery for moderate-severe cases and mild cases that show progressive deterioration [4]. However, reliance on the mJOA is problematic in several ways, as scores can be affected by other medical conditions, interobserver reliability is limited [5,6], and it remains unclear how to best assess patients for neurological deterioration, although comprehensive clinical assessments and quantitative microstructural MRI have been proposed [7,8].

Our current understanding of the complex anatomy and physiology of the spinal cord suggests that more accurate measurements of spinal cord function may be necessary to optimize surgical clinical decision making, the design of clinical trials, and the refinement of future CPGs. The current study aims to analyze the existing literature to determine what neurological, functional, or quality of life (QoL) outcome measures have been utilized to quantify impairment in DCM, for the purpose of identifying research trends, practice patterns, and gaps in our current knowledge.

2. Materials and Methods

A systematic review of the literature was performed in accordance with the Preferred Reporting Items for Systematic Reviews and Meta-Analyses (PRISMA) guidelines and the Cochrane Handbook of Systematic Reviews of Interventions [9,10], and was registered with PROSPERO (CRD42022307161). An electronic database search was performed in PubMed, Embase, and MEDLINE. Search terms were formulated with the assistance of an academic librarian using PubMed and the search strategy was adjusted for the other databases (Supplementary Material S1).

The inclusion criteria were as follows: original research studies (randomized controlled trials—RCTs, cohort studies, case series, cross-sectional and case-control studies) with at least 100 human subjects with a diagnosis of DCM, prospectively collected data (allowing for retrospective analysis of prospectively collected data), English language, and the use at least 1 quantitative/numeric outcome measure that assessed neurological, functional, or quality of life status (Table 1). DCM was defined as a degenerative pathology causing extrinsic spinal cord compression, including CSM, OPLL, OLF, and disc herniations. For the purposes of this study, functional outcome measures were defined as self-reported or administered questionnaires, scores, or ordinal scales that describe high-level functional impairments; neurological outcome measures were defined as physical testing of specific neurological functions, such as power, coordinated movements, sensation, gait, and balance; quality of life measures were defined as questionnaires that evaluated overall wellbeing. Binary measures (i.e., present/absent) were not considered quantitative, but ordinal measures with three or more levels were included. Exclusion criteria were review articles, retrospective studies, case reports, letters the editor, meta-analyses, cadaveric studies, biomechanical studies, commentaries, conference abstracts, editorials, studies with insufficient data, duplicate cohorts, and inclusion of other pathologies (tumor, inflammatory, trauma, and infection).

Table 1. Summary of design elements of the systematic review, in population, intervention, comparison, outcomes, and study design (PICOS) format.

PICOS Element	Criteria Used in Systematic Review
Population	• Studies that analyzed patients with DCM, defined as degenerative pathology causing extrinsic spinal cord compression, including CSM, OPLL, OLF, and disc herniations. • Studies were excluded if they included patients with other pathologies, including neoplastic, infectious, inflammatory, and trauma, or if they included patients without signs of myelopathy (e.g., only neck pain or radiculopathy)
Intervention	• No specific intervention was required for inclusion in this review.
Comparison	• No specific comparison was required for inclusion in this review.
Outcomes	• Functional outcome measures, defined as self-reported or administered questionnaires, scores, or ordinal scales that describe high-level impairments. • Neurological outcome measures, defined as physical tests of specific neurological functions. • Quality of Life outcome measures, defined as overall measures of wellness • Excluded outcome measures: pain, range-of-motion, radiographic, electrophysiologic, and non-quantitative measures
Study Design	• Prospective collection of data • ≥100 patients with a diagnosis of DCM • Original research studies including RCTs, cohort studies, case series, and case-control studies • English language • Measured at least 1 quantitative outcome measure

Abbreviations: CSM: cervical spondylotic myelopathy; DCM: degenerative cervical myelopathy; OLF: ossified ligamentum flavum; OPLL: ossified posterior longitudinal ligament; PICOS: population, intervention, comparison, outcomes, study design; RCT: randomized controlled trial.

Three reviewers independently evaluated the search results, including performing title and abstract reviews, full-text reviews, and data extraction. Covidence (Covidence A/S, Melbourne, Australia) was used to manage citations at each step of the process. The data extracted for each study included: citation, title, year, type of study (RCT, cohort study, case series, or case-control), population studied (DCM, CSM, OPLL, disc herniation), and quantitative functional, neurological, and QoL outcome measures utilized.

Statistical analysis was performed using R v4.0.2 (R Foundation for Statistical Computing, Vienna, Austria). Data were tabulated and summary statistics were calculated for each category of outcome measures. To assess for recent trends, *post-hoc* analyses arbitrarily compared studies published in the past five years (2017 or later) and those published before 2017 using Student's t tests for numeric variables and z tests for proportions. Results were considered statistically significant for $p < 0.05$ due to the exploratory nature of this study.

3. Results

The electronic database search yielded a total of 1958 unique citations, of which 362 studies were retained after title and abstract review (Figure 1). After full-text review, 148 studies met the eligibility criteria and were included in this study (Supplementary Material S2). Of all included studies, there were 84 (57%) cohort studies, 39 (26%) case series,

14 (10%) RCTs, and 11 (7%) cross-sectional studies (Figure 2). Sixty-six (45%) of the studies were multicenter or involved shared databases. The majority of studies (52%) utilized CSM as the preferred terminology to refer to their study population, whereas 44 (30%) used DCM, and 13 (9%) utilized OPLL, cervical spondylosis, or cervical compression myelopathy (Figure 2).

A total of 349 outcome measures were utilized by the 148 included studies, with an average of 2.36 outcome measures per study. Fifty-eight studies (39%) utilized only a single outcome measure, 28 (19%) used 2 measures, 27 (18%) used 3 measures, 25 (17%) used 4 measures, while 10 (6.8%) utilized 5 or more outcome measures (Figure 3). Of all outcome measures, 92% (320/349) were questionnaires or ordinal scales (functional or QoL), whereas objective physical testing of neurological function (strength, gait, balance, dexterity, or sensation) made up 8% (29/349).

Functional outcome measures were the most common type of instrument employed, with all studies employing at least one of these measures and an average of 1.68 measures per study. The most frequently used functional assessments were JOA (71), mJOA (66), the Neck Disability Index (NDI) (54), and the Nurick grade (39) (Figure 4, Table 2). A total of 11 other measures were used including JOA-CMEQ, the Myelopathy Disability Index (MDI) (3), the Geriatric Locomotive Function Scale (GLFS-5), overactive bladder symptom score (OBSS), and the Cooper scale.

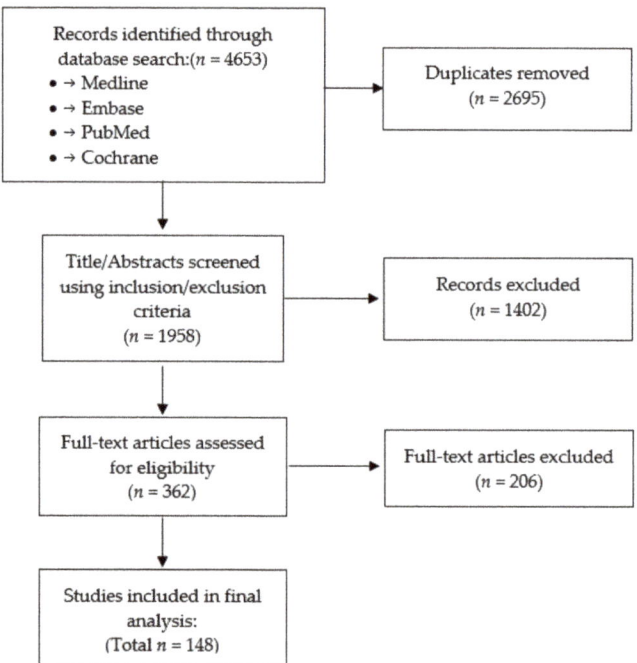

Figure 1. PRISMA flow diagram of systematic review. Abbreviations: PRISMA: Preferred Reporting Items for Systematic Reviews and Meta-Analyses.

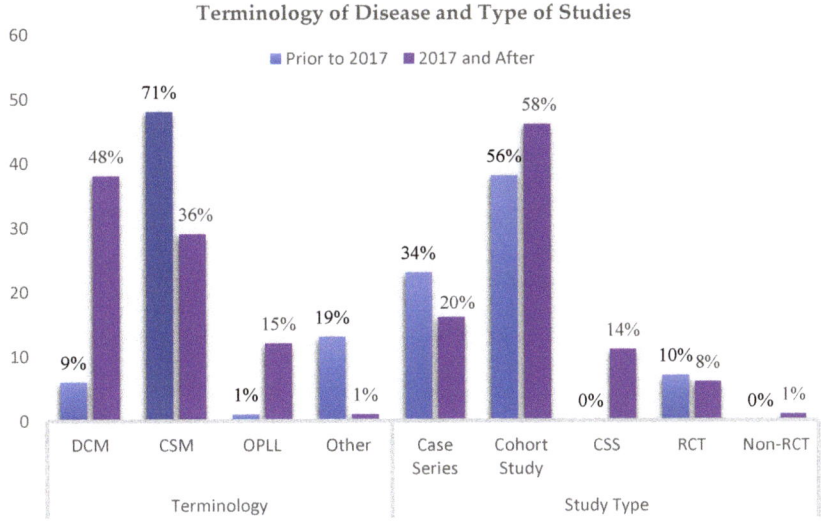

Figure 2. Terminology of Disease and Type of Study prior to 2017 ($n = 68$) compared to 2017 and after ($n = 80$). Abbreviations: DCM: Degenerative Cervical Myelopathy; CSM: Cervical Spondylotic Myelopathy; OPLL: Ossification of Posterior Longitudinal Ligament; CSS: Cross-Sectional Study; RCT: Randomized Controlled Trial.

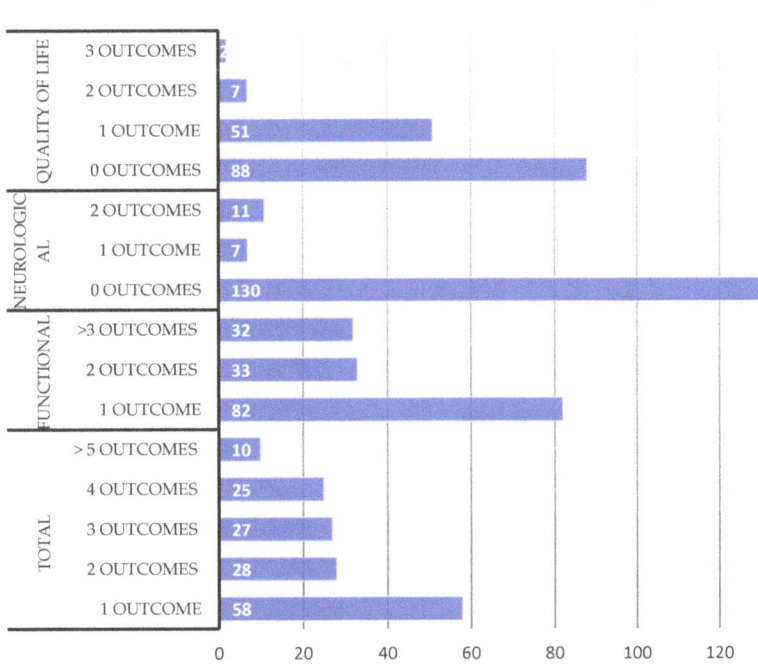

Figure 3. The number of total, functional, neurological, and quality of life outcome measures utilized per study in the identified literature.

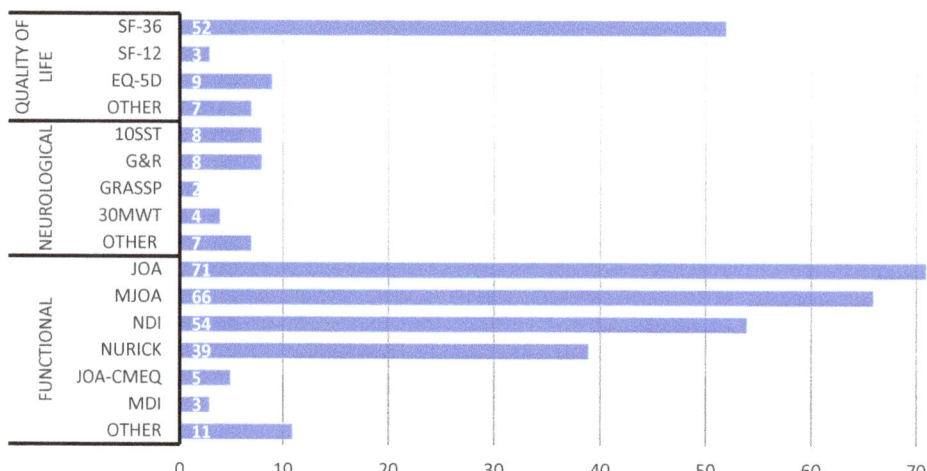

Figure 4. Outcome measures classified into functional, neurological, and quality of life. Abbreviations: SF-36/SF-12: Short Form 36 or 12; EQ-5D: EuroQol-5 Dimension Survey; 10SST: 10 s step test; G&R: 10 s Grip and Release; GRASSP: Graded Redefined Assessment of Strength, Sensibility, and Prehension; 30MWT: 30-m walk test; NDI: Neck Disability Index; MDI: Myelopathy Disability Index; JOA-CMEQ: Japanese Orthopedic Association Cervical Myelopathy Evaluation Questionnaire.

Table 2. Subjective and objective measurements of specific spinal cord functions or pathways in the existing literature. The number of studies that used each measure are in parentheses. Subjective assessments included functional or QoL questionnaires or ordinal scales, whereas objective assessments were defined as physical measurements of specific neurological functions.

Category of Spinal Cord Function	Specific Function or Pathway	Subjective Assessments (e.g., Questionnaires)	Objective Assessments (e.g., Physical examination)
Motor	Non-specific	SF-36 (52) NDI (54) EQ-5D (9) JOA-CMEQ (5) MDI (3) SF-12 (3) GLFS-5 (1) FIM (1)	<none>
	Strength	SF-36 (52) JOA-CMEQ (5) MDI (3) EMS (1) Ranawat (1)	GRASSP (2) MRC (1) Berg Balance (1) Grip dynamometer (1) ISNCSCI LEMS (1)
	Hand dexterity	JOA (71) mJOA (66) JOA-CMEQ (5) EMS (1)	G&R (8) GRASSP (2)

Table 2. Cont.

Category of Spinal Cord Function	Specific Function or Pathway	Subjective Assessments (e.g., Questionnaires)	Objective Assessments (e.g., Physical examination)
	Gait	JOA (71) mJOA (66) SF-36 (52) Nurick (39) EQ-5D (9) JOA-CMEQ (5) MDI (3) SF-12 (3) Cooper (1) GLFS-5 (1) EMS (1) Ranawat (1)	10SST (8) 30MWT (4) 10MWT (1) 10MRT (1) EGA (1)
	Balance	<none>	10SST (8) BBS (1)
Sensory	Non-specific	JOA (71) mJOA (66) JOA-CMEQ (5)	<none>
	Dorsal columns (light touch, vibration, proprioception)	<none>	<none>
	Spinothalamic (pin prick, temperature, pressure)	<none>	GRASSP (2) PPT (1)
Autonomic	Bladder	JOA (71) mJOA (66) JOA-CMEQ (5) OBSS (1)	<none>
	Bowel	<none>	<none>
	Respiratory	<none>	<none>
	Sexual	<none>	<none>

Abbreviations: FIM: Functional Independence Measure; MRC: Medical Research Council; EMS: European Myelopathy Score; GLFS-5: Geriatric Locomotive Function Scale; 10MWT: 10m Walk Test; 30MWT: 30m Walk Test; 10 MRT: 10m Run Test; 10SST: 10s step test), EGA: Electronic Gait Analysis; PPT: Pain Perception Testing; OBSS: Overactive Bladder Symptom Score; BBS: Berg Balance Scale; ISNCSCI LEMS: International Standards for Neurological Classification of Spinal Cord Injury Lower Extremity Motor Score.

Neurological outcome measures were infrequently utilized, with 0.20 measured per study, while 130/148 studies (88%) did not report any objective neurological measurements. The 17 studies tested lower extremity motor function, including the 10-s step test (10SST) in 8 studies, 30m walk test (30MWT) in 4 studies, 10m walk test (10MWT) in 2 studies, and Berg Balance Scale (BBS) in 1 study (Figure 4, Table 2). Electronic gait analysis (EGA) was used by two studies and assessed parameters including stride length, velocity, stability ratio (single-stance to double stance), and variability of a self-paced walk. Upper extremity motor function was measured in 8 studies using the 10s grip and release (G&R) test and 2 studies utilized Graded Redefined Assessment of Strength, Sensibility, and Prehension (GRASSP). The assessment of sensation was only performed in 3 studies, including 2 that used GRASSP and 1 that used Pain Perception Thresholds (PPT) using the PainVision PS-2100 system.

The assessment of QoL was performed with moderate frequency, with 41% (60) of studies using such measures, with an average of 0.48 measures per study. The most used instruments were SF-36 (52), EQ-5D (9), and SF-12 (3) (Figure 4, Table 2). All of the quality-of-life measures were patient-reported surveys.

Comparing recent studies published in the last 5 years (2017–2021, inclusive, $n = 68$) with older studies ($n = 80$), the average number of neurological outcome measures used has increased from 0.06 to 0.31 ($p = 0.005$). There was no difference in the number of total (2.18 vs. 2.51, $p = 0.1$), functional (1.63 vs. 1.73 $p = 0.55$), or QoL (0.49 vs. 0.48) outcome measures employed. In the past 5 years, increased use of upper extremity motor ($p = 0.01$) and lower extremity motor testing ($p = 0.01$) was observed, whereas the use of other outcome measures was similar to earlier studies. Among studies published prior to 2017, CSM was the most common terminology used to refer to the patient population (71%), but its use has declined to 36% among studies published in the past 5 years ($p < 0.001$). In contrast, the term DCM has increased in use from 9% to 48% ($p < 0.001$). Studies focused on OPLL have also proportionally increased in the past 5 years from 1% to 15% ($p = 0.001$).

4. Discussion

This study provides a comprehensive review of how spinal cord function is quantified in large prospective studies of degenerative cervical myelopathy and assesses the recent trends in chosen outcome measures. The most frequently utilized instruments were functional outcome measures, which we defined as subjective scores that describe high-level impairments. Versions of the mJOA and JOA scores were used in a total of 91% (135/148) of studies, suggesting that the DCM research community has reached a consensus on the use of these measures as the primary outcomes of interest. The 1994 version of the JOA was the most popular outcome measure for East Asian populations that utilize chopsticks [11], whereas the 1991 mJOA described by Benzel was the primary measure used elsewhere [12]. The NDI, which is the cervical analogue to the widely used Oswestry Disability Index (ODI) for lower back pain, was the third most common measure utilized [13]. Interestingly, all three of these outcome measures are subjective questionnaires based on patients' self-assessments, which are subject to response, recall, and confirmation biases. These scores are also highly affected by other disabilities (e.g., knee arthritis for gait function). Furthermore, each of these scores make an unvalidated assumption of linearity and equivalence over multiple ordinal scales (e.g., 1 point on mJOA sensation is equivalent to 1 point on gait function), and they all employ terminology such as mild, moderate, or severe impairment without objective definitions. The Nurick grade was also moderately popular and is arguably somewhat more objective, providing specific criteria for each of its six levels. However, Nurick is narrowly focused on gait and does not quantify the most common deficits experienced in DCM, namely upper extremity incoordination, weakness, and numbness. Quality of life measures were employed in 41% of studies, adding important information on the overall impact of DCM, but these were universally patient-reported questionnaires that are also highly subjective and affected by comorbidities, age, and other factors. Interestingly, objective neurological assessments based on physical testing of function were performed in only 12% of studies. In addition, approximately half of studies utilized only one to two outcome measures. In the past five years, the use of objective neurological measures has increased modestly, but otherwise no major differences were detected in the number of outcome measures used, indicating that little has changed in the design of recent studies. Overall, the body of DCM literature is largely deficient in the assessment of spinal cord function, as the vast majority of studies do not obtain any objective data, nor do they perform comprehensive measurements commensurate with the complexity of the spinal cord and the deficits caused by DCM.

The results of this systematic review are consistent with a 2013 study by Kalsi-Ryan et al., which reported a narrative literature review of outcome measures used in CSM [14]. Due to the selection of CSM as the population of interest, their results were potentially biased toward Western populations, showing Nurick (34%) and mJOA (31%) as the most commonly employed measures. In keeping with our conclusions, their study found a paucity of objective data in CSM studies and concluded by recommending one additional questionnaire (QuickDASH) and 5 objective neurological measures (Berg Balance Scale, 30MWT, GRASSP, grip dynamometer, and electronic gait analysis). Our results are also consistent with a 2016 systematic review by Davies et al. [15], which investigated the selection of post-operative outcome measures, categorized in terms of function, complications, quality of life, pain, and imaging. Their review found similar results in 108 studies with slightly different inclusion criteria (prospective studies with ≥50 subjects or retrospective with ≥200), with 90% of studies reporting functional outcomes and 29% reporting QoL measures, and a preponderance of JOA (46%) and mJOA (19%) use. Furthermore, they found only scant use of objective physical testing measures, such as grip and release (1%), 30m walking test (1%), grip strength (1%), and mean locomotion score (1%). While our review overlaps considerably with the previous reviews by Kalsi-Ryan et al. and Davies et al., approximately half of the studies we identified were published after these reviews, indicating that DCM is a highly active area of research. Furthermore, our study differs from these previous works in that we specifically sought to look at the measurement of each specific function controlled by the spinal cord to determine how well previous studies have captured this information, and to identify knowledge gaps for the design of future studies and novel measurement tools.

In stark contrast to the DCM body of literature, traumatic SCI studies have unanimously adopted the ISNCSCI (formerly ASIA) exam as the primary outcome measure [16]. This comprehensive exam of motor and sensory function has several advantages, including high reliability and objective interpretation of findings, but it is time consuming and must be performed by a trained clinician, which limits its practicality for routine office use in the more common condition of DCM. It also is not sensitive to subtle spinal cord dysfunction, including hand incoordination, gait imbalance, and bladder dysfunction. However, a broad spectrum of measures that capture all aspects of motor, sensory, and autonomic impairments have also been developed and validated for SCI patients, including SCIM, FIM, WISCI, and numerous others [17,18]. This rich foundation of outcome measures, including subjective and objective data, allows for a thorough assessment of SCI patients in research studies and clinical management. However, the deficits incurred in traumatic SCI are typically more severe than encountered in DCM, highlighting the need to develop practical and tailored assessments for DCM.

The spinal cord is anatomically complex and has a myriad of functions, including motor control (simple movements, coordination, gait, and balance), sensation (pain, temperature, light touch, pressure, vibration, and proprioception), and various autonomic functions (respiratory, bladder, bowel, and sexual function). Furthermore, emerging evidence indicates that the spinal cord itself contains much of the circuitry for these functions, containing complex neuronal networks and sensorimotor feedback loops that control coordinated movements, central pattern generators, and homeostatic mechanisms. In this context, it seems almost absurd to quantify the entirety of spinal cord function in 4 questions, but the mJOA does exactly this with ordinal scales for motor dysfunction of upper extremities, lower extremities, upper extremity sensation, and bladder dysfunction. However, this simplistic approach at least addresses the most common deficits in DCM. The 1994 version of the JOA has slightly more breadth, including questions on motor function of hands, elbows, and shoulders, and sensory function in the UE, trunk, and LE. The NDI includes two questions on pain (neck pain, headaches) and eight questions regarding various functions, such as working, driving, and reading, but these are non-specific for cervical myelopathy and easily affected by comorbidities or other impairments. QuickDASH is a questionnaire developed for upper extremity function that is potentially more suited to detect deficits in myelopathy, but also non-specific. GRASSP-Myelopathy is a shortened version of the original GRASSP assessment for SCI that is tailored to DCM, measuring sensations using monofilaments (pressure, carried via the spinothalamic pathway), hand dexterity, and upper extremity strength [19]. In the current review of DCM outcome measures, there were no instruments that measured sensory modalities, such as pin pricks, temperature, light touch, vibration, or proprioception, or respiratory, bowel, or sexual function. Ideally, DCM outcome measures could be designed that are comprehensive, sensitive to mild pathology, responsive to changes, specific to myelopathy (rather than other neurological or physical deficits), valid, reliable, and objective. However, the design of such instruments is extremely challenging and needs to strike a balance between being comprehensive and practical. Given the current lack of such measures, we strongly endorse the use of multiple subjective and objective measures for future studies, clinical management, and CPGs, such as JOA or mJOA, NDI, QuickDASH, SF-36 or EQ-5D, grip strength, hand dexterity, multi-modal sensory testing, hand intrinsic power, gait, and balance testing.

This study was subject to several limitations. This review focused only on quantitative functional, neurological, and QoL outcome measures, omitting pain, range of motion, imaging, electrophysiological, and non-quantitative (binary or qualitative) outcomes that are potentially of interest. This limitation was intentional to focus this review narrowly on spinal cord function, while the excluded outcomes have numerous complexities that would benefit from their own detailed exploration. For example, pain may occur as a result of myelopathy, but also has many other potential sources, such as the nerve roots (radiculopathy), joints and ligaments (arthropathy), vertebrae (spondylosis), and muscles (myopathy and spasm). The exclusion of binary variables was necessary as a vast number of studies reported the presence or absence of symptoms and signs, which would have required careful full-text reviews to identify and led the inclusion of many additional studies. However, such binary variables are routinely used in clinical decision making (e.g., the presence of hyperreflexia, dysdiadochokinesia, or gait ataxia) and may constitute useful measurements. We also excluded retrospective and smaller prospective studies due to resource limitations and the length of the manuscript, as these studies often suffer from less thoughtful design, but we may have missed important contributions and additional outcome measures. Another limitation of this study is the English language requirement, which possibly excluded international studies, potentially biasing the results and missing useful outcomes. In addition, we created definitions for "neurological" and "functional" outcome measures to differentiate these terms, but these have variable and overlapping use in the literature. Finally, we describe physical testing of neurological function as "objective", but these tests involve varying degrees of subjectivity (e.g., grading power from 0 to 5) and are also indirect, or surrogate, measures of spinal cord function as they also depend on the brain, peripheral nerves, and musculoskeletal systems to perform physical tasks. Electrophysiology of the spinal cord arguably offers the most "objective" measures, but has only modest sensitivity for myelopathy, cannot test complex functions (e.g., hand dexterity), and is not widely used in practice [20].

In summary, this systematic review of DCM outcome measures revealed that the majority of large prospective studies utilize a small number of outcome measures. Measurements typically include functional and QoL questionnaires, but frequently lack any objective confirmation of neurological impairment, limiting their accuracy and comprehensiveness in measuring spinal cord function. Novel outcome measures should be developed and validated that incorporate subjective and objective information and encompass the numerous functions of the spinal cord, weighting them according to their importance to patients. However, spinal cord function is difficult to measure, as it depends intrinsically on the brain, peripheral nervous system, and other body systems for its input and output, and there is a lack of ground truth information to compare novel outcome measures against. A concerted effort is needed to augment existing methods and develop new tools for quantifying disease in DCM, for the purpose of improving diagnosis, measuring severity, and monitoring patients for deterioration. Such an effort will facilitate improved clinical decision-making and standardization of practice, in addition to improving the robustness and validity of clinical research studies.

Supplementary Materials: The following supporting information can be downloaded at: https://www.mdpi.com/article/10.3390/jcm11051441/s1, Supplementary Material S1: Electronic database search terms; Supplementary Material S2: Reference list of studies included in systematic review.

Author Contributions: Conceptualization: A.R.M.; methodology: K.H.S., T.M.P., and A.R.M.; formal analysis: K.H.S., T.M.P. and A.R.M.; investigation, K.H.S., T.MP, A.O.U., J.Y. and M.B.; data curation: K.H.S., T.M.P., A.O.U., J.Y. and M.B.; writing—original draft preparation: K.H.S. and T.M.P.; writing—

review and editing: K.H.S., T.M.P., A.O.U., J.Y., M.B. and A.R.M.; supervision: A.R.M.; project administration: A.R.M. All authors have read and agreed to the published version of the manuscript.

Funding: This research received no external funding.

Institutional Review Board Statement: Not applicable.

Informed Consent Statement: Not applicable.

Data Availability Statement: All data supporting reported results can be found within the manuscript.

Acknowledgments: Martin received startup research support through the Department of Neurological Surgery, University of California, Davis.

Conflicts of Interest: The authors declare no conflict of interest.

References

1. Tetreault, L.A.; Karadimas, S.; Wilson, J.R.; Arnold, P.M.; Kurpad, S.; Dettori, J.R.; Fehlings, M.G. The Natural History of Degenerative Cervical Myelopathy and the Rate of Hospitalization Following Spinal Cord Injury: An Updated Systematic Review. *Global. Spine J.* **2017**, *7* (Suppl. S3), 28S–34S. [CrossRef] [PubMed]
2. Nurick, S. The pathogenesis of the spinal cord disorder associated with cervical spondylosis. *Brain* **1972**, *95*, 87–100. [CrossRef] [PubMed]
3. Tetreault, L.; Kopjar, B.; Nouri, A.; Arnold, P.; Barbagallo, G.; Bartels, R.; Qiang, Z.; Singh, A.; Zileli, M.; Vaccaro, A.; et al. The modified Japanese Orthopaedic Association scale: Establishing criteria for mild, moderate and severe impairment in patients with degenerative cervical myelopathy. *Eur. Spine J.* **2017**, *26*, 78–84. [CrossRef] [PubMed]
4. Fehlings, M.G.; Tetreault, L.A.; Riew, K.D.; Middleton, J.W.; Aarabi, B.; Arnold, P.M.; Brodke, D.S.; Burns, A.S.; Carette, S.; Chen, R.; et al. A Clinical Practice Guideline for the Management of Patients With Degenerative Cervical Myelopathy: Recommendations for Patients With Mild, Moderate, and Severe Disease and Nonmyelopathic Patients With Evidence of Cord Compression. *Global. Spine J.* **2017**, *7* (Suppl. S3), 70S–83S. [CrossRef] [PubMed]
5. Bartels, R.H.; Verbeek, A.L.; Benzel, E.C.; Fehlings, M.G.; Guiot, B.H. Validation of a translated version of the modified Japanese orthopaedic association score to assess outcomes in cervical spondylotic myelopathy: An approach to globalize outcomes assessment tools. *Neurosurgery* **2010**, *66*, 1013–1016. [CrossRef]
6. Martin, A.R.; Jentzsch, T.; Wilson, J.; Moghaddamjou, A.; Jiang, F.; Rienmueller, A.; Badhiwala, J.H.; Akbar, M.A.; Nater, A.; Oitment, C.; et al. Inter-rater Reliability of the Modified Japanese Orthopedic Association Score in Degenerative Cervical Myelopathy: A Cross-sectional Study. *Spine* **2021**, *46*, 1063–1069. [CrossRef]
7. Martin, A.R.; De Leener, B.; Cohen-Adad, J.; Kalsi-Ryan, S.; Cadotte, D.W.; Wilson, J.R.; Tetreault, L.; Nouri, A.; Crawley, A.; Mikulis, D.J.; et al. Monitoring for myelopathic progression with multiparametric quantitative MRI. *PLoS ONE* **2018**, *13*, e0195733. [CrossRef]
8. Martin, A.R.; Kalsi-Ryan, S.; Akbar, M.A.; Rienmueller, A.C.; Badhiwala, J.H.; Wilson, J.R.; Tetreault, L.A.; Nouri, A.; Massicotte, E.M.; Fehlings, M.G. Clinical outcomes of nonoperatively managed degenerative cervical myelopathy: An ambispective longitudinal cohort study in 117 patients. *J. Neurosurg. Spine* **2021**, *34*, 821–829. [CrossRef]
9. Higgins, J.P.T.; Thomas, J.; Chandler, J.; Cumpston, M.; Li, T.; Page, M.J.; Welch, V.A. (Eds.) Cochrane Handbook for Systematic Reviews of Interventions Version 6.2 (Updated February 2021). Cochrane. 2021. Available online: www.training.cochrane.org/handbook (accessed on 13 November 2021).
10. Moher, D.; Shamseer, L.; Clarke, M.; Ghersi, D.; Liberati, A.; Petticrew, M.; Shekelle, P.; Stewart, L.A.; Group, P.-P. Preferred reporting items for systematic review and meta-analysis protocols (PRISMA-P) 2015 statement. *Syst. Rev.* **2015**, *4*, 1. [CrossRef]
11. Japanese Orthopaedic Association. Scoring system for cervical myelopathy. *Nippon Seikeigeka Gakkai Zasshi* **1994**, *68*, 490–503.
12. Benzel, E.C.; Lancon, J.; Kesterson, L.; Hadden, T. Cervical laminectomy and dentate ligament section for cervical spondylotic myelopathy. *J. Spinal Disord.* **1991**, *4*, 286–295. [CrossRef] [PubMed]
13. Vernon, H.; Mior, S. The Neck Disability Index: A study of reliability and validity. *J. Manip. Physiol. Ther.* **1991**, *14*, 409–415.
14. Kalsi-Ryan, S.; Singh, A.; Massicotte, E.M.; Arnold, P.M.; Brodke, D.S.; Norvell, D.C.; Hermsmeyer, J.T.; Fehlings, M.G. Ancillary outcome measures for assessment of individuals with cervical spondylotic myelopathy. *Spine* **2013**, *38* (Suppl. S1), S111–S122. [CrossRef] [PubMed]
15. Davies, B.M.; McHugh, M.; Elgheriani, A.; Kolias, A.G.; Tetreault, L.A.; Hutchinson, P.J.; Fehlings, M.G.; Kotter, M.R. Reported Outcome Measures in Degenerative Cervical Myelopathy: A Systematic Review. *PLoS ONE* **2016**, *11*, e0157263. [CrossRef] [PubMed]
16. Kirshblum, S.C.; Burns, S.P.; Biering-Sorensen, F.; Donovan, W.; Graves, D.E.; Jha, A.; Johansen, M.; Jones, L.; Krassioukov, A.; Mulcahey, M.J.; et al. International standards for neurological classification of spinal cord injury (revised 2011). *J. Spinal Cord Med.* **2011**, *34*, 535–546. [CrossRef] [PubMed]
17. Wecht, J.M.; Krassioukov, A.V.; Alexander, M.; Handrakis, J.P.; McKenna, S.L.; Kennelly, M.; Trbovich, M.; Biering-Sorensen, F.; Burns, S.; Elliott, S.L.; et al. International Standards to document Autonomic Function following SCI (ISAFSCI): Second Edition. *Top. Spinal Cord Inj. Rehabil.* **2021**, *27*, 23–49. [CrossRef] [PubMed]

18. Alexander, M.S.; Anderson, K.D.; Biering-Sorensen, F.; Blight, A.R.; Brannon, R.; Bryce, T.N.; Creasey, G.; Catz, A.; Curt, A.; Donovan, W.; et al. Outcome measures in spinal cord injury: Recent assessments and recommendations for future directions. *Spinal Cord* **2009**, *47*, 582–591. [CrossRef] [PubMed]
19. Kalsi-Ryan, S.; Riehm, L.E.; Tetreault, L.; Martin, A.R.; Teoderascu, F.; Massicotte, E.; Curt, A.; Verrier, M.C.; Velstra, I.M.; Fehlings, M.G. Characteristics of Upper Limb Impairment Related to Degenerative Cervical Myelopathy: Development of a Sensitive Hand Assessment (Graded Redefined Assessment of Strength, Sensibility, and Prehension Version Myelopathy). *Neurosurgery* **2020**, *86*, E292–E299. [CrossRef] [PubMed]
20. Martin, A.R.; Tetreault, L.; Nouri, A.; Curt, A.; Freund, P.; Rahimi-Movaghar, V.; Wilson, J.R.; Fehlings, M.G.; Kwon, B.K.; Harrop, J.S.; et al. Imaging and Electrophysiology for Degenerative Cervical Myelopathy [AO Spine RECODE-DCM Research Priority Number 9]. *Global. Spine J.* **2022**, *12* (Suppl. S1), 130S–146S. [CrossRef] [PubMed]

MDPI
St. Alban-Anlage 66
4052 Basel
Switzerland
Tel. +41 61 683 77 34
Fax +41 61 302 89 18
www.mdpi.com

Journal of Clinical Medicine Editorial Office
E-mail: jcm@mdpi.com
www.mdpi.com/journal/jcm

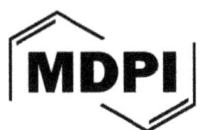

www.ingramcontent.com/pod-product-compliance
Lightning Source LLC
LaVergne TN
LVHW070431100526
838202LV00014B/1574